INFORMATION TECHNOLOGY IN MEDICAL DIAGNOSTICS

PROCEEDINGS OF THE XIIITH CONFERENCE WD 2016, LUBLIN, POLAND, 11–13 JUNE 2016 AND THE XIIITH INTERNATIONAL CONFERENCE – MEASUREMENT AND CONTROL IN COMPLEX SYSTEMS, MCCS- 2016, VINNITSIA, UKRAINE 3–6 OCTOBER 2016

Information Technology in Medical Diagnostics

Editors

Waldemar Wójcik & Andrzej Smolarz

Electrical Engineering and Computer Science Faculty, Lublin University of Technology, Lublin, Poland

CRC Press
Taylor & Francis Group
Boca Raton London New York Leiden

CRC Press is an imprint of the
Taylor & Francis Group, an **informa** business
A BALKEMA BOOK

CRC Press/Balkema is an imprint of the Taylor & Francis Group, an informa business

Typeset by V Publishing Solutions Pvt Ltd., Chennai, India
Printed and Bound by CPI Group (UK) Ltd, Croydon, CR0 4YY

Published by: CRC Press/Balkema
Schipholweg 107C, 2316 XC Leiden, The Netherlands
e-mail: Pub.NL@taylorandfrancis.com
www.crcpress.com – www.taylorandfrancis.com

ISBN: 978-1-138-29929-0 (Hbk)
ISBN: 978-1-315-09805-0 (eBook)

Table of contents

Preface

For many centuries, people have tried to learn about the state of their health. Initially, in the pre-technological period, they had to rely only on their senses. Then there were simple tools to help the human senses. The discovery of X-rays, which allowed people to look "inside" the body, turned out to be a major breakthrough. Contemporary medical diagnostics is increasingly being assisted by information technology that allows, for example, thorough image tissue analysis or pathology differentiation. They also allow very early preventive diagnostics. Influenced by information technology, "classic" diagnostic techniques change and new ones arise.

We present to you a collection of carefully selected distinguished extended presentations from two conferences: XIII Conference WD2016 11–13. June 2016 held during IT days in Lublin, Poland and the XIII International Conference–Measurement and control in complex systems, MCCS-2016 held 3–6 October in Vinnitsia, Ukraine. This volume shows the latest developments in information technology that directly or indirectly use nature patterns to apply them in the medical and technical diagnostics. The individual chapters present separate, closed issues that result from cooperation between scientists from Poland, Ukraine and Kazakhstan. They address problems of application of new methods of image processing for analysis of medical images, new methods of classification of medical data as well as new medical imaging methods. An interesting fact is that some of the presented technologies are inspired by the functioning of living organisms. Moreover, the same methods can be used both for medical diagnostics and technical diagnostics.

This set of articles on technological issues interwoven with medical and biological problems is of interest not only to academics and engineers, but also to professionals involved in biomedical engineering, seeking solutions for the problems that cannot be solved thanks to "traditional" technologies. We hope that the book will contribute to better use of the latest research results in practice. We are convinced that the experience and knowledge of the authors of the chapters have influenced the value of this book. Finally, we would like to express our appreciation to all who have helped to prepare this book: Mr. Jerzy Warakomski for improving the linguistic side of the book, as well as all the anonymous reviewers who not only evaluated papers, but often made valuable suggestions helping authors and editors to improve the scientific standard of this book.

Waldemar Wójcik & Andrzej Smolarz
Lublin, March 2017

About the editors

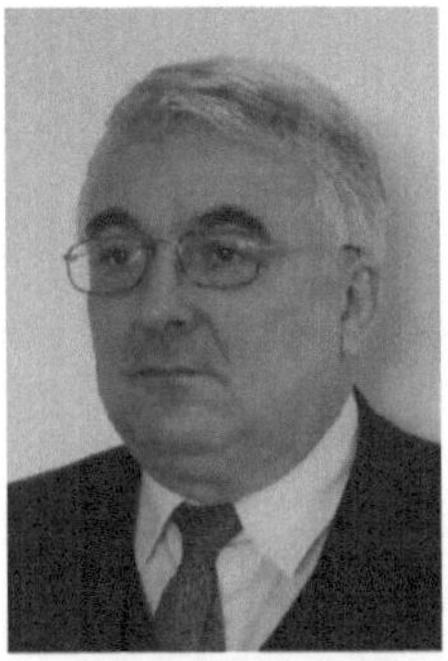

Waldemar Wójcik was born in Poland, 1949. He is Director of the Institute of Electronics and Information Technology, former long-time dean of the Faculty of Electrical Engineering and Computer Science at Lublin University of Technology. Doctor Honoris Causa of five universities in Ukraine and Kazakhstan. He obtained his Ph.D. in 1985 at the Lublin University of Technology, and D.Sc. in 2002 at the National University Lviv Polytechnic, Ukraine. In 2009 he obtained a title of professor granted by the President of Poland. In his research he mainly deals with process control, optoelectronics, digital data analysis and also heat processes or solid state physics. Particular attention is paid to the use optoelectronic technology in the monitoring and diagnostics of thermal processes. He is a member of Optoelectronics Section of the Committee of Electronics and Telecommunications of the Polish Academy of Sciences; Metrology Section of the Committee of Metrology and Scientific Equipment of the Polish Academy of Sciences and many other scientific organisations of Poland as well as Europe and Asia. In total, he has published 53 books, over 400 papers, and authored several patents. He is also a member of the editorial board of numerous international and national scientific and technical journals.

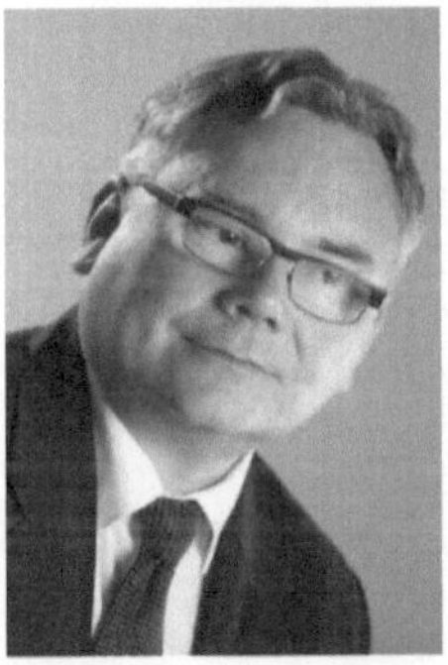

Andrzej Smolarz (Ph.D., D.Sc. Eng.) graduated from Lublin University of Technology Faculty of Electrical Engineering. During 28 years of professional work he has reached the position of associated professor at his Alma Mater in the Institute of Electronics and Information Technology. He has also worked as a Research Fellow at The Laboratory of Research in Fluid Dynamics and Combustion Technologies (LIFTEC by its Spanish acronym) a joint center between the Spanish Scientific Research Council (CSIC) and University of Zaragoza. His research field of interest covers wide variety of optical methods in industrial diagnostics and control as well as applications of artificial intelligence methods in industrial diagnostics. Author of more than 100 publications in this research area.

CHAPTER 1

Recognition of textured objects using optimal inverse resonant filtration

R.N. Kvyetnyy & O.Yu. Sofina
Vinnytsia National Technical University, Vinnytsia, Ukraine

Y.A. Bunyak
WIN-interactive, Vinnytsia, Ukraine

W. Wójcik & A. Kotyra
Lublin University of Technology, Lublin, Poland

B. Akhmetov
Kazakh National Research Technical University after K.I. Satpaev, Almaty, Kazakhstan

1 INTRODUCTION

Recognition of textured objects is one of the main challenges for vision-based measurements and control systems. One of the main problem is choosing properly defined features that would extract image objects from the background. The texture features may be characterized by their statistical, structural and dynamic properties. The latest methods of texture analysis are presented in (Randen & Husoy 1998, Radke et al. 2005, Haralick et al. 1973, Xie 2008).

Statistical based methods use both parametric and nonparametric models of the image textures such as Bayes analysis, Hidden Markov Models, Regression, Linear Autoregression (AR), Nonlinear Autoregression (NAR), and Autoregression with Moving Average (ARMA) Randen & Husoy 1998, Radke et al. 2005, Haralick et al. 1973, Xie 2008, Celeux et al. 2003, Lazebnik 2003, Zhang & Wu 2008, Sayadi et al. 2008). The statistical nonparametric methods are generally nonlinear and not always return textured image pattern estimates that would be invariant to spatial transforms of the image. Correlation methods can be implemented with arithmetic structures. The most commonly used method of this class is the co-occurrence matrix method (Radke et al. 2005, Haralick et al. 1973, Partio et al. 2007). Further development of the correlation method includes definition of a nonlinear metric that relates with geometry of textures (Clarenz et sl. 2004, Fu & Huang 2008).

The newest methods of object recognition are based on image transforms in the spatial-frequency domain, where spectral parameters of the image have simple statistics within a narrow range (Randen & Husoy 1998, Li et al. 2006.). These methods combine statistical models and spatial-frequency representation as 1D and 2D wavelets (Huang & Aviyente 2006) as well as the classic Gabor functions (Palm & Lehmann 2002, Vyas & Rege 2006).

The wavelet and Gabor spectra represent local textures geometric features with a minimal number of significant coefficients. However, it does not represent periodicity of the texture because both wavelets and Gabor functions have shift-variant spectrum. This problem was partially overcome by the introduction of the Complex Wavelet Transform (CWT) (Kingsbury 2001). CWT transfers the spatial domain into a frequency-phase domain and suppresses the spectrum aliasing that appears as a result of texture variations. CWT was also used to obtain the rotate-invariant transform (Hill et al. 2000).

A need to present textures with a minimal number of parameters has driven the development of new transforms, many of which are combined of the existing ones. For example,

Radon transform combined with Fourier or wavelet transforms provides the possibility of image representation in a frequency-angle domain that has a much lower dimension for it is affine-invariant (Yarman & Yazici 2006, Liu et al. 2009).

In many cases, the exact texture shape description is not necessary. It applies especially when a texture is dynamic and both spatial and temporal changes are more important than the local surface pattern characteristics.

Combining the eigenvector decomposition (EVD) of texture kernel with filters that are resonant to certain image eigen modes maintains compact texture description (Ade 1983). For EVD is computationally expensive, Independent Component Analysis (ICA) (Coltuc et al. 2007, Khaparde et al. 2008), Empirical Mode Decomposition (EMD) (Nunes et al. 2003, Chang-zhen et al. 2006, Yang & Yang 2009) and Singular Values Decomposition (SVD) (Wall et al. 2003, Soatto et al. 2003, Costantini et al. 2008) can be applied as well. The purpose of applying the mentioned decompositions is both size and dimension reduction of texture parameters as it does in the case of Principal Component Analysis (PCA). PCA makes a projection of a textured image into a subspace configured by the most significant parameters. Usually the decompositions are used for full image transformation that makes their application difficult in real time systems.

Another implementation of PCA and EMD is based on the applying of filter bank that can be synthesized by Fourier and wavelet transform. The problems with texture analysis using filters bank arise from the sequence of task, such as decomposition, classification of the spectral components and recognition.

Filtering procedures can be implemented with matrix transformations or convolution, which can be done by components pattern analysis with thresholding, clustering, segmentation and modeling techniques (Randen & Husoy 1998, Radke et al. 2005, Haralick et al. 1973, Xie 2008). In the case of dynamic textures, decompositions require also on dynamic models based on discrete differential equations (Soatto et al. 2003, Costantini et al 2008, Fujita & Nayar 2003). Although the synthesis of the model is computationally expensive, however implementation itself does not require significant amount of computational power and thus can be executed in real time using a standard DSP processor or arithmetic array (Costantini et al 2008).

The correlation matrix and other integral matrices, such as Wigner integral are used as objects of the decomposition because they represent the dynamic properties of a large image in compact form. The asymptotic correlation matrix of a stationary process has Toeplitz structure and its eigenvectors are harmonic (Marple 1987). A textured image can be considered as a 2D stationary process with the block-Toeplitz correlation matrix. Therefore, harmonic decomposition is a natural approximation of EVD or EMD. The parameters of harmonics should match the periods of a texture pixels and gray scale spatial variations. Such harmonics are considered as eigen or resonant considering the texture structure.

The eigen-harmonic decomposition (EHD) is based on planar and spherical functions that have been used for compact presentation of textured images as well as human facial images in some articles (Huang & Chan 2004, Pattichis & Bovik 2006).

The demands of textured pattern recognition invariance are not restricted by shift and rotation invariance. Demands for recognition of textured object are extended and can be formulated as follows.

- The method should be invariant to scaling perturbations of target object to identify different resolutions of the same image objects.
- The isometry invariance. This includes changes of brightness, rotations, mirror operations, color rotations and inversions.
- Similarity. The recognition filters (methods) of similar images should be also similar. That approach needs a notion of similarity expressed in a well-defined manner. Similarity of images may be measured with Euclidean distances.

- The recognition filter should have a shorter representation than the associated object image.

These are the natural requirements if recognition filters (methods) of objects that are presented in metric spaces are considered. One of the novel approach to invariant object recognition is the interpretation images as Riemannian manifolds (Kimmel et al. 1999). In the context of image classification, it is motivated by the fact that most content preserving operations are isometrics, i.e. this map and its inverse preserve the arc length of all curves (Peinecke et al. 2007). This includes changes of brightness, rotations, mirror operations, color rotations and inversions.

A brief survey of textured image analysis methods enables to put forward the following conclusions:

- Dynamic model based methods of texture analysis and synthesis are the most effective. They can be used for analysis of static, dynamic and quasi-regular textures. The models may be created using a fragment of the image. The remainder of the image of an arbitrary size can be restored by the model operator using a generation process.
- Object recognition on a textured background may be accomplished by comparative analysis of the original and generated by the model images.
- An implementation of the structured object recognition with the inverse model of object scheme results in a process of texture generation. Usually, the generating process can be described with white noise (Soatto et al. 2003), therefore the recognition method may operate as a whitening filter, similarly to AR, NAR, and ARMA. Variations of the retrieval generating signal can be described by simple statistical parameters as mean value and dispersion. The parameters can be applied as indicators of the target object.
- Autoregressive models are not suitable for object recognition because they indirectly reflect signal frequency spectrum. It is difficult to find a single valued solution for the estimation of whitening filter parameters for they relate to the second order moments of texture signals. The solution to this problem will be considered with the use of linear inverse filtration suppressing a textured object structure. At the same time, it keeps signal fluctuations of the other objects without changing their energy. This class of inverse problem can be solved using first order moments of the textured image signals.
- The dynamic models are usually synthesized using Fourier transform or the decompositions mentioned above. The survey of previous research reveals that transforms and decompositions applying depends on the image type: full format, or only a typical fragment (known as texture kernel or as texton) (Charalampidis 2006). For the case when for a full format image wavelet and Radon transforms combined with Fourier transform are applied the results obtained are appropriate. When a texton uses wavelet transforms, SVD ignores the structural information because it is not shift-invariant. It has been shown that SVD and its multidimensional generalization are effective for dynamic model synthesis (Soatto et al. 2003, Costantini et al 2008).
- The wavelet transforms have approximate and restricted shift invariance and cannot represent periodicity because they are intended for analysis of transient signals. EVD and EMD can represent texture periodicity as well as local kernel structure, however, the functional basis for these decompositions does not have analytical definition and is variant in respect to image shift. This feature complicates their use for interpolation of the image fragment when the exact texture period is unknown or periodically pulsating (such as for example marine surface).
- In contrast to the mentioned above decompositions, EHD has simple analytical definition and joins capabilities to approximation and interpolation of 2D fields (Bunyak 1998). Therefore, EHD is an appropriate function basis for the design of a linear inverse filter. The filter suppresses the approximation of texture structure in the form of eigen harmonic series. The harmonics in this series have resonant frequencies in respect to the image signal.

An elimination of these harmonics makes the texture signal simpler and easier for recognizing. This filter can be defined as the Inverse Resonant Filter (IRF).

Texture modeling and recognition with properties of invariance to space and scale perturbation can be made by including transforms of initial image into its invariant projections as surface curvature and Beltrami flow (Kimmel et al. 1999, Peinecke et al. 2007). Applying EHD the approach discussed is useful because the projections can transform mismatch for harmonic approximation step like image signal into sequence of fluctuations which associate with feature of step level change.

2 OBJECT RECOGNITION PROBLEM STATEMENT AS THE PROBLEM OF OPTIMAL FILTRATION

The problem of object filtration can be formulated as follows. Let in the space Ω is given an image X which includes an object O: $O \in \Omega_O \subset \Omega$ as subset Ω_O of Ω. The aim is to define a linear or non-linear transform

$$F(O; x \in X : x \in \Omega_O) = E, \tag{1.1}$$

where E is a signal of object presence indicator. At the same time, the next condition should be satisfied simultaneously with equation (1.1):

$$F(O; x \in X : x \notin \Omega_O) \neq E. \tag{1.2}$$

Recognition of some objects can be made using conditions (1.1) and (1.2):

$$F(O_i; x \in X : x \in \Omega_{O_i}) = E, \quad F(O_i; x \in X : x \notin \Omega_{O_i}) \neq E, \tag{1.3}$$

$$F(O_i; x \in X : x \in \Omega_{O_i}) = E_i, \quad F(O_i; x \in X : x \notin \Omega_{O_i}) \neq E. \tag{1.4}$$

Equation (1.3) defines filters of some different objects O_i without their classification. It can be applied especially when the objects compile textured background and should be eliminated by the filter. The condition (1.4) defines the filter for retrieving textured objects O_i with their classification.

There are several approaches to solve problems denoted by equations (1.1)–(1.4), which can be separated in two classes, reversible and not-reversible methods. Statistical and some spectral methods give the indicator E parameters set not appropriate for initial object reconstruction compiles the second class. The deficiency of this methods class is absence of the feedback for control object changes by compare target object with its model. The feedback is inherent to reversible methods class. In this case it is meaning that there is inverse to filter $F(\cdot)$ operator $\Psi(\cdot)$, such that

$$\Psi(O; E : E \in \Omega_O) \cong X : X \in \Omega_O. \tag{1.5}$$

The expression (1.5) is the problem of the object modeling by using its characteristic O and indicator signal E. Evidently, this problem is inverse in respect to (1.1).

Object recognition characteristic relates with errors of the object model (1.5)

$$X - \Psi(O; E) = N(X) \tag{1.6}$$

and filter (1.1)

$$E - F(O;X) = N(E) \tag{1.7}$$

A functional *I* can be defined

$$I = \arg\min_{\Psi,F}\left\{\int_O \left(X - \Psi(O;E)\right)^2 d\Omega + \int_O \left(E - F(O;X)\right)^2 d\Omega + \int_O Reg(N;F;\Psi)\,d\Omega\right\}, \tag{1.8}$$

where $N(\cdot)$ is error noise, $Reg(\cdot)$ is a regularization functional of additional restrictions on error shape (minimal variation or minimal surface). Euler-Lagrange variation of the functional (1.8) relatively parameters of the object filter and object model gives an optimal structure of object recognition.

Let consider the framework given by equations (1.1)–(1.8) when recognition filter and model filter are linear and are implemented as convolutions:

$$\tilde{H} * X = E : X \subset \Omega_O, \tag{1.9}$$

$$H * X = X : X \subset \Omega_O. \tag{1.10}$$

Variation of two first components in (1.8) with account of (1.9) and (1.10) yields the following expression.

$$\left(X - H * E\right) * E + \left(X - G * X\right) * X \approx 0 \tag{1.11}$$

where variation of the regularization functional is omitted. The δ-function or Heaviside step function, uncorrelated white noise can be used as the object indicator. Then up to a constant factor $H * E(x, y) * E(x, y) \sim H$. The convolutions $E(x, y) * E(x, y)$ are presented with different signs and therefore can be eliminated. Thus, the equation for optimal object filter and model operators' characteristics can be obtained:

$$H - \tilde{H} * R_{XX} \cong 0, \tag{1.12}$$

where R_{XX} denotes correlation matrix of the object signal. If it is satisfied the equation $\tilde{H} * H \cong \mathrm{I}$, where I is the trivial operator, then convolution (1.12) with H and $\tilde{H}$ shows that:

$$H * H \cong R_{XX} \tag{1.13}$$

and

$$I - \tilde{H} * \tilde{H} * R_{XX} \cong 0. \tag{1.14}$$

The expression (1.13) indicates that *H* is an object forming filter surge characteristic. It is well known as Wiener–Khintchine filter (Wiener 1964, Khintchine 1934). The filter creates correlative relations of the object model by convolution with generating process in a manner of white noise or Heaviside step function. The expression (1.14) means that optimal recognition filter eliminates signal components which form correlative relations. In the other words, filter is resonant with respect to object texture shape. Since it eliminates components it can be defined as inverse resonant filter. The expression (1.14) reveals the evident fact that the white noise which correlation has the form of I does not contain any object. The problem is to define principal components of an object texture that can be eliminated by linear convolution. The main demand to IRF properties is invariance to object space location and initial phase of its texture shape. This demand can be formulated as the shift invariance. It points on choice of a method for retrieval of principal components of the object model. The shift invariance is inherent to harmonic functions under condition, that they are resonant with respect to object shape.

3 HARMONIC MODEL OF TEXTURED IMAGE

An ideal textured image of size $N \cdot P \times M \cdot Q$ can be represented as a tensor product of two matrices,

$$D = T \otimes B, \tag{1.15}$$

where matrix T of size $N \times M$ includes unit elements with insignificant fluctuations and matrix B of size $P \times Q$ is the texture kernel. Rank of matrix (1.15) equals to the rank of the kernel matrix. Therefore, it can be represented by EVD and SVD using P left vectors and Q right vectors. The same representation is possible with the use of Discrete Fourier Transform (DFT) (Elliot & Rao 1983). The matrix T can be decomposed as:

$$T = F_N diag[10 \ldots 0] F_M^H, \tag{1.16}$$

where $F_N = (1/N)[z_i^k]_{i,k=0,\ldots N-1}$; $z_i^k = \exp(-i2\pi ik/N)$ is DFT operator whose size is pointed by low indexes. The kernel matrix has the following spectral decomposition:

$$B = F_P A_{FB} F_Q^H \tag{1.17}$$

where A_{FB} is the spectral matrix of the kernel B in the basis F. The substitution of expression (1.16) and (1.17) into (1.15) yields the following decomposition of the textured matrix:

$$\begin{aligned} D &= (F_N \otimes F_Q)(diag[1\ 0\ \ldots\ 0] \otimes A_{FB})(F_Q^H \otimes F_M^H) = \\ & F_{NP} diag[A_{FB}\ 0\ \ldots\ 0] F_{MQ}^H. \end{aligned} \tag{1.18}$$

In the expression given above associativity of the tensor product was used as well as $F_{NP} = F_N \otimes F_P, F_{MQ} = F_M \otimes F_Q$. It shows that DFT contains the same information as EVD and SVD on the condition that the basis is exactly aligned with texture pattern. Additionally, DFT representation of (1.18) is invariant with respect to image initial point shift. The textured matrix (1.15) initial point causes the cyclical shift of the kernel matrices. The shifted matrix relates with the original matrix B by simple expression:

$$B^{t,\tau} = C_P^t B C_Q^{\tau H}, \tag{1.19}$$

where $B^{t,\tau}$ denotes shifted matrix along t rows and τ columns, C_P – cyclical shift operator (CSO) of size $P \times P$ (Elliot & Rao 1983). The following expression is the well-known CSO spectral decomposition:

$$\begin{aligned} C_P^t &= F_P diag[z_1^t\ \ldots\ z_P^t] F_P^H, \\ C_Q^t &= F_Q diag[z_1^t\ \ldots\ z_Q^t] F_Q^H. \end{aligned} \tag{1.20}$$

Considering the expressions (1.3)–(1.6) the texture matrix (1.15) with shifted kernel matrices given by equation (1.19) can be represented as:

$$D^{t,\tau} = T \otimes B^{t,\tau} = F_{NP} diag\left[diag[z_1^t\ \ldots\ z_P^t] A_{FB} diag[z_1^{\tau *}\ \ldots\ z_Q^{\tau *}]\ 0\ \ldots\ 0\right] F_{MQ}^H, \tag{1.21}$$

where * denotes complex conjugation. The spectral factorization of the textured image matrix (1.18) and (1.21), shows that the power spectrum of the kernel matrix is invariant to transforms by CSO (1.20) because the spectrum matrix of the shifted kernel (1.19) differs from the original by phase multiplies.

The main problem of spectral factorization in canonical manner, as shown in (1.18) and (1.21), is the alignment of DFT with texture structure. There are known methods of texture period estimation based on algebraic geometry and complex EMD (Muhly & Solel 1999, Gu et al. 2004). Another method is based on adaptation of the EHD to texture structure, idealized or real. This adaptation can be made by determining the shift transform that is natural for a given texture (Soatto et al. 2003). The eigen vectors system of the shift transform can then serve as a generalized harmonic basis for texture presentation Following this approach, linear shift instead of cyclic shift (1.19) can be substituted. This operation transfers rows (or columns) of the image matrix linearly on one step. Each new row or column is a linear combination of adjacent rows (columns). The new rows and columns are the approximate model of real image rows and columns that appear because of image translation. The Linear Shift Operator (LSO) has the form of a Frobenius matrix

$$K_P \begin{bmatrix} 0 & 1 & \dots & 0 \\ \vdots & \vdots & \ddots & \vdots \\ 0 & 0 & \dots & 1 \\ -a_P & -a_{P-1} & \dots & -a_1 \end{bmatrix} \tag{1.22}$$

and its characteristic polynomial,

$$1+\sum_{i=1}^{P} a_i z^i = 0 \tag{1.23}$$

has the roots $z_i = 1\dots P$, that have exponential form in analytical presentation: $z_i = \exp(\iota 2\pi f_i)$, where f_i denotes eigen or resonant frequencies. Linear shift operator can be defined for two image coordinates. The spectral factorization of LSO has the form of equation (1.20) and can be written for both coordinates as:

$$\begin{aligned} K^t_{xP} &= Z_{xP} diag\left[z^t_{x1} \dots z^t_{xP}\right] Z^{\#}_{xP}, \\ K^{\tau}_{yQ} &= Z_{yQ} diag\left[z^{\tau}_{y1} \dots z^{\tau}_{yQ}\right] Z^{\#}_{yQ}. \end{aligned} \tag{1.24}$$

where $Z_{xP} = \left[z^t_{xi}\right]^{t=0\dots P-1}_{i=1\dots P}$, $Z_{yQ} = \left[z^t_{yi}\right]^{t=0\dots Q-1}_{i=1\dots Q}$, # is the pseudoinverse. The shifted linear kernel matrix can be presented by EHD in the following manner,

$$\begin{aligned} & B^{t,\tau} = K^t_P B K^{\tau T}_Q = \\ & Z_{xP} diag\left[z^t_{x1} \dots z^t_{xP}\right] Z^{\#}_{xP} Z_{xP} A_{ZB} Z^T_{yQ} Z^{\#T}_{yQ} diag\left[z^{\tau}_{y1} \dots z^{\tau}_{yQ}\right] Z^T_{yQ} = \\ & Z_{xP} diag\left[z^t_{x1} \dots z^t_{xP}\right] A_{ZB} diag\left[z^{\tau}_{y1} \dots z^{\tau}_{yQ}\right] Z^T_{yQ} \end{aligned} \tag{1.25}$$

where T denotes transposition, and A_{ZB} is the spectral matrix of the matrix B in the basis Z,

$$A_{ZB} = \tilde{Z}^{\#}_{xP} B \tilde{Z}^{\#T}_{yQ}. \tag{1.26}$$

Expression (1.25) shows the spectrum invariance to linear shift operations that is equivalent to equation (1.21). The kernel periodicity in a textured image is defined by the condition

$$B^{mP,nQ} = B, \tag{1.27}$$

where m and n are arbitrary integer values. The condition mentioned above allows representation of the full image D by overdetermined matrices $\tilde{Z}_{xP} = \left[z^t_{xi}\right]^{t=0\dots NP-1}_{i=1\dots P}$, $\tilde{Z}_{yQ} = \left[z^t_{yi}\right]^{t=0\dots MQ-1}_{i=1\dots Q}$ with the spectral matrix (1.26),

$$D \approx \tilde{Z}_{xP} A_{ZB} \tilde{Z}_{yQ}^{T}. \tag{1.28}$$

Expression (1.28) is analogous to (1.18) but it is approximate because the pseudoinverse of the overdetermined matrices yields approximate results.

Linear shift is natural for many models of textured images, both static and dynamic. Therefore, the EHD provides appropriate representation of the image model. The parameters of the LSO (1.22) should be estimated in accordance with the dynamic properties of texture. As it follows from condition (1.27), the shift operations do not change the texture signal energy. Therefore, the shift operator is unitary. The operator (1.22) is unitary if its characteristic polynomial (1.23) roots lie on the unit circle in the complex domain. It is important the problem to define the LSO order P and Q for both coordinates.

The spectral presentation (1.28) is basing on the linear shift model of the data matrix in the form of two LSO (1.22) associated with the coordinates. The roots of the characteristic polynomial (1.23) are using for generation of the functions basis of the discrete Fourier transform. Such spectral presentation may be used if the texture is homogeneous. In other case estimation of the EHD component should accounts full texture image matrix. For that purpose, 2D generalization of the LSO may be used:

$$K_{P\times Q}^{(2)} = K_{xP} \otimes K_{yQ}. \tag{1.29}$$

The evaluation of the 2D LSO parameters in the manner of product of two polynomials associated with coordinates has nonlinear feature (Barbieri & Barone 1992). As it was shown in (Bunyak 1996), the parameters of the characteristic polynomials (1.23) associated with the coordinates and approximation of the polynomials product can be estimated by using linear extended equations based on the LSO (1.29). The roots of the polynomials products are useful for definition of the 2D harmonics parameters.

4 DESIGN OF OPTIMAL INVERSE RESONANT FILTER

Linear version of the object recognition pattern given by equation (1.1) is the inverse problem with respect to object signal model in the manner of forming filter (1.10). It means restoration of the originating signal matrix $E = \left[e_{i,k}\right]_{i=0\ldots M-1}^{k=0\ldots N-1}$ using measurement data $D = \left[d_{i,k}\right]_{i=0\ldots M-1}^{k=0\ldots N-1}$ of size $M \times N$ in the object region of the image under the assumption that mentioned matrices are connected by some linear operator with unknown transient characteristic $H = \left[h_{m,n}\right]_{m=0\ldots P-1}^{n=0\ldots Q-1}$. The measured data matrix includes samples of additive noise $\xi_{i,k}$ associated with texture model error. Formally the model can be written in the discrete manner as the convolution equation:

$$d_{i,k} = \sum\nolimits_{m=0}^{P-1} \sum\nolimits_{n=0}^{Q-1} h_{m,n} e_{i-m,k-n} + \xi_{i,k}. \tag{1.30}$$

There is classical Wiener solution of the inverse problem for the model defined by equation (1.30) using Fourier transform (Marple 1987, Wiener 1964). However, such an approach is acceptable when noise is observed separately and the image statistical parameters are known. When the noise is not considered, the Wiener approach may give unstable or singular solutions. To overcome this problem regularization methods are used that are based on PCA with SVD or EMD of the measured data.

Equation (1.30) can be considered as a linear dynamic model of the textured object image D which is initiated by the generating process E of the known form. The model is like the ones that were considered in (Soatto et al. 2003, Costantini et al. 2008, Fujita & Nayar 2003). The generating process is the object presence indicator. It should have simple form which is easy for recognition purposes.

The filter has a much smaller size comparing to object image size. Therefore, the problems of the direct and inverse transient response evaluation need regularization. Let the 2D Heaviside step function:

$$e_{i,k} = \begin{cases} 1, & (i \geq 0^+) \wedge (k \geq 0^+), \\ 0.5, & i = 0, \quad k = 0, \\ 0, & (i \leq 0^+) \wedge (k \leq 0^+) \end{cases} \tag{1.31}$$

is the generating process in (1.30). The textured object image is specified in range $(i \geq 0^+) \wedge (k \geq 0^+)$ and is a response of linear dynamic system (1.30) to the excitation (1.31). Let consider the problem of generating signal reconstruction using an inverse filter with transient characteristic $\tilde{h}_{m,n}$. Within the image being considered, the generating signal has constant value E. Therefore, the problem appears in the following way:

$$\sum_{m=0}^{P-1} \sum_{n=0}^{Q-1} \tilde{h}_{i+m,k+n} d_{m,n} = E + \varsigma_{i,k}, \tag{1.32}$$

where $\varsigma_{i,k}$ represents error noise. The dispersion value of the noise in (1.32) serves as a criterion for filter matching with object texture.

There exit some approaches of solving the problem (1.17). It is possible to compile equation (1.32) for shifted data matrices

$$\sum_{m=0}^{P-1} \sum_{n=0}^{Q-1} \tilde{h}_{i+m,k+n} d_{m+t,n+\tau} \cong E : \forall d_{m+t,n+\tau} \in O \subset \Omega \tag{1.33}$$

and find the minimum square solution of (1.33) with respect to transient characteristic $\tilde{h}_{m,n}$ elements by pseudoinverse of the extended data matrix. But such a solution will be not shift invariant. It obtains the shift invariance upon the condition that it is presented in shift invariant functions basis.

Let the elements of the object image matrix are presented by EHD (1.27) as the following series:

$$d_{i,k} = \sum_{m=1}^{P} \sum_{n=1}^{Q} A_{m,n} z_{xm}^{i} z_{yn}^{k} + \varepsilon_{i,k} \tag{1.34}$$

where $A_{m,n}$ represents the amplitudes of the two-dimensional harmonic functions $z_{xm}^{i} z_{yn}^{k}$, $\varepsilon_{i,k}$ is the approximation error which has much less dispersion than signal power. The resonant frequencies f_{xm}, f_{yn} are the main parameters of the harmonic functions $z_{xm}^{i} = \exp(\iota 2\pi f_{xm} i)$ and $z_{yn}^{k} = \exp(\iota 2\pi f_{yn} k)$ in (1.34). Their values characterize eigen fluctuations of the target object surface associated with the coordinate axes OX and OY. The set of frequencies relates with roots of characteristic polynomial (1.23) of the texture dynamic model (1.30).

It is not necessary to use a full textured object image for series (1.34) parameters determination. Some base region $D : B \subset D$ of the size $n_x \times n_y; n_x > 2P; n_y > 2Q$ is sufficient. This region should cover the texture kernel B. The EHD of the base region is equivalent to (1.27) and it can be represented in the matrix form as:

$$D \approx Z_x A Z_y^T, \tag{1.35}$$

$$A = Z_x^{\#} D Z_y^{T\#}, \tag{1.36}$$

where $A = \left[A_{ik}\right]_{i=1\ldots P}^{k=1\ldots Q}$, $Z_{x(y)} = \left[z_{x(y)i}^{k}\right]_{i=1\ldots P(Q)}^{k=0\ldots n_{x(y)}-1}$.

Attention should be paid to shift invariance of the direct and pseudo-inverted EHD bases because it is important for the spectral presentation (1.35)–(1.36). The t-shifted along the space coordinate matrix $Z_x^t = Z_x diag\left[z_{x1}^t \ldots z_{xP}^t\right]$ in pseudo-inverted manner has the form of t-shifted matrix $Z_x^{\#t} = diag\left[z_{x1}^{-t}...z_{xP}^{-t}\right]Z_x^{\#}$, too. Therefore, the pseudo-inverted matrix $Z_x^{\#t} = diag\left[z_{x1}^{-t}...z_{xP}^{-t}\right]Z_x^{\#}$ is also shift invariant.

By analogy to (1.35) and (1.36), EHD of transient characteristic can be found

$$h_{i,k} = \sum_{m=0}^{P-1}\sum_{n=0}^{Q-1} H_{m,n} z_{xm}^{i} z_{yn}^{k}. \tag{1.37}$$

Substituting equations (1.34)–(1.37) into (1.30) and neglecting the error yields the following spectral decomposition.

$$\begin{aligned} d_{i,k} &\cong \sum_{m=1}^{P}\sum_{n=1}^{Q}\sum_{t=0}^{P-1}\sum_{\tau=0}^{Q-1} H_{m,n} z_{xm}^{i+t} z_{yn}^{k+\tau} e_{t,\tau} = \\ &\sum_{m=1}^{P}\sum_{n=1}^{Q} H_{m,n} z_{xm}^{i} z_{yn}^{k} \sum_{t=0}^{P-1}\sum_{\tau=0}^{Q-1} e_{t,\tau} z_{xm}^{t} z_{yn}^{\tau} = \sum_{m=1}^{P}\sum_{n=1}^{Q} H_{m,n} E_{m,n} z_{xm}^{i} z_{yn}^{k} \end{aligned} \tag{1.38}$$

where

$$E_{m,n} = \sum_{i=0}^{P-1}\sum_{k=0}^{Q-1} e_{i,k} z_{xm}^{i} z_{yn}^{k} = \sum_{i=0}^{P-1}\sum_{k=0}^{Q-1} e_{i,k} z_{xm}^{i} z_{yn}^{k} \tag{1.39}$$

in accordance with (1.31). As it follows from expressions (1.30), (1.38), $A_{m,n} \approx H_{m,n} E_{m,n}$ and the IRF spectrum is

$$\tilde{H}_{m,n} \cong H_{m,n}^{-1} = E_{m,n} A_{m,n}^{-1}. \tag{1.40}$$

The transient characteristic of IRF (1.32) for object texture recognition can be defined using equation

$$\tilde{H} = \left[h_{i,k} = \sum_{m=1}^{P}\sum_{n=1}^{Q} E_{m,n} A_{m,n}^{-1} z_{xm}^{i} z_{yn}^{k}\right]_{i=0\ldots P-1;\, k=0\ldots Q-1.} \tag{1.41}$$

The scheme (1.35)–(1.41) implements the approach to filter design basing on Fourier transform. It differs from the well-known classic schema by using EHD instead usual discrete Fourier transform. Eigen-harmonic decomposition allows avoid of small amplitudes $A_{m,n}$ influence because all eigen fluctuations have comparative value levels. This creates the effect of the regularization of the solution (12).

In the given above scheme, the base equations (1.34), (1.37) and (1.38) are approximate. Therefore, approach discussed provides an estimate of the aim transient characteristic. It needs optimization in accordance with a criterion of quality. The main influence factor is variation of data spectrum because the recognizing objects are only similar to template object which was used for filter designing. As the elements of $E_{m,n}$ in (1.39) are not varied by data fluctuations directly, the better way is to define the transient characteristic of the forming filter as $H_{m,n} \cong E_{m,n}^{-1} A_{m,n}$ and then evaluate the inverse filter using the condition

$$\tilde{\mathbf{h}}^{T} \cdot \mathbf{H} \cong [0\ldots010\ldots0], \tag{1.42}$$

where $\mathbf{H}$ is the matrix which is equivalent to convolution operation with vector $\tilde{\mathbf{h}}$.

$$\mathbf{H} = \begin{bmatrix} \mathbf{H}_0\mathbf{H}_1 & \ldots & \mathbf{H}_{P-1}\mathbf{0} & \ldots & \mathbf{0} \\ \mathbf{0} & \mathbf{H}_0\mathbf{H}_1 & \ldots\mathbf{H}_{P-1} & \ldots & \mathbf{0} \\ \vdots & & \ddots & & \vdots \\ \mathbf{0} & \ldots\mathbf{0} & \mathbf{H}_0\mathbf{H}_1 & \ldots & \mathbf{H}_{P-1} \end{bmatrix} \quad \mathbf{H}_k = h\begin{bmatrix} h_{k,0}h_{k,1} & \ldots & h_{k,Q-1}0 & \ldots & 0 \\ 0 & h_{k,0}h_{k,1} & \ldots h_{k,Q-1} & \ldots & 0 \\ \vdots & & \ddots & & \vdots \\ 0 & \ldots 0 & h_{k,0}h_{k,1} & \ldots & h_{k,Q-1} \end{bmatrix} \tag{1.43}$$

where **0** denotes null matrix. The vector $\tilde{\mathbf{h}}$ is the lexicographical presentation of matrix $\tilde{H}$ (1.41). The solution of equation (1.42) can be founded by the least squares method (Marple 1987).

$$\tilde{\mathbf{h}}^T \cong \left(\mathbf{H}\cdot\mathbf{H}^T\right)^{-1}\left(\mathbf{H}\right)_M, \tag{1.44}$$

where $M = (2PQ-1)/2$.

The approximate solution (1.44) is not optimal because it is not shit invariant and includes fluctuations that are enforced by inversion.

Using expressions (1.42) and (1.43), it is possible to define the functional for IRF spectrum optimization as

$$I_{\tilde{h}} = \arg\min_{\tilde{H}} \left\{ \begin{array}{l} \sum_{i,k\in O}\left\| \sum_{m=1}^{P}\sum_{n=1}^{Q}\sum_{t=0}^{n_x-P}\sum_{\tau=0}^{n_y-Q}\tilde{H}_{m,n} z_{xm}^{i+t} z_{yn}^{k+\tau} h_{t,\tau} - \delta_{i,i_0}\delta_{k,k_0}\right\|^2 + \\ \lambda\cdot Reg\left(\tilde{H}\right) \end{array} \right\}, \tag{1.45}$$

where (i_0, k_0) is a central point in object region, *Reg* denotes regularization functional, λ is parameter that sets additional restrictions on the function $\tilde{H}$ surface. The functional is applied for finding minimal surface. It provides minimization of fluctuations and serves main part of the characteristic feature. The surface area of the function $H(x,y)$ is defined as (Kimmel et al. 1999):

$$\Sigma_H = \int_O \sqrt{1 + H_x^2 + H_y^2}\,(x,y)\,dxdy, \tag{1.46}$$

where $H_x = \delta H(x,y)/\delta x$ and $H_y = \delta H(x,y)/\delta y$. In the spectral domain, the surface area expressed as the regularization functional can be written in the following form:

$$Reg\left(\tilde{H}\right) = \sum_{i,k\in O}\sqrt{1+\left(\sum_{m,n}\tilde{H}_{m,n} dz_{xm} z_{xm}^i z_{yn}^k\right)^2 + \left(\sum_{m,n}\tilde{H}_{m,n} dz_{ym} z_{xm}^i z_{yn}^k\right)^2}, \tag{1.47}$$

where $dz_{x(y)m} = 0.5(z_{x(y)m} - z_{x(y)m}^{-1})$ are spectrum coefficients introduced by discrete derivatives of the harmonic functions. Euler-Lagrange variational derivative of the functional (1.45) and surface area (1.47) looks as the following equation (all indexes serve numbering like in (1.45)).

$$\begin{array}{l} \dfrac{\partial I_{\tilde{h}}}{\partial \tilde{H}_{u,v}} = \sum_{m,n}\tilde{H}_{m,n}\Big(2\sum_{i,k\in O}\sum_{t,\tau}h_{t,\tau}\sum_{i,k\in O} z_{xm}^{i+t} z_{yn}^{k+\tau}\sum_{t',\tau'}h_{t',\tau'} z_{xu}^{i+t'} z_{yu}^{k+\tau'} - \\ \qquad \lambda\left(dz_{xm}dz_{xu} + dz_{ym}dz_{yu}\right)\sum_{i,k\in O} z_{xm}^i z_{yn}^k z_{xu}^i z_{yv}^k Reg\left(\tilde{H}\right)^{-1}\Big) - \\ \sum_{i,k\in O}\sum_{t',\tau'}h_{t',\tau'} z_{xu}^{i+t'} z_{yu}^{k+\tau'} = 0 \end{array} \tag{1.48}$$

The *PQ* expressions (1.48) create the system of equations for iterative evaluation of the IRF transient characteristic optimal spectrum $\tilde{H}$ elements,

$$\sum_{m,n}\tilde{H}_{m,n}^{(p)}\Psi_{u,v,m,n}\left(\tilde{H}^{(p-1)}\right) = \psi_{u,v}; \quad u = 0,\ldots P-1; \quad v = 0,\ldots Q-1; \tag{1.49}$$

where

$$\begin{array}{l} \Psi_{u,v,m,n} = \Big(2\sum_{i,k\in O}\sum_{t,\tau}h_{t,\tau}\sum_{i,k\in O} z_{xm}^{i+t} z_{yn}^{k+\tau}\sum_{t',\tau'}h_{t',\tau'} z_{xu}^{i+t'} z_{yu}^{k+\tau'} - \\ \qquad \lambda\left(dz_{xm}dz_{xu} + dz_{ym}dz_{yu}\right)\sum_{i,k\in O} z_{xm}^i z_{yn}^k z_{xu}^i z_{yv}^k Reg\left(\tilde{H}^{(p-1)}\right)^{-1}\Big), \\ \psi_{u,v} = \sum_{i,k\in O}\sum_{t,\tau}h_{t',\tau'} z_{xu}^{i+t} z_{yu}^{k+\tau}, \end{array}$$

$\tilde{H}^{(p)}_{m,n}$ is the result of p-th iteration step, $\tilde{H}^{(0)}_{m,n} = \tilde{H}_{m,n}$ in (1.40) or $\tilde{H}^{(0)}_{m,n}$ can be obtained by EHD of the (1.44). The solution of the (1.49) is

$$\sum\nolimits_{m,n} \tilde{H}^{(p)}_{m,n} \Psi^{-1}_{u,v,m,n} \left(\tilde{H}^{(p-1)}\right) \psi_{m,n}; \quad u = 0, \dots P-1; \quad v = 0, \dots Q-1. \tag{1.50}$$

The regularization parameter λ can be chosen with the convergence condition of the q first iterations:

$$\sum\nolimits_{u,v=0} \left\| \tilde{H}^{(t+1)}_{u,v} - \tilde{H}^{(t)}_{u,v} \right\|^2 \theta \le \sum\nolimits_{u,v=0} \left\| \tilde{H}^{(t)}_{u,v} - \tilde{H}^{(t-1)}_{u,v} \right\|^2, \tag{1.51}$$

where $t = 1, 2, \dots, q, \theta$ – a positive value. The iteration process can be stopped if

$$\sum\nolimits_{u,v} \left\| \tilde{H}^{(t+1)}_{u,v} - \tilde{H}^{(t)}_{u,v} \right\|^2 \le \varepsilon_{\tilde{H}}, \tag{1.52}$$

where $\varepsilon_{\tilde{H}}$ is a small value.

The optimization of the inverse resonant filter transient characteristic may be made in coordinates space. But in this case on each step of iterations the operation of projection in to EHD spectrum space is necessary for serving of the IRF shift invariance. The projection consists in direct and inverse Fourier transforms (1.36) and (1.35). Because the basis of EHD is not complete this operation is not trivial.

The next step of the optimal IRF transient characteristic evaluation is its normalization in accordance with the condition:

$$\tilde{\mathbf{h}}^T \cdot \mathbf{H} \cong \mathbf{h}^T \cdot \tilde{\mathbf{H}} \tag{1.53}$$

Let the both parts of eq. (1.53) be multiplied by $\mathbf{H}^T$. Then, similarly as in (1.44), one can define vector

$$\tilde{\mathbf{h}}^{(k+1)T} = \mathbf{h}^{(k)T} \left(\tilde{\mathbf{H}} \cdot \mathbf{H}^T\right)\left(\mathbf{H} \cdot \mathbf{H}^T\right)^{-1}. \tag{1.54}$$

The vector obtained can be considered as the next in the series of iterations. The right side of the expression (1.54) includes the matrix $\tilde{\mathbf{H}}$ that is compiled in the previous step. The iterative process is continuing until the condition

$$\sum\nolimits_{i,k} \left\| h^{(t+1)}_{u,v} - \tilde{H}^{(t)}_{u,v} \right\|^2 \le \varepsilon_{\tilde{H}} \tag{1.55}$$

will be met ($\varepsilon_{\tilde{H}} \sim 10^{-8} \dots 10^{-10}$).

The procedures of optimization in spectral domain and the presented above the normalization procedure can be rearranged in their sequence. The equations (1.45) and (1.54) show that in case of normalization, the influence of the forming filter transient characteristic is more significant than in the case when the optimization takes place in spectral domain. Therefore, if the forming filter is given with high level of trust then the normalization should be the last operation. If not, then it should be first one or omitted.

The alternative to the IRF is so called auto-regression with shifted mean (ARSM) (Marple 1987) which can be written as

$$\sum\nolimits_{m=1}^{P} \sum\nolimits_{n=1}^{Q} a_{m,n} d_{i-m,k-n} = d_{i,k} + E + \varsigma_{i,k}, \tag{1.56}$$

where $a_{m,n}$ are the parameters of the model, E is the shift of the mean of the error noise $\varsigma_{i,k}$. The similarity of the models (1.32) and (1.56) is evident. The ARSM is shift invariant that follows from the way it is defined. Generally, it cannot be presented as series of harmonics, in contrast to IRF. The difference will be explained with object recognition examples.

5 CREATION OF FUNCTIONS BASIS FOR EIGEN HARMONIC DECOMPOSITION

The first step of designing inverse resonant filter is eigen harmonic decomposition of the target textured object template. There are known some approaches to 2D nonlinear spectral analyses. The simplest way is the estimation of the LSO parameters and its characteristic polynomial (1.23) roots for two space coordinates. This approach gives appropriate result, if the 2D signal is uniform. Otherwise, the full matrix of 2D data should be used. The following approaches to 2D EHD are developed: 2D-MUSIC (Multiple Signal Classification) (Marple 1987), 2D-ESPRIT (Estimation of Signal Parameter via Rotational Invariance Techniques) (Rouquette & Najim 2001), 2D-Matrices Pencil Method (MPM) (Hua 1992), Total Least Squares (TLS) version of MPM (Bunyak 1995), and 2D-Linear Prediction Method (LPM) using the 2D generalization of the LSO (1.22) as (1.28) (Barbieri & Barone1992, Bunyak 1996). In the case of texture EHD, it is necessary to consider important restrictions to the model parameters:

The texture model is considering as a response on excitement (1.31) of the linear dynamic system (1.30). Texture stationarity implies the condition of periodicity which is defined by equation (1.26). Therefore, the eigen modes in (1.34) should have a trivial dumping factor. It implies the roots of the model's characteristic polynomial (1.23) must be placed on the unit circle. In the other words, the dynamic model must have unitary symmetry in respect to the linear shift operations.

- Texture might not be a smooth function. Therefore, the EHD method should not be sensitive to image signal breaks.
- The inverse problem solution in spectral domain of the EHD requires the determination of the principal eigen mode numbers to exclude the unstable results.
- A high order filter is required when background texture is complicated, quasi-regular, or corrupted by noise spikes.
- The last two requirements above are mutually inconsistent when used to determine the IRF order. This conflict requires designing of a spectral basis that would be adapted to the specific image signal properties if high order inverse filtration is to be performed.

5.1 *Estimation of texture resonant spectrum*

The examined methods of spectral parameter estimation are based on a correlative relation between two mutually shifted data sets. Linear parameterization of this relation yields the linear prediction (LP) model and its various implementations. LP based methods are sensitive to signal phase. Usually, this sensitivity becomes apparent in splitting of spectral lines (Marple 1987). Therefore, there is a need to design methods that are not sensitive to image signal phase brake. An approach will be considered that based on 1D data harmonic decomposition and an approach based on 2D data harmonic decomposition.

5.1.1 *The linear symmetry method*

The product of sample matrices $X_0 = \left[x_{i+k}\right]_{i=0\ldots P-1, k=0\ldots N-P-1}$ and X_0^T forms the correlation matrix of size $P \times P$

$$R_P = X_0 X_0^T. \tag{1.57}$$

The same product of matrices $X_1 = \left[x_{i+k+1}\right]_{i=0\ldots P-1, k=0\ldots N-P-1}$ and X_1^T gives also the correlation matrix. These matrices and matrices in eq. (1.57) are related by LSO (1.22):

$$X_1 X_1^T = K_P X_0 X_0^T K_P^T = K_P R_P K_P^T \tag{1.58}$$

If a data set is infinitely long, then the product (1.58) is equal to (1.57). Then, the following equation can be written

$$R_P = K_P R_P K_P^T \tag{1.59}$$

which defines the linear symmetry (LS) in (Bunyak & Bunyak 2007) of the correlation matrix. The usual LP model like (1.56) is shift invariant, relatively to data first moments in the manner of data samples. The LS supplement the LP model by the condition of invariance to shift operations of the second moments—correlation samples. This restriction on the data model is imposed with the aim to reduce sensitivity to data breaks. As it was shown in (Bunyak & Bunyak 2007) this additional symmetry removes LP model dependence on signal initial phase. Equation (1.59) provides unitarity of the LSO because the similarity transformation does not change the correlation matrix energy. It can be easy proved that transformation (1.59) is valid on the condition that the correlation matrix has Toeplitz structure. This allows to use the correlation function for evaluation model LS parameters as well as in Levinson-Durbin algorithm (Marple 1987). Though, when data set is short the Toeplitz structure corrupts spectrum. Therefore, the solution of the LS equation is considered which gives unitarity LSO and uses the correlation matrix (1.57).

Let the expression of the last row and column transforms in equation (1.59) will be considered under condition the correlation matrix is Toeplitz and is signed by correlation function vector $[r_i]_{i=0...P-1}$. To simplify the expressions, the following designations will be applied: $\alpha_i = -\alpha_{P-i}, i = 0 \ldots P-1$. Then the equation for first $p-1$ elements has the next form.

$$\sum_{i=0}^{k} r_{k-i+1}\alpha_i + \sum_{i=0}^{P-k-2} r_i \alpha_{i+k+1} = r_{P-1-k} \tag{1.60}$$

where $k = 0 \ldots p-2$. The equation for the last element is as follows:

$$\sum_{i=0}^{k} r_{k-i+1}\alpha_i \left(\sum_{i=0}^{k-1} r_{k-i}\alpha_i + \sum_{i=0}^{P-k-1} r_i \alpha_{i+k} \right) = r_0 \tag{1.61}$$

The system of equations (1.60)–(1.61) contains the nonlinear equation (1.61), relatively to P^2 squares of the desired values. Therefore, it does not have unique solution. One of them can be found by the approach basing on the reference element method.

The reference element should be chosen as the most sensitive to influence of the polynomial (1.9) roots. It is known that:

$$-\alpha_i = \alpha_{P-1} = \sum_{i=1}^{P} (z_i + \delta z_i); \quad -\alpha_P = \alpha_0 = \prod_{i=1}^{P} (z_i + \delta z_i) \tag{1.62}$$

If $|z_i| \leq 1$ then it is evident from equation (1.62) that $-a_1 = a_{P-1}$ is mostly sensitive to variations $|\delta z| << 1$ because the rest coefficients are combinations of sums of multiplicative components. The multiplicative components include second other variations and weighted variations.

Let select in $P-1$ equations (1.60) the components related with α_{P-1} and carry them from the left to the right side. The obtained equations system in the matrix form can be written as

$$\begin{bmatrix} r_1 & r_0 & \cdots & r_{P-3} \\ r_0 & r_1 & \cdots & r_{P-4} \\ \vdots & \vdots & \ddots & \vdots \\ r_{P-3} & r_{P-4} & \cdots & r_1 \end{bmatrix} \cdot \begin{bmatrix} \alpha_0 \\ \alpha_1 \\ \vdots \\ \alpha_{P-1} \end{bmatrix} = \begin{bmatrix} r_{P-1} - \alpha_{P-1} r_{P-2} \\ r_{P-2} - \alpha_{P-1} r_{P-3} \\ \vdots \\ r_1 - \alpha_{P-1} r_0 \end{bmatrix}. \tag{1.63}$$

The Toeplitz matrix in (1.63) can be changed by associated elements of the matrix like (1.57). Then, instead of the exact equation (1.63) the approximate expression will be obtained:

$$\begin{bmatrix} r_{1,0} & r_{1,1} & \cdots & r_{1,p-2} \\ r_{2,0} & r_{2,1} & \cdots & r_{2,P-2} \\ \vdots & \vdots & \ddots & \vdots \\ r_{p-1,0} & r_{p-1,1} & \cdots & r_{p-1,p-2} \end{bmatrix} \cdot \begin{bmatrix} \alpha_0 \\ \alpha_1 \\ \vdots \\ \alpha_{p-2} \end{bmatrix} \cong \begin{bmatrix} r_{0,p-1} - \alpha_{p-1} r_{1,p-1} \\ r_{1,p-1} - \alpha_{p-1} r_{2,p-1} \\ \vdots \\ r_{p-2,p-1} - \alpha_{p-1} r_{1,p-10} \end{bmatrix}. \tag{1.64}$$

Let $[\rho_{i,k}]_{i,k=0...P-2}$ is the inverse matrix with respect to matrix in left part of (1.64). Then the solution of the system (1.64) can be presented as:

$$\alpha_i = b_i - \alpha_{p-1} g_i, \tag{1.65}$$

where $b_i = \sum_{k=0}^{P-2} \rho_{i,k} r_{i,p-1}$; $g_i = \sum_{k=0}^{P-2} \rho_{i,k} r_{i+1,p-1}$. The nonlinear equation (1.64) generalized for arbitrary correlation matrix has the following form

$$\sum_{i,k=0}^{P-1} \alpha_i \alpha_k r_{i,k} \cong r_{P-1,P-1}. \tag{1.66}$$

The substitution of eq. (1.65) into (1.66) yields square equation

$$a\alpha_{p-1}^2 + b\alpha_{p-1} + c = 0. \tag{1.67}$$

The minimal sensitivity to variations has the extremum of the (1.67). Therefore,

$$\alpha_{P-1} = -b/2a \tag{1.68}$$

where

$$a = \sum_{i=0}^{P-2} \left(\sum_{k=0}^{P-2} g_i g_k r_{i,k} - 2 g_i r_{i,p-1} \right) + r_{p-1,p-1},$$
$$b = \sum_{i=0}^{P-2} \left(2 b_i r_{i,p-1} - \sum_{k=0}^{P-2} (b_i g_k + b_k g_i) \right).$$

The numerical experiments have shown that the solution in the form of (1.65) and (1.68) corresponds to unitary model of the signal. The element should fulfil $\alpha_0 = -a_p \cong 1$ with accuracy of $\sim 10^{-10}$.

An arbitrary arrow and column of the target object image matrix can be used for definition of LSO (1.22) parameters and roots of the characteristic polynomial (1.23) if the image signal is homogeneous. In the other case the components of a 2D correlation matrix are more descriptive. The 2D correlation matrix of the object image region is expressed as

$$R^{(2)} = \left[r^{(2)}_{i_x,k_x,i_y,k_y} \right]_{i_x,k_x=0...P-1}^{i_y,k_y=0...Q-1} = \left[\sum_{m=0}^{n_x-P} \sum_{n=0}^{n_y-Q} d_{m+i_x,n+i_y} d_{m+k_x,n+k_y} \right]_{i_x,k_x=0...P-1}^{i_y,k_y=0...Q-1}. \tag{1.69}$$

The correlation matrices that characterize data along coordinates may be defined as

$$R_x^{(2)} = \left[r^{(2)}_{i_x,k_x,0,0} \right]_{i_x,k_x=0...P-1}^{i_y,k_y=0}$$
$$R_y^{(2)} = \left[r^{(2)}_{0,0,i_y,k_y} \right]_{i_x,k_x=0}^{i_y,k_y=0...Q-1}. \tag{1.70}$$

These matrices can be used as R_p in expression (1.57) for estimation of the two LSO parameters.

5.1.2 *The 2D Correlation Matrix Splitting Method (CMSM)*
When texture is dynamic the correlation matrices (1.57), (1.70) do not reflect image variability, therefore the 2D correlation matrix (1.69) should be used for estimation of the texture resonant frequencies. The methods of the mentioned above 2D eigen-harmonic decomposition differs by data type employed. The MUSIC and ESPRIT methods use second data moments, MPM uses first data moments and 2D LPM uses first and second data moments. 2D EHD method is based on first moment data shift of the dynamic model, which transforms the data along coordinates. Generalization of these approaches will be considered on SVD platform. This decomposition allows to select a principal part of an image signal and omit weak fluctuations. What is more, it allows splitting data on mutually shifted matrix pencils in orthogonal vector space. The matrix pencils create an eigenvalues problem that can be solved by TLS approach. The eigenvalues are equal to roots of polynomial (1.38). The eigenvalues problem may be written for 2D data $d_{m,n}$ of size $M \times N$ as matrix pencils (Hua 1992, Bunyak 1995):

$$D_x^{(2)} - z_x D^{(2)}; \quad D_y^{(2)} - z_y D^{(2)}, \tag{1.71}$$

where:

$$D_{x(y)}^{(2)} = \left[D_{i+k+x}^{(y)} \right]_{i=0\ldots M-L-1}^{k=0\ldots L-1},$$
$$D_{i+k+x}^{(y)} = \left[d_{i+k+x,m+n+y} \right]_{n=0\ldots M-L-1}^{m=0\ldots L-1},$$

z is the spectral parameter, L is the splitting parameter. If the 2D data include $P/2$ real harmonics and do not contain noise, value $P \le L$, the rank of matrix pencils (15) is equal to P, the data can be presented by P vectors of the SVD. If z_x and z_y are equal to the matrix pencils eigenvalues, then the expressions (15) are equal to zero. In order to solve the eigenvalues problem, the following matrices can be used relatively to x and y coordinates,

$$Z_{Ex(y)}^{(2)} = \left(D^{(2)} \right)^{\#} D_{x(y)}^{(2)}. \tag{1.72}$$

Singular value decomposition can be used for the operation of pseudoinverse in eq. (1.72) by using the P largest singular values and corresponding them eigen vectors. As we mentioned above, the textured image object dynamic model needs in unitary shift transform by the matrix in left part (1.72) as well as by LSO (1.22). This condition may be supported by including into (1.72) direct and backward shift transforms to eliminate influence of the dumping factors of the spectral parameters in the case of data matrices splitting. The data matrices in (1.72) can be accomplished by inverse direction components as $[D^{(2)} J T^{(2)}]$, where J is matrix with unitary cross-diagonal.

The correlation matrix $R^{(2)} = [D^{(2)} J T^{(2)}]^T [D^{(2)} J T^{(2)}]$ can be found by multiplying the matrices in the left side of equation (1.72) by the transposed matrices. Its singular value decomposition can be written as the follows

$$R^{(2)} = U \cdot \Xi \cdot V^T \tag{1.73}$$

where U and V are matrices of the left and right orthogonal eigenvectors, Ξ is the diagonal matrix of the singular values. Applying expression (1.46) the matrix (1.45) may be rewritten as

$$Z_{Ex(y)}^{(2)} = \left(U_0^H U_0 \right)^{-1} U_0^H U_{x(y)}, \tag{1.74}$$

where matrices U_0, $U_{x(y)}$ have M vectors which correspond to M largest singular values in decomposition (1.73). Their rows correspond to reciprocally shifted matrices $D^{(2)}$ and $D_{x(y)}^{(2)}$, The matrix U_0 is the basis matrix of expression (1.74), the shifted matrix $U_{x(y)}$ has structure that depends on the direction of the shift: toward x yields U_x; toward y yields U_y. The basic matrix U_0 is formed by extracting from matrix U the last $M - L - 1$-th rows and each $N - L - 1$-th rows starting from the last row. The matrix U_x is formed by extracting from matrix U in (1.73) the first $M - L - 1$ rows. The matrix U_y is formed by each $N - L - 1$ row of matrix U, starting from the first row. The inversion of the matrix $D^{(2)}_{x(y)}$ may be executed by iteration operation (Marple 1987),

$$F_k = F_{k-1} + \frac{\left(F_{k-1}\mathbf{u}_{\alpha}^{H}\right)\left(\mathbf{u}_{\alpha}F_{k-1}\right)}{1+\mathbf{u}_{\alpha}F_{k-1}\mathbf{u}_{\alpha}^{H}}, \tag{1.75}$$

where $U_0 = I_M$ is the identity matrix of size M, and $\mathbf{u}_{\alpha}$ is the vector of α-th row of the matrix U first M vectors, the indices α denote the set of rows that extracted as was described above. If all extracted rows are used sequentially in (1.75), then the last matrix F_k is equal to $\left(U_0^H U_0\right)^{-1}$. The eigenvalues z_{xi}, z_{yi} $(i = 1 \ldots M)$ can be defined as eigenvalues of the matrices (1.71), (1.72), (1.74), which are modified depending on shift direction.

As it follows from the method description, the number of principal harmonic components of the textured image signal EHD is defined by the rank of the matrices in (1.72). Singular value decomposition allows to define harmonics number carefully if $L \geq M \geq P$. The chosen M vectors correspond to largest singular values and therefore the method is not sensitive to phase brakes and noise spikes which usually relate with vectors of the small singular values. This property confirms the earlier made conclusion that alignment with texture EHD is equivalent to SVD and EVD.

5.2 *Creation of a function basis for high order EHD*

The matrix operator of DFT of size $N \times N$ can be presented as a multiplication of simpler matrices on condition that N is a composite number, for example $N = m^n$, where m, n are arbitrary integer constants. The factorized presentation gives the algorithm of Fast Fourier Transform (FFT) (Marple 1987, Elliot & Rao 1983). As it was presented in (Bunyak 1989)

$$\begin{gathered} F_N(k,x) = \prod_{i=1}^{n} W_i(k,x) = \prod_{i=1}^{n}\left(V_m(v_i) \otimes I_{m^{n-i}}\left(k^i,x^i\right)\right) \otimes \left(\Omega_m\left(m^{i-1}k^i,v_i,u_i\right) \otimes I_{m^{i-1}}\right) \\ k = k^i + \sum_{j=1}^{i} v_j m^{n-j};\ x = m^i x^i + \sum_{j=1}^{i} u_j m^{j-1}; \end{gathered} \tag{1.76}$$

where $I_{m^{n-i}}\left(k^i, x^i\right)$ is a unitary diagonal matrix with numbered rows and columns corresponding to k^i and x^i, k^i, $x^i = 0, 1, \ldots N/m^i - 1$. The matrix $I_{m^{n-i}}$ index means its size, $u^i = 0, 1, \ldots m - 1$, x^i are the numbers of data vector elements which are multiplied by the phase rotating matrix

$$\Omega_m\left(k^i, v_i, u_i\right) = \left[\exp\left(-\iota\frac{2\pi}{N}\left(k^i + v_i\frac{N}{m}\right)u_i\right)\right], \tag{1.77}$$

where the indices $v_i = 0,1,\ldots m - 1$ together with k^i are the number of result vector elements. The factorization (1.76) can be generalized for any N that is a product of arbitrary integer values. If $N = p \times m^{n-1}$ the matrix (1.77) for $i = 1$ in (1.76) is follows:

$$\Omega_p\left(k^1, v_1, u_1\right) = \left[\exp\left(-\iota\frac{2\pi}{N}\left(\frac{v_1 u_1}{p} + \frac{k^1 v_1}{N}\right)\right)\right]. \tag{1.78}$$

The first term of the sum in the exponent factor in (1.78) creates elements of the DFT operator of size $N = p$. The second term is the modulation coefficient which serves to extend low order DFT.

The DFT operator in the base of texture eigen harmonics is presented by matrices $Z^{\#}_{x(y)}$, $Z_{x(y)}$ in (1.35), (1.36). The matrices can be extended by such way as is extended phase rotating matrix (1.77) in the Fourier operator (1.76). For this let change the first term of the sum in (1.78) by elements which are analogues to the matrix $Z_{x(y)}$. Then, the following phase rotating matrix can be obtained:

$$\Omega_{zp}\left(k^1, v_1, u_1\right) = \left[z^{u_1}_{v_1+1} \exp\left(-\imath 2\pi \frac{k^1 v_1}{N} \right) \right]_{u_1, v_1 0, \ldots, p-1} . \tag{1.79}$$

Substitution of the matrix (1.79) into equation (1.76) yields the operator of DFT with the eigen kernel (EK) associated with the textured object image signal. The signal is characterized by series of resonant frequencies $f_1 \ldots f_p$. The equation can be written in factored form

$$F_{zN}(k,x) = \prod\nolimits_{i=2}^{n} W_i(k,x) \cdot W_Z(k,x); \tag{1.80}$$

$$W_z(k,x) = \left(I_{m^{n-1}}\left(k^1, x^1\right) \otimes \Omega_{zp}\left(k^1, v_1, u_1\right) \right);$$

$$\begin{cases} i = 1 : k = k^1 + v_1 m^{n-1}; \quad x = px^1 + u_1 \\ i > 1 : k = k^i + \sum_{j=1}^{i} v_1 p m^{n-j-1}; \quad x = v_1 p m^{n-1} + \sum_{j=1}^{i} u_1 p m^{j-2} \end{cases} .$$

Discrete Fourier transform expressed as eq. 1.80 is equivalent to $F_{zN} = F_{N/p} \otimes Z_p$. The inverse discrete Fourier transform with eigen kernel is similar to equation (1.80) with phase rotating matrix:

$$\Omega_p^{-1}\left(k^1, v_1, u_1\right) = \left[\overline{z}_{v_1 u_1} \exp\left(\imath \frac{2\pi k^1 v_1}{N} \right) \right]_{v_1, u_1 0, \ldots, p-1} , \tag{1.81}$$

where $\overline{z}_{v_1 u_1}$ are the elements of a matrix $Z^{\#}$ like the matrices in (1.21) of $p \times p$ size.

Discrete Fourier Transform with Eigen Kernel (DFTEK) implements both PCA and EMD. The p main components can be selected using the EHD and they can be considering as principal components. These p empirical modes are splintered on N/p aliquot quasi-harmonic components and together they create the DFTEK. The textured image signals usually are quasi-periodical, but not exactly harmonic. Therefore, the DFTEK spectrum is numerically valid and informative. Application of DFTEK for inverse problem solution and high-order filtering is well-founded. DFTEK is not exactly orthogonal and has a partly multiplicative functions basis.

6 IMPLEMENTATION AND EXPERIMENTAL ANALYSIS OF THE IRF

Inverse resonant filter can be realized in spatial domain by convolution of image data with transient characteristic (1.41) or with obtained by the transform (1.37) optimized characteristic (1.49). This operation needs $P \times Q$ multiplications and accumulations per pixel. Another approach is based on filtration in the spectral domain. This approach may be significantly more effective but it has some particularities which will be considered bellow.

Filtration in spectral domain includes definition an image fragment of the size $P \times Q$ with spectrum A in accordance to equation (1.36). The fragment is then multiplied using the elements of the filter spectrum (1.40) or (1.49), and then the filtered values are calculated according to equation (1.35). These operations need $2(P + Q) + 1$ complex MACC operations per pixel. Therefore, the filtration in spectral domain has higher efficiency in comparison with the filtration in spatial domain when filter order $P(Q) \geq 64$.

IRF realization will be considered in spectral domain on an example textured object of the size 288 × 768 pixels on textured background as shown in Figure 1.1a. The task is to recognize the texture of dried up riverbed and remove it. The accompanying problem is to detect the foreign object. One color component of the image signal is presented in Figure 1.1b. As it seen in the figure, the signal amplitude of the foreign object is analogous to the background signal and differs by another dynamic and statistical features. The analysis of inverse correlation matrices (Bunyak & Bunyak 2007) has revealed that IRF order can be chosen as $P \times Q = 32 \times 32$. The base region of size $n_x \times n_y = 64 \times 64$ was chosen in the upper left corner of the image for evaluation of IRF transient characteristic. The result of filtration is presented in Figure 1.1c. According to equation (1.32) the figure shows variability in the neighborhood $E = 1$. Because the background texture is heterogeneous there is a surface displacement that is larger in the corner comparing to base region. The dispersion of the filter error noise in the object base region was applied to perform statistical analysis of the filtered signal. It was estimated in the form of the following equation

$$\sigma_\varsigma^2 = \frac{1}{n_x n_y}\sum_{i=0}^{n_x-1}\sum_{j=0}^{n_y-1}\left(\tilde{d}_{i,j}-E\right)^2 \qquad (1.82)$$

where $\tilde{d}_{i,j} = E + \varsigma_{i,k}$ represents the filtered image signal values. The dispersion is the parameter of the target textured object pattern as well as the transient characteristics of the IRF (1.41) or (1.49).

It is possible to generate an image $G : d_{i,k}^{(t)} \in G;\ t = 1,2,3$ by filtration of the image $D : d_{i,k}^{(t)} \in D$ using IRF which contains mapped objects defined by the following logical filter:

$$\begin{aligned} &\textbf{if} \quad \bigcup_{t=1}^{3}\left(\left|\tilde{d}_{i,j}-E\right| > 3\sigma_\varsigma^{(t)}\right)\sigma_\varsigma^2 \\ &\textbf{then} \quad g_{i,k}^{(t)} = d_{i,k}^{(t)} \\ &\textbf{else} \quad g_{i,k}^{(t)} = 0; \quad t = 1,2,3\,. \end{aligned} \qquad (1.83)$$

The upper indices in the brackets point to color components. The dispersion was estimated for each color component. The result of filtering (G) is presented in Figure 1.1d. It contains the mapped object, and unwanted fragments of the background differing slightly from the

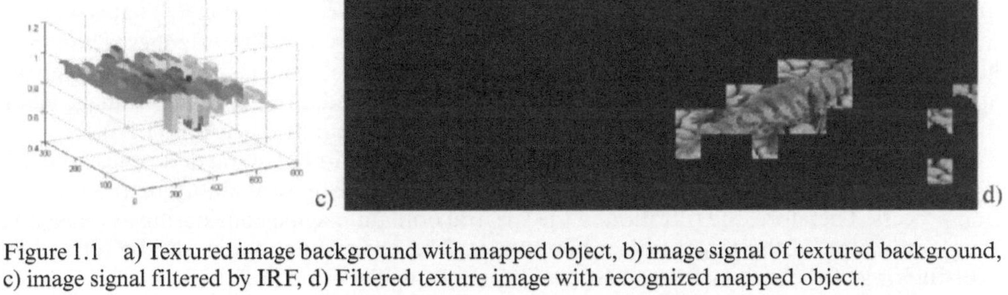

Figure 1.1 a) Textured image background with mapped object, b) image signal of textured background, c) image signal filtered by IRF, d) Filtered texture image with recognized mapped object.

base region pattern. The appearance of unwanted fragments is also caused by the image fragment spectrum differing in phase from the base region spectrum. The phase equalization of spectrum fragments can be performed in order to eliminate the unwanted objects.

Let the spectrum matrix (1.36) of the object base region be denoted by $A^{(0)}$. The approximation given by equation (1.35) of some shifted fragment can be written with phase displacement functions as it is shown in equation (1.25).

$$D' = Z_x diag\left[e^{\phi_{x1'}} \ldots e^{\phi_{xP}}\right] A^{(0)} diag\left[e^{\phi_{y1'}} \ldots e^{\phi_{yQ}}\right] Z_y^T. \quad (1.84)$$

The phase coefficients in eq. (1.59) can be found using least square method by minimizing the following functional:

$$I = \underset{\Phi}{\arg\min} \sum_{i=1}^{P} \sum_{k=1}^{Q} \left(A_{i,k} \Phi_{xi} \Phi_{yk} - A_{i,k}^{0}\right)^2, \quad (1.85)$$

where $\Phi_i = \exp(\phi_i)$. The variation of the functional the functional above

$$\frac{\partial I}{\partial \Phi_{x(y)i}} = 0; \quad i = 1 \ldots P(Q)$$

gives the system of nonlinear equations:

$$\begin{aligned} \Phi_{xi} &= \frac{\sum_{k=1}^{Q} A_{i,k} A_{i,k}^{(0)} \Phi_{yk}}{\sum_{k=1}^{Q} A_{i,k}^2 \Phi_{yk}^2}; \quad i = 1 \ldots P \\ \Phi_{yk} &= \frac{\sum_{k=1}^{P} A_{i,k} A_{i,k}^{(0)} \Phi_{xi}}{\sum_{k=1}^{P} A_{i,k}^2 \Phi_{xi}^2}; \quad k = 1 \ldots Q \end{aligned} \quad (1.86)$$

The system can be simply solved with iterative method. The initial values of the phase displacement functions on the right side of both equations (1.86) are trivial: $\Phi_{x(y)i}^{(0)} = 1$. The first and next iterations give the sequence of values $\Phi_{x(y)i}^{(k)}$, $k = 1, 2, \ldots$. If the sequence match the condition

$$\sum_i \left|\Phi_{x(y)i}^{(k)} - \Phi_{x(y)i}^{(k-1)}\right| \approx \sum_i \left|\Phi_{x(y)i}^{(k-1)} - \Phi_{x(y)i}^{(k-2)}\right|, \quad (1.87)$$

the iteration process can be stopped. The resulting values $\Phi_{x(y)i}^{(k)}$ are then applied for spectrum redefinition as it was done in equation (1.84). If condition given by equation (1.87) is not fulfilled, system of equation (1.86) has no solution and the phase multipliers are not applied.

The image signal filtered by the inverse filter with phase equalization in agreement with equations (1.84)–(1.87) is presented in Figure 1.2a. In comparison with the signal in Figure 1.1c, the signal surface is smoother, however some spikes can be noticed. That is why the target object image in Figure 1.2b is recognized without substantial error zones. Though, it has solitary chaotic error pixels. From the point of view of object classification such errors are less important than those in Figure 1.1c and can be ignored. For the example image being discussed, not more than 5 iterations were used to solve system of equations (1.86).

Figure 1.1c and 1.2b show that filtration in spectral domain has some deficiencies. Image zones can be recognized with some space step. It reduces resolution ability of the recognition process. Therefore, the filtration in the spectral domain may be considering as a fast and rough estimator of the target object boundaries. The object boundaries can be refined by post-filtering of the recognized and adjoined zones using the same IRF in the spatial domain.

Figure 1.2 a) Image signal filtered by the inverse filter with spectrum phase equalization, b) object image filtered by the inverse filter with spectrum phase equalization.

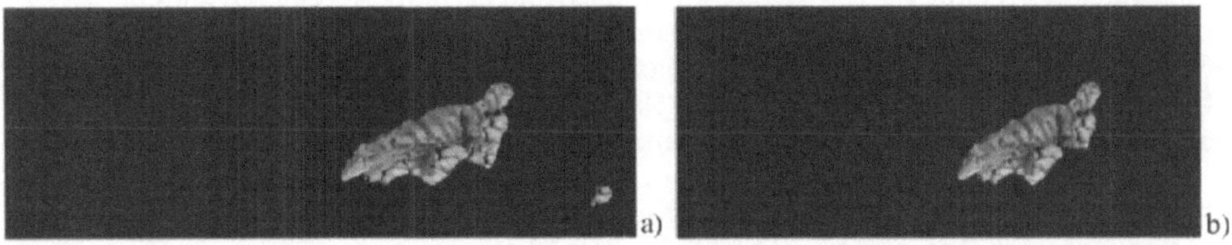

Figure 1.3 a) Result of image post-filtration in spatial domain of the image presented in Figure 1.1c; b) result of image post-filtration in spatial domain of the image presented in Figure 1.2b.

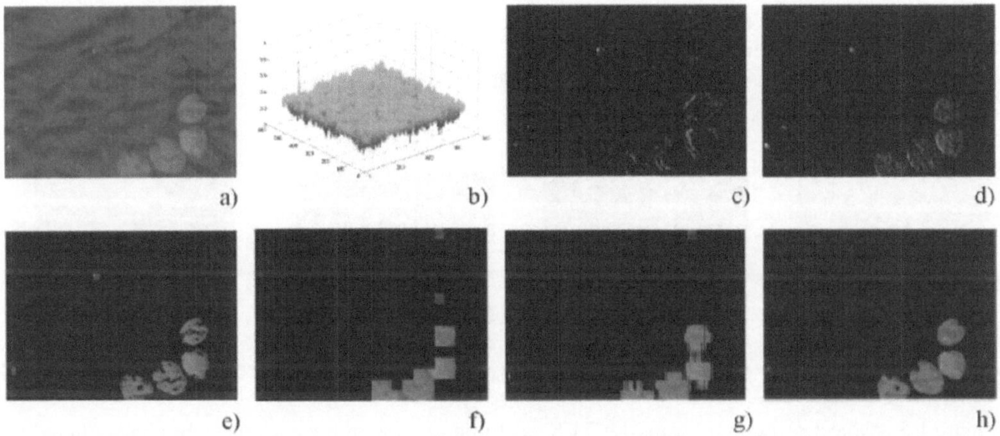

Figure 1.4 a) Initial image, b) one color signal, c) the results of filtration by AR, d) by AR with shifted mean (1.56), e) by IRF (1.26), f) by IRF in spectral domain, g) by IRF in spectral domain with phase equalization, h) by the post filtration by the optimal IRF (1.49).

The results of post-filtering of nontrivial zones of the images in Figures 1.1c and 1.2b are shown in Figures 1.3a and 1.3b, respectively.

The example presented in Figure 1.4 reveals ability of inverse resonant filters in recognizing dynamic textures and sensitivity to small objects. The texture presented in Figure 1.4a) can be considered as spatial dynamic because its each fragment is a result of dynamic change or extension of an adjacent fragment. The fragments are similar but not the same as it can be noticed in Figure 1.4b). The mapped objects signal slowly differs from the background texture signal. Figures 1.4c)–d) shows that alternative to inverse resonant filter usual AR filter and AR filter with shifted mean of 16th order give unsatisfactory results. As it can be seen in Figure 1.4e), inverse resonant filter of 16th order allows to recognize target texture as well as small (white points) and slow mapped objects. The region of 64×64 pixels in the left upper corner of the initial image for evaluation of the filters parameters. Fast filtration in the spectral domain (Figs. 1.4f–g) produces similar results but with rough object boundaries and some errors. The result of the post filtration of selected and adjoining zones of the image by optimal IRF is shown in Figure 1.4h. The filter allows to specify mapped objects boundaries and eliminate improper objects in all color components.

The example in Figure 1.5 shows implementation of high order filtration using discrete Fourier transform with eigen kernel. The multi-component image in Figure 1.5 a) of 2496×3072 pixels includes target textured background of wheat grains. The image contains several zones where wet grains, oat and rye grains with fuzzy boundaries are present. For texture recognition, a filter of order of $P \times Q = 96 \times 96$ was applied and decomposed as $P(Q) = p \times m^n = 6 \times 2^4$. To generate DFTEK basis, three pairs of complex roots of the characteristic polynomial of 96th order were used that correspond to maximal amplitudes of the spectrum (1.21). Results of the filtration are presented in Figures 1.5b)–d). The results of the filtration using EHD of 96th order have same quality but up to 7 times more MACC complex operations are needed.

In the case of the first two examples, linear symmetry of correlation matrices (1.70) was used for estimation of linear shift operator parameters as well as for synthesis of eigen-harmonic decomposition basis. 2D CMSM method was used to estimate the 96 principal harmonic components of the target texture model.

A bank of inverse resonant filters can be used for classification of textured components of multicomponent image. The example of the filter bank is shown in Figure 1.6. Three filters of 16th order were designed for the corresponding textured images in Figures 1.6b), d), f), which then were used for filtration of the initial image shown in Figure 1.6a). The results of the optimal filtration are shown in Figures 1.6c), e), g). As it can be observed, the target textured objects are recognized and the image presented in Figure 1.6a) can be split into separate components.

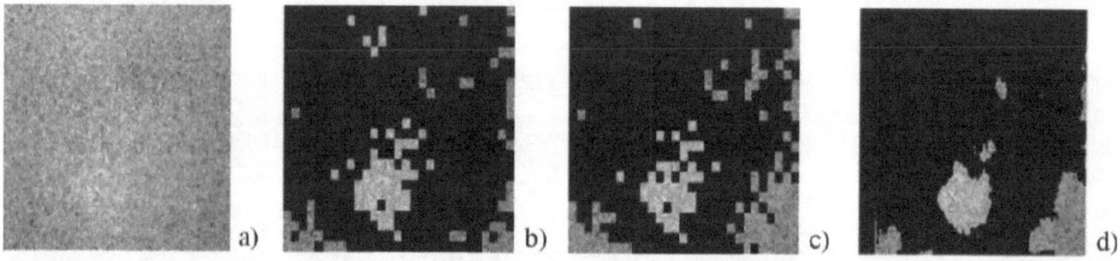

Figure 1.5 Object recognition using DFTEK. a) Initial multi-component image, b) image filtered in spectral domain, c) in spectral domain with phase alignment, d) post-filtration of previous image in spatial domain.

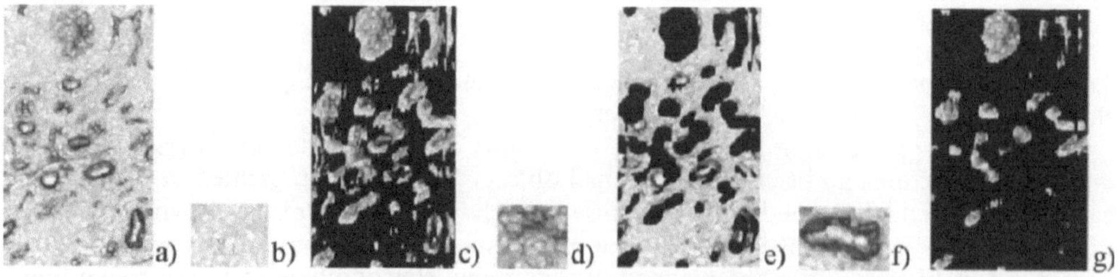

Figure 1.6 Filtration of the multicomponent texture a) by IRF bank of the textures b), d), f) which gives the result images c), e), g) where the corresponding textures are eliminated.

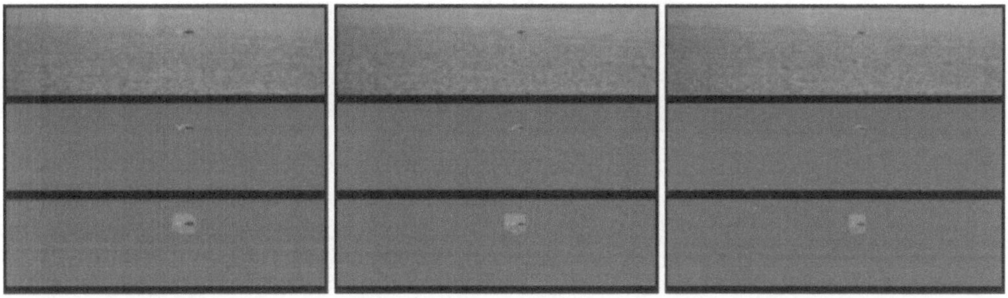

Figure 1.7 Three consecutive fragment of the dynamic time and space varying texture as the marine surface (high row) are filtered by the IRF (middle row) and correlation filter (1.63) (low row) for robust recognition of the foreign object.

When texture is varying both in time and space and is characterizing by non-stationary surges, the application of simple statistical analysis and logical filtration given by equations (1.82), (1.83) will not provide high quality filtration and recognition. If texture tracking is continuous, it is possible to remove false mapped objects by binary correlation of the objects, which are found in the consequent frames.

The method of filtration by binary correlation includes (Podobna et al. 2009):

- Estimation of the objects size and its geometrical center.
- Evaluation of the correlation coefficients between objects in L consecutive frames:

$$r = \frac{\sum_{t=0}^{L-1}\sum_{i,j\in S_x\times S_y}\left\{g_{i,j}^{[0]}>0\right\}\wedge\left\{g_{i,j}^{[t]}<0\right\}}{\sum_{t=0}^{L-1}\sum_{i,j\in S_x\times S_y}\left\{g_{i,j}^{[t]}>0\right\}} \tag{1.88}$$

where $\left\{g_{i,j}^{[0]}>0\right\}\wedge\left\{g_{i,j}^{[t]}<0\right\}$ denotes logical function "AND". If the condition in the brackets is true then the value is equal to one, otherwise the value is zero, $S_x \times S_y$ is the object location. The numbers in the square brackets point to the frame number.

- If the correlation coefficient (1.88) exceeds the threshold level then the object is true, otherwise it is false.
- A true object is refined with its immediate surrounding background for further classification.
- The L frames running time should be much smaller in comparison to the moving time of the object of interest within the location rectangle $S_x \times S_y$.

An example consecutive frames of marine surface filtering are shown in Figure 1.5. As it can be noticed in the upper row, the texture of marine surface is heterogeneous. Therefore, the filtration was made by filters bank of fore IRF for fore separated image zones along the vertical coordinate. Full frame is 200 × 600 pixels. A base region of 32 × 32 pixels for design the IRF of 8th order in each zone was chosen in its upper left corner. It was used CMSM. Binary correlative filter defined by equation (1.88) with $L = 3$ and $r = 0.3$ was applied. Some errors remained after applying IRF and logical filtration as shown in the middle row of Figure 1.5. They were successfully removed with correlative filtration.

7 CONCLUSIONS

Most of the current textured image modeling methods focus on decompositions and integral transforms that provide the most informative parameters and reflect both spatial and temporal properties of the texture. These methods are founded on texture symmetry in respect to shift and rotate transforms. The symmetry means that there exists character of a texture pattern transform that reflects its changes in space or time domain. Such a type of dynamic transform can be represented by linear shift operator that models step changes of texture pattern as well as its periodicity. The eigenvectors of LSO can serve as a basis for eigen-harmonic decomposition of the texture with invariance to shift transforms.

The problem of object recognition against a textured background can be solved by elimination of the background by IRF if the background is presented as a response of the dynamic model on exciting signal of simple form. The classification of the exiting signal pattern is sufficiently simpler than classification of the original image.

It was shown in equation (1.14) that if the inverse filtration is resonant in respect to texture pattern than such filter is optimal. The term "resonant" has many meanings. In general, this is equivalence of a target object to some templates of pattern. The most known is the resonance with harmonic fluctuations.

The next step of the filtration optimizing is evaluation of the optimal transient characteristic (1.49) in spectral domain. Although EHD basis provides a mathematically correct solution of the inverse problem with a certain number of estimated harmonic principal components, the elements of the amplitude matrix in equation (1.36) and their inverse values are sensitive to empirical data chaotic fluctuations. Therefore, the optimization of the found spectrum (1.41) needs for enforcing of main harmonic components. This is achieved with additional restrictions on the form of the spectral matrix in equations (1.45) – (1.47). The restriction of minimal surface allows select principal spectral components. It needed up to 5 iterations (1.49) to achieve the condition provided by (1.52). The next step of optimization (1.53) is rather a verification of the transient characteristic inversion. The condition (1.55) is satisfied after 2 iterations of (1.54).

The couple of transforms defined by equations (1.35) and (1.36) play the key role in filter design. They relay with precise estimation of LSO and its eigenvalues which mean the parameters of the texture pattern eigen fluctuations. The numerical experiments have shown that IRF carefully eliminates fluctuations if the series (1.35) approximates the texture surface with error level not exceed – 40 dB in respect to image signal power. This criterion can serve for choosing of the method of harmonic decomposition, correlation matrices (1.69) or (1.70), target of approximation—original image or its reflexes in the manner of flat plane projection, curvature or Laplace-Beltrami flow and others.

The inverse filter designed and implemented using EHD of the texture acquires the same invariance to space transforms that the EHD provides. Therefore, the filtration in spectral domain is preferable for higher order filtration. Presence of mapped object in a texture fragment corrupts an arbitrary number of the pattern spectral components. Therefore, the filtration in spectral domain resolution ability is determined by fragment size which is equivalent to filter order. On the other side, as it was shown with computation examples, the resolution can be improved by optimization of resonant interaction of the filter and texture fragments by phase aligning (1.84). The phase alignment is unitary operation which does not change image signal power. This procedure also reduces sensitivity of the filter to weak variations in the textured image structure.

The filtration in spectral domain was optimized in respect to number of computations by generation of DFTEK basis in the manner of factorized fast transform (1.80). The using of the DFTEK instead of the usual EHD does not essentially change the quality of filtration. The computational advantage depends from DFTEK structure and can be significant in comparison with EHD.

The optimized scheme of the objects recognition includes the next stages:

- fast rough filtration in spectral domain;
- statistical analysis and selection nontrivial zones;

- filtration in space domain using convolution with transient characteristic of the nontrivial zones and adjacent ones to them;
- statistical analysis of the obtained signal for exact texture bound recognition.

The considered above method of textured image filtration and mapped object recognition differs from other known method by following features: each texture is characterized by its unique filter; it is feasible filter implementation in real time using graphic processor units; regulation of resolution and quality is provided; invariance to image movement induced changes; based on principal harmonic decomposition that is more convenient than EMD, or EVD, because it has an analytical form. Therefore, it may be adapted to any image and image sample fragment.

REFERENCES

Ade, F. 1983. Characterization of texture by "eigenfilter". *Signal Processing* 5: 451–457.

Barbieri, M.M. & Barone, P.A. 1992. Two-dimensional Prony's method for spectral estimation. *IEEE Trans* SP-40(11): 2747–2756.

Bunyak, O. & Bunyak, Y.A. 2007. Location and Estimation Parameters of Weak Wave Packets in Noise. *IEEE Instrumentation and Measurement Technology Conference – IMTC-2007 Warsaw May 1–3*, New Jersey: IEEE.

Bunyak, Y.A. 1989. The class of discrete orthogonal sub-exponential functions. *J. of Communication Technology and Electronics* 34(6): 1300–1303.

Bunyak, Y.A. 1995. Estimation of radiation sources angular coordinates by the method of antenna array data samples matrices factorization. *J. of Communication Technology and Electronics* 40(1): 87–94.

Bunyak, Y.A. 1996. Two-dimensional spectral analysis on method of maximum likelihood on base of the linear symmetry of correlation matrix. *Radioelectronics and Communication Systems* 39(4): 65–75.

Bunyak, Y.A. 1998. Harmonic analysis of wave fields. *J. of Communication Technology and Electronics.* 43(3): 239–243.

Celeux, G. Forbes, F. Peyrard, N. 2003. EM procedures using meanfield-like approximations for Markov model-based image segmentation. *Pattern Recognition* 36(1): 131–144.

Chang-zhen, X. Jun-yi, X. Jian-cheng, Z. Dong-xu, Q. 2006. Texture classification based on EMD and FFT. *Journal of Zhejiang University SCIENCE* 7(9): 1516–1521.

Charalampidis, D. 2006. Texture synthesis: textons revisited. *IEEE Trans. on Image Processing* 15(3): 777–787.

Clarenz, U. Diewald, U. Rumpf, M. 2004. Processing textured surfaces via anisotropic geometric diffusion. *IEEE Trans. on Image Processing* 13(2): 248–261.

Coltuc, D. Fournel, T. Becker, J.M. Jourlin, M.A. 2007. Multiresolution Independent Component Analysis for textile images, *Anti-counterfeit Image Analysis Methods: A Special Session of ICSXII IOP Journal of Physics: Conference Series* 77:1–11.

Costantini, R. Sbaiz, L. Susstrunk, S. 2008. Higher Order SVD Analysis for Dynamic Texture Synthesis. *IEEE Trans. on Image Processing* 17(1): 42–52.

Elliot D.F. & Rao, R. 1983. *Fast Transforms: Algorithms, Analysis and Applications*. New York: Academic Press.

Fu, Y. & Huang, T.S. 2008. Image Classification Using Correlation Tensor Analysis. *IEEE Trans. on Image Processing* 17(2): 226–234.

Fujita K. & Nayar, S.K. 2003. Recognition of Dynamic Textures using Impulse Responses of State Variables. *Pattern Recognition* 31: 1496–1509.

Gu, X. Wang, Y. Yau S-T. 2004. Computing Conformal Invariants: Period Matrices. *Communications in information and systems* 3(3): 153–170.

Haralick, R. Shanmugam, K. Dinstein I. 1973. Textural features for image classification. *IEEE Transactions on Systems, Man, and Cybernetics* 3(6): 610–621.

Hill, P.R. Bull, D.R. Canagarajah, C.N. 2000. Rotationally Invariant Texture Features using the Dual-Tree Complex Wavelet Transform. *Proc. Int'l Conf. Image Process.* 3: 901–904.

Hua, Y. 1992. Estimating two-dimensional frequencies by matrix enhancement and matrix pencil. *IEEE Trans* SP-40(9): 2267–2280.

Huang, K. & Aviyente, S. 2006. Information-theoretic wavelet packet subband selection for texture classification. *Signal Processing* 86: 1410–1420.

Huang, Y. & Chan, K.L. 2004. Texture decomposition by harmonics extraction from higher order statistics. *IEEE Transactions on Image Processing* 13(1): 1–14.

Khaparde, A. Deekshatulu, B.L. Madhavilatha, M. Farheen, Z. Kumari, S. 2008. Content Based Image Retrieval Using Independent Component Analysis, *IJCSNS International Journal of Computer Science and Network Security* 8(4): 327–332.

Khintchine, A. 1934. Korrelationstheorie der stationären stochastichen prozesse. *Matematische Annalen* 109(1): 604–615.

Kimmel, R. Sochen N.A. Malladi, R. 1999. On the Geometry of Texture. *Proc. International Conference on Curves and Surfaces [4th], Saint-Malo, 1–7 July 1999*. Nashville: Vanderbilt University Press.

Kingsbury, N.G. 2001. Complex wavelets for shift invariant analysis and filtering of signals. *Journal of Applied and Computational Harmonic Analysis* 10(3): 234–253.

Lazebnik, S. Schmid, C. Ponce, J. 2003. Affine-invariant local descriptors and neighborhood statistics for texture recognition. *In Proc. ICCV* 6: 221–229, 2003.

Li, H. Liu, G. Zhang, Z. 2006. A new texture generation method based on pseudo-DCT coefficients. *IEEE Trans. on Image Processing* 15(5): 1300–1312.

Liu, G. Lin, Z. Yu, Y. 2009. Radon Representation-Based Feature Descriptor for Texture Classification. *IEEE Trans. on Image Processing* 18: 921–928.

Marple, S.L. 1987. *Digital Spectral Analysis with Applications*. New Jersey: Prentice-Hall.

Muhly, P.S. & Solel, B. 1999. Tensor Algebras, Induced Representations and the Wold Decomposition. *Canad. J. Math* 51(4): 850–880.

Nunes, J.C. Niang, O. Bouaoune, Y. Delechelle, E. Bunel, P. 2003. Bidimensional Empirical Mode Decomposition Modified for Texture Analysis. *Proc. 13th Scandinavian Conference, SCIA 2003, Halmstad, Sweden, June 29–July 2*: 171–177.

Palm, C. & Lehmann, T.M. 2002. Classification of color textures by Gabor filtering. *Machine Graphics & Vision* 11(2/3): 195–219.

Partio, M. Cramariuc, B. Gabbouj, M. 2007. An Ordinal Co-occurrence Matrix Framework for Texture Retrieval. *EURASIP Journal on Image and Video Processing*. Article ID 17358:1–15.

Pattichis M.S. & Bovik, A.C. 2006. Analyzing Image Structure By Multidimensional Frequency Modulation. *IEEE Trans. on Pattern Analysis and Machine Intelligence* 5: 1–36.

Peinecke, N. Wolter, F.-E. Reuter, M. 2007. Laplace spectra as fingerprints for image recognition. *Computer-Aided Design* 39: 460–476.

Podobna, Y. Kvetnyy, R. Schoonmaker, J. Bunyak, Y. Sofina, O. Boucher, C. Contarino, V. 2009. A cooperative effort to develop a real time marine mammal detection and tracking system, *Proc. AUVSI's Unmanned Systems Europe, La Spezia 20–22 April 2009*. La Spezia: Curran Associates.

Radke, R.J. Andra, S. Al-Kofahi, O. Roysam, B. 2005. Image change detection algorithms: a systematic survey. *IEEE Trans. on Image Processing* 14(3): 294–307.

Randen, T. & Husoy, J.H. 1998. Filtering for Texture Classification: A Comparative Study. *IEEE Trans. Pattern Analysis and Machine Intelligence* 21(4): 291–310.

Rouquette, S. & Najim, M. 2001. Estimation of Frequencies and Damping Factors by Two-Dimensional ESPRIT Type Methods. *IEEE Trans. on Signal Processing.* 49(1): 128–137.

Sayadi, M. Sakrani, S. Fnaiech, F. Cheriet, M. 2008. Gray-level Texture Characterization Based on a New Adaptive Nonlinear Auto-Regressive Filter. *Electronic Letters on Computer Vision and Image Analysis* 7(1): 40–53.

Soatto, S. Doretto, G. Wu, Y.N. 2003. Dynamic Textures. *International Journal of Computer Vision* 51: 91–109.

Vyas, V.S. & Rege, P. 2006. Automated Texture Analysis with Gabor filter. *GVIP Journal* 6(1): 35–41.

Wall, M.E. Rechtsteiner, A. Rocha, L.M. 2003. Singular value decomposition and principal component analysis. In D.P. Berrar, W. Dubitzky, M. Granzow (ed.) *A Practical Approach to Microarray Data Analysis* Norwell: Kluwer.

Wiener, N. 1964. *Time series.* Cambridge: M.I.T. Press.

Xie, X. 2008. A Review of Recent Advances in Surface Defect Detection using Texture Analysis Techniques. *Electronic Letters on Computer Vision and Image Analysis* 7(3): 1–22.

Yang, Z. & Yang, L. 2009. Decomposition Based on Classical Empirical Mode Decomposition and Radon Transform. *Proceedings of the International MultiConference of Engineers and Computer Scientists* 1:471–476.

Yarman, C.E. & Yazici, B. 2006. An Inversion Method for the Exponential Radon Transform Based on the Harmonic Analysis of the Euclidean Motion Group. *Proc. of SPIE,* 6142: 61424 A-1–61424 A-8.

Zhang X. & Wu X. 2008. Image Interpolation by Adaptive 2-D Autoregressive Modeling and Soft-Decision Estimation. *IEEE Trans. on Image Processing* 17(6): 887–896.

CHAPTER 2

Approximation of bidirectional reflectance distribution function for highly efficient shading

O.N. Romanyuk, S.V. Pavlov, S.O. Romanyuk & S.V. Tymchyk
Vinnytsia National Technical University, Vinnytsia, Ukraine

P. Komada & J. Sikora
Lublin University of Technology, Lublin, Poland

A. Burlibay
Kazakh University of Railways and Communications, Almaty, Kazakhstan

M. Kalimoldayev
Institute of Information and Computational Technologies, Almaty, Kazakhstan

1 INTRODUCTION

In the synthesis and rendering of synthetic scenes it is necessary to solve the complex problem of the need of high quality vs. the need for high speed. It is a trade-off between providing high realism of the scene and a producing it at a required frame rate, especially for real-time applications.

As hardware and computational power develops further, the demand for realism in computer generated images also increases. Today, it is easy to program Phong shading (Hern 2005, Hill 2002, Phong 1975) on the GPU. However, not all graphics devices have such hardware. It is not always feasible to have a battery consuming device in a cell phone or other types of PDA's. Not all costumers are willing to pay for advanced graphics hardware on these devices either. Therefore, there is still a need for efficient software implementations of graphics algorithms for increased realism, or even hardware implementations that are very small and simple to its nature.

The most complicated and resource-intensive computing at the rendering stage takes place in the shading of 3-D objects, which have volume effect created by colour gradation.

The color intensity and coordinates are detected for every pixel on the surface in the process of shading. Taking into consideration, that high resolution displays are used for representing realistic images, the shading process takes a lot of time. Especially it reveals when illumination models are used, this one which represent specular constituent of the colour. That's why the question of increasing shading productivity in computer graphic systems is very urgent one.

2 ANALYSIS OF EXISTING APPROACHES TO BRDF APPROXIMATION AND PROBLEM FORMULATION

The intensity of pixels' color according to Phong method (Foley et al. 1996) is detected by using the following formula:

$$I = I_a k_a + I_l \left(k_d \cos\psi + k_s \cos^n \lambda\right), \tag{2.1}$$

where I_a, I_l – intensities of sparse and direct light sources correspondingly, k_a, k_d, k_s – sparse, diffusive and reflecting light coefficients, ψ – angle between the direction of light and normal vector $\vec{N}$, λ – angle between the direction of reflected light and the observer, n – surface brightness coefficient, $\cos^n \lambda$ – Bidirectional Reflectance Distribution Function (BRDF) which represents surface optical properties.

In shading of the surfaces, the most resource-intensive procedure is computation of $\cos^n \gamma$, which is used in Phong and Blinn illumination models (Anandan 1989, Hern et al. 2005). It is to be mentioned, that n varies from 0 to 1.

On BRDF models creation one must consider the most exacting requirements for the highlight epicentre representation (Hast 2003, Kautz 2000, Schlick 1994). For the peripheral regions, which are responsible for blooming zones formation it's necessary to provide monotonous color intensity fading to exclude artifact (Foley 1996, Levoy 1996). At the same time, there're no especial accuracy requirements towards color intensity determination within these zones (Hast 2003, Schlick 1994).

Among most successful achievements in BRDF approximation following are to be mentioned:

- The Schlick Approximation (Rogers D. 2001);
- An approximation by Taylor series suggest by Lyon in (Hast et al. 2003).
- An approximation by the $\cos^k(\sqrt{n/k} \cdot \lambda)$ function (Hill 2002);
- An approximation by the 2-degree polynomial (Romanyuk 2008).

Schlick in (Rogers 2001) proposed approximation of the function $\cos^n \gamma$, which is used for computing intensity of the mirror constituent of the color in Phong and Blinn illumination models, with the following function:

$$\cos\gamma / (n - n\cos\gamma + \cos\gamma).$$

Analysis showed this approach to provide satisfactory quality only for highlight's epicenter representation and is hardly applicable for hardware implementation.

Function $\cos^n \gamma$ is expanded into Taylor series using a method proposed by Lion in (Hill 2002). Instead of the angle λ between reflected light and observer, the length of chord between mentioned vectors is used:

$$\gamma = \left|\vec{D}\right| = \left|\vec{N} - \vec{H}\right|.$$

Expression $1/\sqrt{\vec{N} \cdot \vec{N}}$, which is used for normalizing of normal vector $\vec{N}$, is also expanded into Taylor series. Only first three terms are used. This allows exclusion of division and square root operations from computing process. Replacement of the angle with chord length doesn't influence greatly upon accuracy of the calculations for low values of angles. Using limited quantity of Taylor series terms doesn't allow to perform approximation of normalized vectors $\vec{N}$ and function $\cos^n \lambda$ with necessary accuracy.

Better accuracy of approximation is reached for approximation of function $\cos^n \lambda$ with function (Hast et al. 2003):

$$\cos^k(\sqrt{n/k} \cdot \lambda),$$

where $k = 2, 4, 8, \ldots$ and is selected depending on parameter n. Unfortunately, for this approach it is necessary to define angle λ, which needs time consuming calculation of arcos trigonometric function.

The idea of approximation by 2-degree polynomial is defined in (Romanyuk 2008):

$$\cos^n \gamma = a\cos^2 \gamma + b\cos x\gamma + c,$$

To find *a*, *b*, *c* they use values of $\cos^n \gamma$ at the start and the end points, and at cusp point as well. It's proved that $b = 1 - a$, $c = 0$. The hardware solution has *a* values for every *n* are stored in memory unit, and two other coefficients are computed by simple formulas. This solution allows sufficiently accurate highlight epicenter approximation with relative error no more than 4,5%. Unfortunately, the fast fading of this function at $\gamma \to 0$ leads to sharp borders of the blooming.

Though, approximation approaches mentioned above reached rather satisfactory results, however two pitfalls remain. Namely:

- high value of the approximation error;
- either performing operations with "angle" operand or division operation presence.

Hereby, a persuasive evidence of necessity of more efficient BRDF approximation comes. Finally, we can state a problem: To provide BRDF approximation having high accuracy, low computational complexity and simple hardware implementation for *a*, *b*, *c* coefficients.

3 APPROXIMATION OF BRDF BY THE 3-DEGREE POLYNOMIAL

It is proposed to approximate BRDF by the 3-degree polynomial (Romanyuk 2007) with condition that input operand is a function of cosine between normal vector and $\vec{H}$ vector. Let's approximate BRDF with the following cubic polynomial $f(x)$:

It is proposed to approximate BRDF by the 3-degree polynomial (Romanyuk 2007) with condition that input operand is a function of cosine between normal vector and $\vec{H}$ vector. Let's approximate BRDF with the following cubic polynomial $f(x)$:

$$f(x) = a \cdot \cos(x)^3 + b \cdot \cos(x)^2 + c \cdot \cos(x) + d = \cos(x)^n. \tag{2.2}$$

For finding a, b, c, d coefficients, it is considered, that $\cos(0) = 1$, so that:

$$a + b + c + d = 1. \tag{2.3}$$

If $\cos(x) = 0$ then:

$$d = 0. \tag{2.4}$$

Let's equate the BRDF value and value of cubic polynomial at the point *t*, where $\cos(t)^n = 0.5$. Taking into consideration, that $\cos(t) = \sqrt[n]{0.5}$, we receive:

$$a \cdot \cos(t)^3 + b \cdot \cos(t)^2 + c \cdot \cos(t) + d = 0.5 \tag{2.5}$$

The last equation for finding variables a, b, c, d can be received by equal derivatives of BRDF and proposed cubic polynomial at the point *t*, where $\cos(t)^n = 0.5$.

$$\text{BRDF}' = -n \cdot \cos(x)^{n-1} \cdot \sin(x) \tag{2.6}$$

$$f(x)' = -3 \cdot a \cdot \cos(x)^2 \cdot \sin(x) - 2 \cdot b \cdot \cos(x) \cdot \sin(x) - c \cdot \sin(x) \tag{2.7}$$

Equality of right parts of equations (2.5) and (2.6) and dividing them by $-\sin(x)$ gives:

$$n \cdot \cos(t)^{n-1} = 3 \cdot a \cdot \cos(t)^2 + 2 \cdot b \cdot \cos(t) + c \tag{2.8}$$

The equations (2.3), (2.4), (2.5) and (2.8) create system of equations for defining coefficients of cubic polynomial (2.2):

$$\begin{cases} a+b+c+d=1 \\ d=0 \\ a\cdot\cos(t)^3+b\cdot\cos(t)^2+c\cdot\cos(t)+d=0.5 \\ n\cdot\cos(t)^{n-1}=3\cdot a\cdot\cos(t)^2+2\cdot b\cdot\cos(t)+c \end{cases} \tag{2.9}$$

After some simple mathematical manipulation, the system of two equations is received:

$$\begin{cases} a\cdot\cos(t)^3+b\cdot\cos(t)^2+(1-a-b)\cdot\cos(t)=0.5 \\ n\cdot\cos(t)^{n-1}=3\cdot a\cdot\cos(t)^2+2\cdot b\cdot\cos(t)+(1-a-b), \end{cases} \tag{2.10}$$

where $\cos(t)=\sqrt[n]{0.5}$.

Solution of the system of equations (2.10) is expressed in the following formulas:

$$a=0.5\cdot\frac{-2q+1+2q^2+n\cdot q-n}{q^2\left[-2q+q^2+1\right]} \qquad b=-0.5\frac{4q^3+q^2\cdot n-3q^2-n+1}{(q-1)^2\cdot q^2},$$

where $q=e^{\frac{-0.6931471}{n}}$.

It is advisable to store coefficients a and b for all possible values of n in a permanent memory unit.

An example of BRDF approximation with cubic polynomial is represented in the Figure 2.1. The graphic shows, that using cubic polynomial for highlights fading area is impossible, because increasing of the specular constituent of light is observed instead of its fading.

Modeling has shown that for $\forall n\in[1;\ 256],\ \Rightarrow\ \delta(n)\leq 0.67\%$ (see Fig. 2.2). In comparison with Schlick model of BRDF at this interval relative error is decreased more than 17 times. It is worth to mentioned, that in BRDF approximation the most exacting requirements are set for representation of highlight's epicenter (Rogers 2001), which occurs above cusp. For other areas, it is enough to provide monotonous fading of color intensity, which excludes appearance of artifacts (Rogers 2001, Foley et al. 1996). The requirements to accuracy are not required as a rule (Kautz 2000).

Usage of BRDF approximation with cubic polynomial makes that $\cos^n(x)<0.5$ can lead to such an undesirable result, represented in Figure 2.3. Its kernel cause that BRDF takes negative values even if expression $\cos^n(x)>0.5$.

Let's analyze BRDF like function $gg(x)=\frac{\cos(x)}{a-b\cos(x)}$ if $\cos^n(x)<0.5$ is provided. The coefficients a, b can be found by equating values of $gg(x)$ and $\cos^n(x)$ at the point $x=\arccos\left(\sqrt[n]{0.5}\right)$, and their derivatives at this point as well. Thus, following system of equations is received:

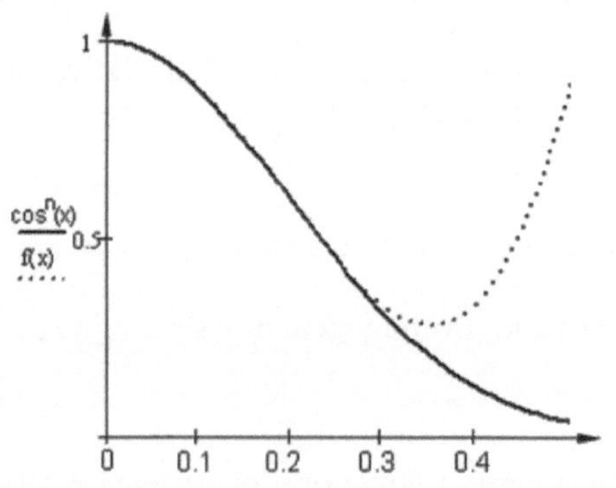

Figure 2.1 An example of BRDF approximation fo $n=25$.

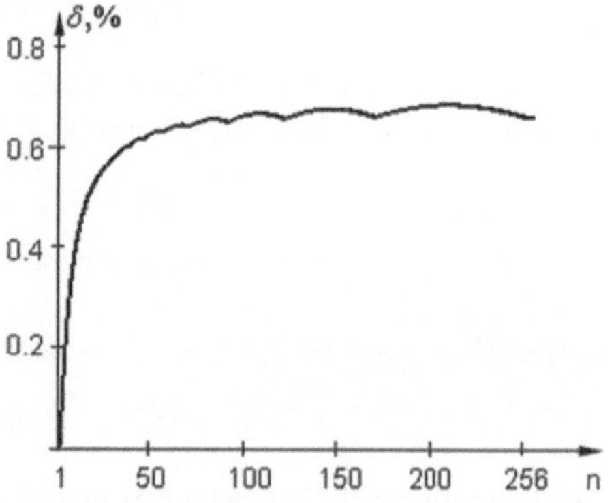

Figure 2.2 The maximal relative error of BRDF approximation.

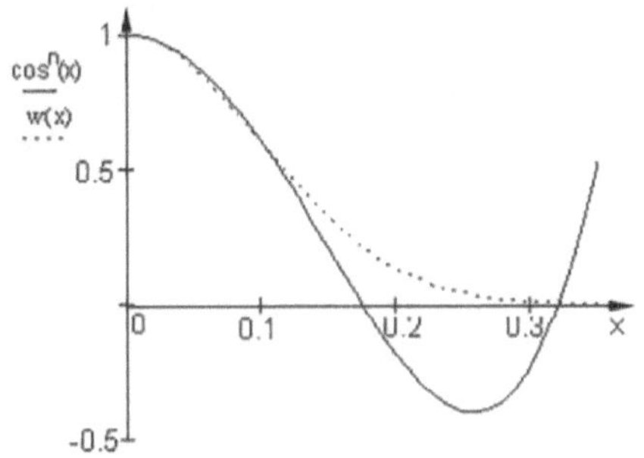

Figure 2.3 The weakness of using cubic approximation.

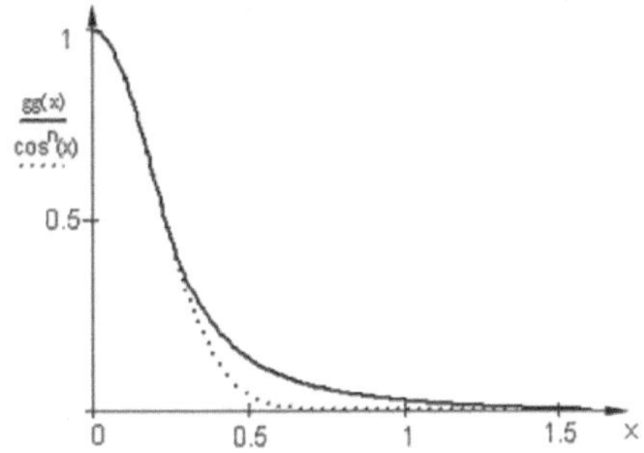

Figure 2.4 An example of BRDF polynomial with functions $f(x)$, $g(x)$ for $n = 25$.

$$\begin{cases} \dfrac{\cos(t)}{a - b\cdot\cos(t)} = 0.5 \\ \dfrac{1}{a - b\cdot\cos(t)} + \dfrac{\cos(t)\cdot b}{(a - b\cdot\cos^2(t))} = n\cdot\cos^{n-1}(t) \end{cases}$$

where $\cos^n(t) = 0.5$.

Let's show, that $b = 2\cdot n - 2, a = 2n\sqrt[n]{0.5}$. The solution of the system of equations is:

$$\begin{pmatrix} a \\ b \end{pmatrix} = \begin{pmatrix} 4\cdot n\cdot\cos^{n+1}(t) \\ 4\cdot n\cdot\cos^n(t) - 2 \end{pmatrix}.$$

Substituting into above equation $\cos^n(t) = 0.5$, and $\cos(t) = \sqrt[n]{0.5}$ leads to:

$$\begin{pmatrix} a \\ b \end{pmatrix} = \begin{pmatrix} 2\cdot n\cdot\sqrt[n]{0.5} \\ 2\cdot n - 2 \end{pmatrix}.$$

Example of BRDF approximation is represented in Figure 2.4.

It is to be mentioned, that relative error of function $g(x)$ representing highlights fading area, doesn't exceed 1% if $0.42 < f(x) < 0.5$, doesn't exceed 3% if $0.37 < f(x) < 0.42$ and is less than 10% if $0.27 < f(x) < 0.37$, what is acceptable.

New BRDF approximation, being proposed in this work, represents highlights on the surface of graphic objects with rather high accuracy, at the same time approximating function operates with cosine of angle between the normal vector $\vec{N}$ and middle vector $\vec{H}$. In comparison with Schlick BRDF considerable reduction of approximation error is reached both in highlight epicenter and fading area representation.

4 APPROXIMATION OF BRDF BY USING LOGARITHMIC FUNCTION

Let's represent function $\cos^n\gamma$ by the equivalent formula $\cos^n\gamma = 2^{n\cdot\log_2(\cos\gamma)}$. Such a representation of the BRDF allows its easy hardware definition, because $n\cdot\log_2(\cos\gamma)$ function could be represented by table and 2^x function – could be approximated. Let's investigate the variation interval of the product $\log_2(\cos\gamma)$ for the highlight epicenter. The distribution function has $\gamma = \operatorname{arctg}\frac{1}{\sqrt{n-1}}$, which separates highlights epicenter from its fading zone. Let's prove, that:

$$\lim_{\gamma\to\operatorname{arctg}\frac{1}{\sqrt{n-1}}} (n\cdot\log_2\cos\gamma) = \log_2\left(\frac{n-1}{n}\right)^{\frac{n}{2}}. \tag{2.11}$$

If we change the function argument γ to its boundary value, we receive:

$$\lim_{\gamma\to\mathrm{arctg}\frac{1}{\sqrt{n-1}}}(n\cdot\log_2\cos\gamma)=n\cdot\log_2\cos\left(\mathrm{arctg}\frac{1}{\sqrt{n-1}}\right). \tag{2.12}$$

According to the well-known formula, we have: $\cos(\mathrm{arctg}\,a)=\frac{1}{\sqrt{1+a^2}}$. So that:

$$\lim_{\gamma\to\mathrm{arctg}\frac{1}{\sqrt{n-1}}}(n\cdot\log_2\cos\gamma)=n\cdot\log_2\frac{1}{\sqrt{1+\dfrac{1}{n-1}}}=n\cdot\log_2\sqrt{\frac{n-1}{n}}=\log_2\left(\frac{n-1}{n}\right)^{\frac{n}{2}}. \tag{2.13}$$

With the received formula, we find, that for $n=2$:

$$\lim_{\gamma\to\mathrm{arctg}\frac{1}{\sqrt{n-1}}}(n\cdot\log_2\cos\gamma)=-1. \tag{2.14}$$

Since $\lim_{n\to\infty}\sqrt{\frac{n-1}{n}}=1$, then for $n\to\infty$ $\lim_{\gamma\to\mathrm{arctg}\frac{1}{\sqrt{n-1}}}(n\cdot\log_2\cos\gamma)=0$.

The maximal value of n is 1000. For this value: $\lim_{\gamma\to\mathrm{arctg}\frac{1}{\sqrt{n-1}}}(n\cdot\log_2\cos\gamma)=0{,}722$.

Thus, for highlight epicenter values of $n\cdot\log_2(\cos\gamma)$ for all n are placed within the interval from -1 to $-0{,}722$.

Let's examine the approximation of the 2^x function by the $f(x)=A\cdot\log_2(1-x)+B$ on the interval – $[-1,0]$. This interval was chosen because it covers not only epicenter of the highlight, but a considerable part of the fading zone either (about 30%). Let's find unknown parameters A and B.

At $x=0$ we have: $A\cdot\log_2(1-x)+B=A\cdot\log_2(1)+B=1$. From the last equation, we see, that $B=1$.

At $x=-1$ we have: $A\cdot\log_2(1-x)+B=A\cdot\log_2(2)+B=\frac{1}{2}$. In as much as $B=1$, then $A=-\frac{1}{2}$. Thus, at the interval $[-1,0]$ we will see:

$$2^x\approx 1-\frac{1}{2}\log_2(1-x). \tag{2.15}$$

Considering (2.15) we receive:

$$\cos^n\gamma=2^{n\log_2(\cos\gamma)}=1-\frac{1}{2}\log_2(1-n\cdot\log_2(\cos\gamma)). \tag{2.16}$$

Let's estimate the $\cos^n\gamma$ approximation error by the following function:

$$\Omega(\gamma,n)=1-\frac{1}{2}\log_2(1-n\cdot\log_2\cos\gamma)$$

An absolute approximation error is:

$$\Delta=\cos^n\gamma-\Omega(\gamma,n).$$

Let's find out maximum of the approximation error. If derivate expression:

$$\cos^n\gamma-1+\frac{1}{2}\log_2(1-n\cdot\log_2\cos\gamma),$$

we have:

$$\frac{\partial \Delta}{\partial \gamma} = -n \cdot \cos^{n-1} \gamma \cdot \sin \gamma + \frac{n \cdot \sin \gamma}{\cos \gamma \cdot \ln^2 2 \cdot \left(1 - n \cdot \frac{\ln(\cos \gamma)}{\ln 2}\right)}.$$

The roots of the expression, which determine extreme, are:

$$\gamma_1 = \arccos\left(\exp\left(\frac{W\left(\frac{-1}{4\ln 2}\right)}{n} + \ln 2\right)\right), \quad \gamma_3 = 0, \quad \gamma_2 = \arccos\left(\exp\left(\frac{W(-1) + \ln 2}{n}\right)\right),$$

where $W()$ is a Lambert function.

It is well known (Hern et al. 2011), that $W(x) = \sum_{n=1}^{\infty} \frac{(-1)^{n-1} n^{n-2}}{(n-1)!} x^n$. Let's find:

$$W\left(\frac{-1}{4\ln 2}\right) = -0{,}814, \qquad W(-1) = -1{,}23.$$

Hence, critical values of the argument occur in the following points:

$$\gamma_1 = 0, \quad \gamma_2 = \arccos\left(\exp\left(\frac{-0.814 + \ln 2}{n}\right)\right), \quad \gamma_3 = \arccos\left(\exp\left(\frac{-1.23 + \ln 2}{n}\right)\right).$$

The analysis showed, that critical points are extremums and they are situated inside the interval: $\left[0, \operatorname{arctg}\frac{1}{\sqrt{n-1}}\right]$ for $\gamma_1 < \gamma_2 < \gamma_3$.

If substitute $\gamma_1 < \gamma_2 < \gamma_3$ into previous equation, we get:

$$|\Delta(\gamma_1)| = 0, \quad |\Delta(\gamma_2)| = 2{,}098 \times 10^{-3}, \quad |\Delta(\gamma_3)| = 1{,}703 \times 10^{-3}.$$

Comparing received data we can state that $\max|\Delta(\gamma)| = 2.098 \times 10^{-3}$ and takes place at $\gamma = \arccos\left(\exp\left(\frac{-0.814 + \ln 2}{n}\right)\right)$. We have also analyzed maximal relative error of BRDF approximation by $\Omega(\gamma, n)$ function for highlight epicenter. Error reaches maximum at the point $\arccos\left(\exp\frac{1 + \ln 2 \cdot W\left(\frac{-1}{4\ln 2}\right)}{n \cdot W\left(\frac{-1}{4\ln 2}\right)}\right)$ and doesn't exceeds 0,29%. That confirms high accuracy of highlight epicenter representation.

The approximation of 2^x function by the different polynomials was also analyzed (Rogers 2001). The usage of one polynomial within whole interval wasn't successful, because at high accuracy of highlight epicenter representation we have artifacts at blooming zone. This happened because approximating curve didn't reach 0-level and changed behavior from decreasing to increasing and this could cause unnatural object illumination. So, we have tried piecewise-functional approximation of BRDF.

Solution is to divide BRDF variation interval into two subintervals and approximate function at each one of them by the quadratic polynomial. Approximating functions have to have equal second-order derivatives at the adherent point. In contrast to spline interpolation, where intervals are defined, this approach supposes adherent point of mentioned functions is to be found. It is necessary generating functions to touch at the connection point, or to have non-significant difference between ordinates for the full BRDF definition. One of the functions is supposed to approximate highlight epicenter with high accuracy, the other one—its blooming zone.

The following formulas for $2^{n \cdot \log_2(\cos \gamma)}$ approximation have been received:

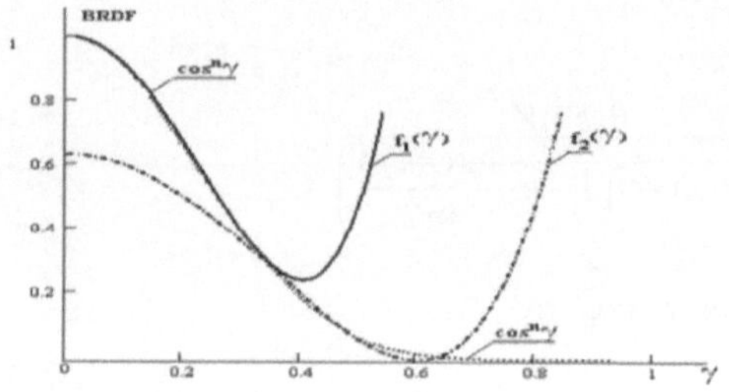

Figure 2.5 Graphic of functions $\cos^n\gamma$, $f_1(\gamma)$, $f_2(\gamma)$ for $n = 10$.

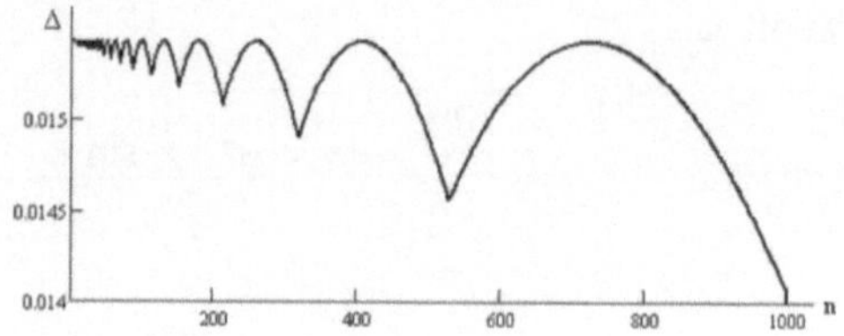

Figure 2.6 Absolute approximation error of functions $\cos^n\gamma, f_1(\gamma), f_2(\gamma)$.

$$f_1(\gamma) = 1 + 0{,}617 \cdot n \cdot \log_2(\cos\gamma) + 0{,}124 \cdot (n \cdot \log_2(\cos\gamma))^2.$$

$$f_2(\gamma) = 0{,}64 + 0{,}227 \cdot n \cdot \log_2(\cos\gamma) + 0{,}02 \cdot (n \cdot \log_2(\cos\gamma))^2.$$

The $f_1(\gamma)$ function was used to reproduce highlight and a part of fading zone, and $f_2(\gamma)$ function—for the blooming zone.

Selection of intervals approximation has the following basics. If level $1/2^q$ is given, then from the equation $\cos^n(\gamma) = 1/2^q$ we could find border value of the angle $\arccos(\exp(-\ln(2) \cdot \frac{q}{n}))$. As a rule $q = 8$. The maximal value of the variable is being searched:

$$n \cdot \log_2 \cos\left(\arccos\left(\exp(-\ln 2) \cdot \frac{8}{n}\right)\right) = 8.$$

Let's find for these functions adherent point and solve the following equation for γ:

$$1 + 0{,}617 \cdot n \cdot \log_2(\cos\gamma) + 0{,}124 \cdot n \cdot \log_2(\cos\gamma)^2 =$$
$$0{,}645 + 0{,}232 \cdot n \cdot \log_2(\cos\gamma) + 0{,}02 \cdot n \cdot \log_2(\cos\gamma)^2.$$

The solution is $\gamma = \arccos\left(\exp\frac{-1.205}{n}\right)$.
The derivative is

$$-0{,}385 \cdot n \cdot \frac{\sin(x)}{\cos(x) \cdot \ln 2} - 0{,}208 \cdot n^2 \cdot \frac{\ln(\cos x)}{(\ln 2)^2} \cdot \frac{\sin(x)}{\cos(x)} = 0.$$

The equation has solution at $\gamma = \arccos(\exp(-1.282/n))$.

Comparing values which was already found we can draw a conclusion, that inflection point and the point, where two function derivatives coincide, are very close to each other, that meets prescribed requirements. The Figure 2.5 depicts $\cos^n\gamma, f_1(\gamma), f_2(\gamma)$ for $n = 10$. Analysis has shown that the absolute approximation error doesn't exceeds 0,0154 (Fig. 2.6), and relative error –2,3%. For the blooming zone, where BRDF value tends to zero the absolute error doesn't exceed 0,05. This confirms rather high accuracy of BRDF approximation.

5 BRDF APPROXIMATION MODELS BASED ON NEW COSINE-DEGREE FUNCTIONS WITH SIMPLE HARDWARE IMPLEMENTATION

Let's try to approximate $\cos^n\gamma$ by the function $W(n, \gamma) = (\zeta \cdot (\cos\gamma - 1) + 1)^m$ under conditions that $0 \le \gamma \le \pi/2$.

This function is suggested because:

a. both functions are based on the cosine function;
b. at $\gamma = 0$, $\cos^n \gamma = (\zeta \cdot (\cos\gamma - 1) + 1)^m = 1$, that satisfies boundary conditions;
c. both functions are positive, when $0 \le \gamma \le \pi/2$ and $m = 2k$, where $k \in N$ ε;
d. $(\zeta \cdot (\cos\gamma - 1) + 1)^m$ function reaches zero value, that is pre-condition of blooming formation;
e. ζ coefficient changes the highlight size.

To determine ζ if $(\zeta \cdot (\cos\gamma - 1) + 1)^m$ we expand $\cos^n \gamma$ into Taylor series and take first 2 terms $\cos^n \gamma \approx 1 - n \cdot \gamma^2 / 2$.

The same procedure on $W(n, \gamma)$ leads to equation:

$$(\zeta \cdot (\cos\gamma - 1) + 1)^m \approx 1 - \zeta \cdot m \cdot x^2.$$

Let's find ζ. Right sides of these formulas are supposed to be equal, so that $\zeta = n/m$. Let's examine the situation, when $m = 2$, then:

$$\cos^n \gamma \approx (n(\cos\gamma - 1)/2 + 1)^2. \tag{2.17}$$

Let's analyze this BRDF model. The comparison with Schlick formula was done. This formula is widespread in computer graphics devices, because of its sufficient accuracy and low computation complexity.

The graphs of the function (2.17) and of Schlick functions on the condition that $n = 100$ are shown in the Figure 2.8.

The Figure 2.7 shows that suggested BRDF model approximates highlight epicenter with sufficient accuracy and monotonously fades to zero after the cusp point. The part of BRDF function above the cusp point is responsible for the highlight epicenter formation. The behavior of this function fits the requirements to BRDF model. The Figure 2.8 shows graphics of maximal relative errors of the approximation of $\cos^n \gamma$ by $W(n, \gamma)$ function for epicenter zone. These figures show the accuracy of epicenter approximation has increased in comparison with Schlick formula.

The $W(n, \gamma)$ function reaches zero value, when $\cos(\gamma) = (n-2)/n$. The function $W(n, \gamma)$ is square of real number—and is never negative. Let's find when derivative of $W(n, \gamma)$ is equal to zero.

$$W_x'(n, \gamma) = -\left(\frac{n}{2}(\cos\gamma - 1) + 1\right) \cdot n \cdot \sin\gamma = 0. \tag{2.18}$$

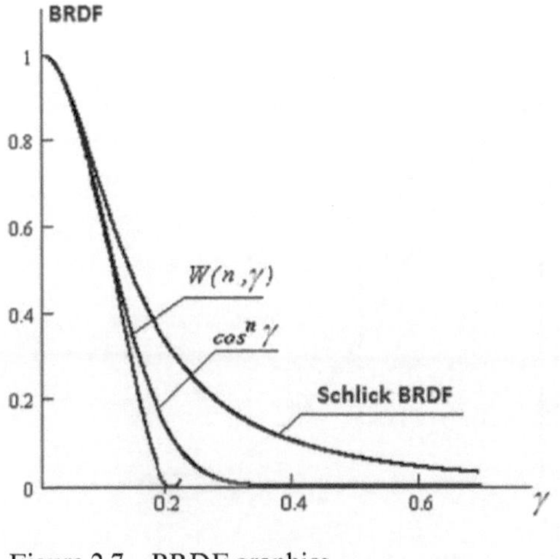

Figure 2.7 BRDF graphics.

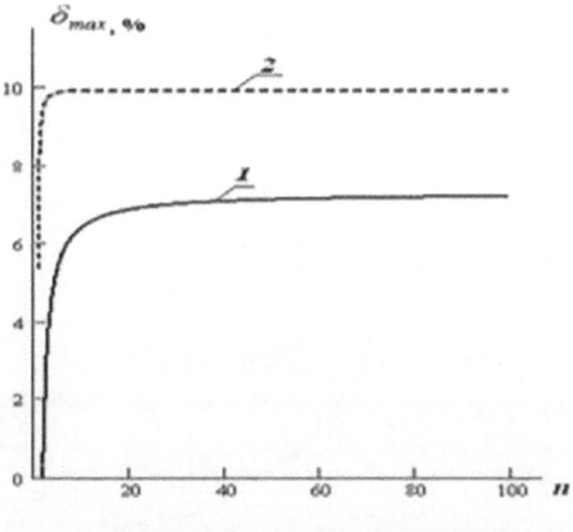

Figure 2.8 The maximal relative error graphics for the higlight epicenter approximation by: 1 – function; 2 – Schlick function.

Let's determine extremum of the function. From the last formula, it is obtained that $\cos(\gamma) = (n-2)/n$. The function $W(n, \gamma)$ signs analysis from the left and right side shows that BRDF reaches zero value at:

$$\gamma = \arccos\left(\frac{n-2}{n}\right).$$

$W(n, \gamma)$ monotonously fades within the interval 0, $\gamma = \arccos((n-2)/n)$, because its derivative with respect to x equals to $-\left(\frac{n}{2}(\cos\gamma - 1) + 1\right) n \sin\gamma$.

In its turn, $n \cdot \sin\gamma$ is positive on interval from 0 to π. $-(n(\cos\gamma - 1) + 1)/2 \leq 0$ is true at the condition that $0 \leq \gamma \leq \arccos((n-2)/n)$. Thus, within interval where function changes from 1 to 0, its derivative hasn't negative values, q. e. d.

Let's examine how the raising of power m influences upon approximation accuracy. Three cases are chosen – $m = 4$, $m = 8$ and $m = 16$:

$$W_1(n,\gamma) = \left(\zeta_1(\cos\gamma - 1) + 1\right)^4,\ W_2(n,\gamma) = \left(\zeta_2(\cos\gamma - 1) + 1\right)^8,\ W_3(n,\gamma) = \left(\zeta_3(\cos\gamma - 1) + 1\right)^{16}$$

Considering the equation $\zeta = n/m$, one can find:

$$\zeta_1 = \frac{n}{4},\ \zeta_1 = \frac{n}{8},\ \zeta_3 = \frac{n}{16}.$$

Considering values of ζ_1, ζ_2 and ζ_3 coefficients, it's possible to find $W_1(n, \gamma), W_2(n, \gamma)$, and $W_3(n, \gamma)$:

$$W_1(n,\gamma) = \left(\frac{n}{4_1}(\cos\gamma - 1) + 1\right)^4,\ W_2(n,\gamma) = \left(\frac{n}{8}(\cos\gamma - 1) + 1\right)^8,\ W_3(n,\gamma) = \left(\frac{n}{16}(\cos\gamma - 1) + 1\right)^{16}$$

Figures 2.9–2.11 show graphics of $\cos^n\gamma, W_1(n, \gamma), W_2(n, \gamma)$ and $W_3(n, \gamma)$ functions when n = 35. The analysis of those graphics leads to conclusion that increasing of m leads to approximation accuracy increase. The modeling helps to determine maximal relative error of the approximation within the range $n \in [1,1000]$. The results of such modeling are presented in Figure 2.12.

It is significant, that special requirements for approximation accuracy are applied only for epicenter zone—part of BRDF from 0 to cusp point. The BRDF values after cusp point determine blooming zone formation.

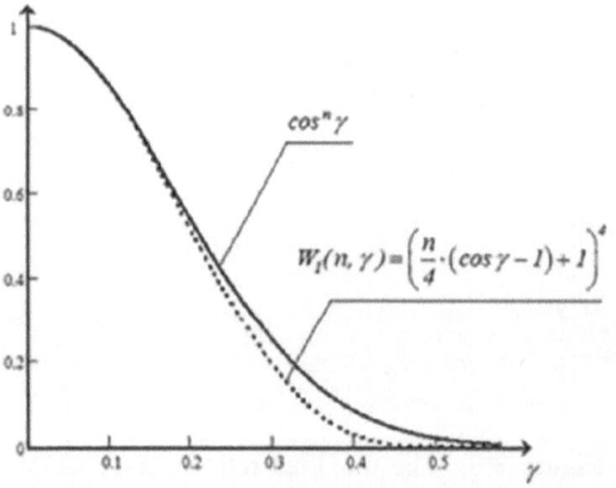

Figure 2.9 Graphics for $\cos^n \gamma$ and $W_1(n, \gamma)$.

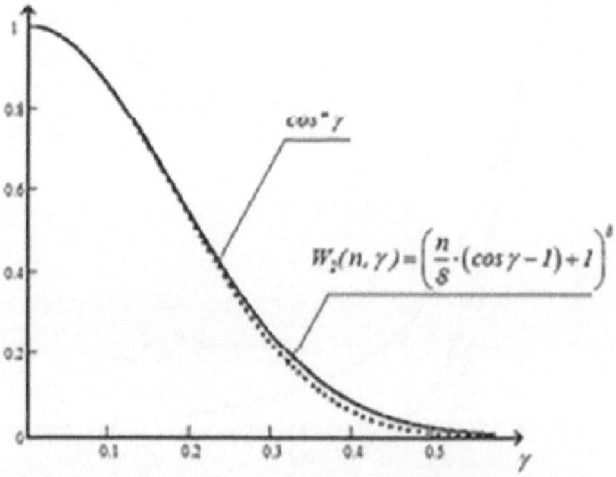

Figure 2.10 Graphics for $\cos^n \gamma$ and $W_2(n, \gamma)$.

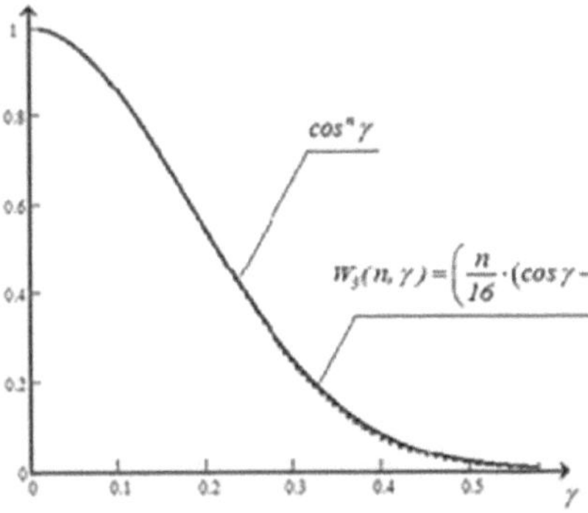

Figure 2.11 Graphics for $\cos^n \gamma$ and $W_3(n, \gamma)$.

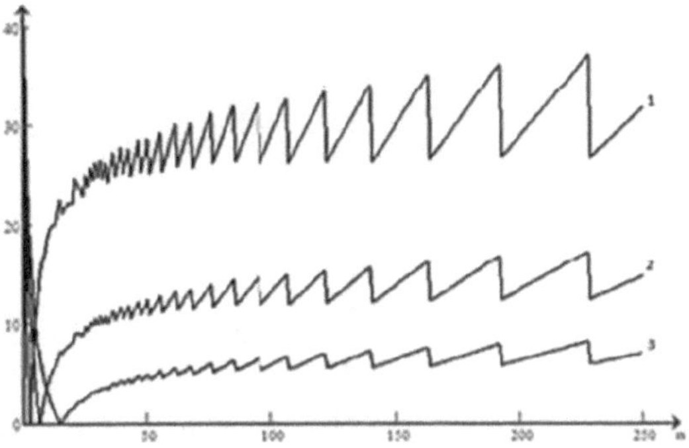

Figure 2.12 Maximal relative error $\cos^n \gamma$ approximation by: 1 – $W_1(n, \gamma)$, 2 – $W_2(n, \gamma)$ and 3 – $W_3(n, \gamma)$.

Table 2.1 Maximal relative errors of functions $W_1(n, \gamma)$, $W_2(n, \gamma)$, $W_3(n, \gamma)$ and Schlick function.

Function	ε,% before the cusp point	ε,% after the cusp point
$W_1(n, \gamma)$	8,0	35,2
$W_2(n, \gamma)$	3,8	16,2
$W_3(n, \gamma)$	1,0	7,6
Schlick	22,4	98,2

The investigation has shown, that maximal relative error of the $\cos^n \gamma$ approximation before the cusp point, within interval $n \in 1,512$ doesn't exceed: 8% – for $W_1(n, \gamma)$, 3,8% – for $W_2(n, \gamma)$ and 1% – for $W_3(n, \gamma)$. The obtained results tell about considerable increase of the approximation accuracy in comparison with Schlick function. The maximal relative error for the Schlick function within this interval is 22,4%.

Function $W_3(n, \gamma)$ has very good approximation quality even for the blooming zone. The maximal relative errors ε values for approximation functions $W_1(n, \gamma), W_2(n, \gamma)$ and of $W_3(n, \gamma)$ within various ranges are collected in Table 2.1. The corresponding relative errors for the Schlick function are also provided in the table.

Figure 2.13 represents graphics of maximal relative error of $W_1(n, \gamma)$, $W_2(n, \gamma)$ and $W_3(n, \gamma)$ functions at blooming zone.

The analysis of these errors leads to conclusion, which result is the best obtained by approximation of $W_3(n, \gamma)$ function.

The relative error of $W_3(n, \gamma)$ in cusp point doesn't exceed 1%, at the same time this error for Schlick formula is more than 22%. To calculate the Schlick BRDF it's necessary to perform one multiplication operation, one dividing operation, one subtraction and one decrement operations. The dividing operation complicates hardware implementation of this formula. The suggested formula $W_3(n, \gamma)$ doesn't contain resource-intensive dividing operations. It's enough to perform only four multiplication operations, shift operation, increment and decrement one.

All these operations have easy hardware implementation. The software implementation $W_3(n, \gamma)$ takes in two times less time than Schlick formula. These facts lead to conclusion, that computation complexity of $W_3(n, \gamma)$ is considerably lower than that of Schlick function. It is important, that all three suggested functions provide better accuracy than Schlick formula.

There're peculiarities of blooming zone formation. The boundary value is chosen to be equal to 2^{-q}, where q is picked depending on the required specular constituent accuracy.

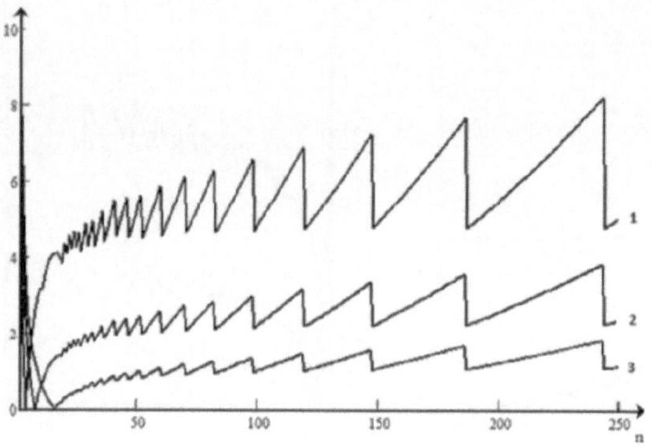

Figure 2.13 Graphics of maximal relative error values for approximation of by functions: 1-, 2- amd 3- for the blooming zone.

Then expression $\cos^n \gamma$ must be computed within the following interval – $2^{-q} \leq \cos^n \gamma \leq 1$, from which:

$$0 \leq \gamma \leq \arccos\left(2^{\left(-\frac{q}{n}\right)}\right) \tag{2.19}$$

For Schlick function we have:

$$2^{-q} \leq \frac{\cos \gamma}{n - n\cos \gamma + \cos \gamma} \leq 1. \tag{2.20}$$

From this we can find that Schlick function is to be calculated only within this interval:

$$0 \leq \gamma \leq \arccos \frac{n}{2^q + n - 1}. \tag{2.21}$$

Let's determine the γ vary interval for suggested BRDF. Solution of the eq. (2.21) allow us to find that:

$$2^{-q} \leq \left(\frac{n}{m}(\cos \gamma - 1) + 1\right)^m \leq 1.$$

$$0 \leq \gamma \leq \arccos\left(\frac{m2^{-q/m} - m + n}{n}\right).$$

The significant disadvantage of Schlick formula is extremely slow fading in blooming zone leading to unnatural object illumination. Vary interval for γ in this case increases.

The ratio $\mathfrak{R}$, defines, in how many times the arguments in $\cos^n \gamma$ and in suggested functions differs under the condition that these functions reach value 2^{-q}. This ratio also determines the highlight sizes correlation.

For $\cos^n \gamma$ and $W_1(\gamma, n)$:

$$\mathfrak{R}_1 = \frac{\arccos(2^{(-q/n)})}{\arccos\left(\frac{4 \cdot 2^{-q/4} - 4 + n}{n}\right)}.$$

For $\cos^n \gamma$ and $W_2(\gamma,n)$:

$$\mathfrak{R}_2 = \frac{\arccos(2^{(-q/n)})}{\arccos\left(\frac{8 \cdot 2^{-q/8} - 8 + n}{n}\right)}.$$

For $\cos^n \gamma$ and $W_3(\gamma,n)$:

$$\mathfrak{R}_3 = \frac{\arccos(2^{(-q/n)})}{\arccos\left(\frac{16 \cdot 2^{-q/16} - 16 + n}{n}\right)}.$$

For $\cos^n \gamma$ and Schlick formula $\mathfrak{R}_3 = \frac{\arccos(2^{(-q/n)})}{\arccos\left(\frac{16 \cdot 2^{-q/16} - 16 + n}{n}\right)}$:

$$\mathfrak{R}_4 = \frac{\arccos(2^{(-q/n)})}{\arccos\left(\frac{n}{2^q + n - 1}\right)}.$$

The suggested BRDF models have:

- Much better approximation accuracy in comparison with Schlick formula.
- More simple hardware implementation in comparison with Schlick formula.

The approximation accuracy is increased more than 22 times for the epicenter zone and more than 14 times for the blooming zone in comparison with Schlick formula. For the hardware implementation of the suggested functions only simple functions are required.

6 A METHOD FOR ACCELERATED COMPUTATION OF COLOR INTENSITIES FOR SCAN-LINE FILLS OF THREE-DIMENSIONAL GRAPHICS OBJECTS

According to the traditional realization of shading specular part of color intensity is calculated by using the following formula:

$$I_{spec} = I_l k_s BRDF,$$

where BRDF can be found by using one of the proposed approximation.

The fastest method for shading is the method introduced by Gouraud (Gouraud 1971). In this method, the color intensities for the vertices are calculated for each triangle of the polygon mesh of the object being shaded. These intensities are linearly interpolated over the polygon during the rasterization process, also known as a scan-line fill, which means that the intensity is linearly interpolated along the edges and then linearly interpolated across each scanline.

The most obvious disadvantages of the Gouraud method are:

1. The method is most suitable for generation of matte surfaces, i.e. diffuse surfaces, which reflect light in all directions. Because of the linear interpolation used in this method, the highlights will be smeared out over the polygon, or perhaps even missed completely if the highlight appears in the center of the polygon. This can happen since the intensity is sampled at the vertices only.
2. Color artifacts might appear when objects are transformed from frame to frame. When an object is rotated, the positions of the polygons will change in a nonlinear way, while the Gouraud method shades the interior in a linear way, since it does not consider the local curvature of the surface. Phong shading handles this in a better way.

3. Furthermore, the Gouraud method only provides C^1 continuity of color intensity values over polygon boundaries, and the famous Mach band effect (Hern et al. 2011) is more obvious for Gouraud than for Phong shading. The reason is once again the linear behavior of the method. The Phong shading intensity curve often approximates the C^2 continuity over polygon boundaries better, even though not perfectly.

In general, the Phong shading method (Rogers 2001) produces more realistic images and handles the three mentioned problems better than Gouraud shading does. The reason for this is that instead of interpolating color values over the polygon, normal vectors are interpolated, which then are used for computing the intensity per pixel using the Phong illumination model.

Of course, the increased shading quality does not come for free. In comparison with the Gouraud method, the Phong method is characterized by a considerably larger computational cost.

The computational complexity of the Phong method limits its wide usage in computer graphics systems aimed at real-time image generation. On the other hand, the usage of the Gouraud method is limited by its poor quality in the generated images as explained above.

As a result, the problem of developing new approaches for shading, which would provide the acceptable compromise between real-time image generation and high quality and realism. Especially for systems which cannot use modern graphics hardware, which are found on most PC's.

One possible approach to solve this problem is to use a second order surface (Hill 2002, Hast et al. 2003) to approximate the true color intensity over the polygon. Thus, it will consider the local curvature of the surface and the mentioned problems with Gouraud shading will be minimized. Such methods are generally much faster than the Phong shading.

The color intensity on a second order surface can be computed by a polynomial:

$$I(x,y) = Ax^2 + By^2 + Cxy + Dx + Ey + F. \tag{2.22}$$

where x, y are the coordinates of the points laying on the surface and $I(x,y)$ is the color intensity.

The equation shows that it is necessary to determine six unknown coefficients A, B, C, D, E, F. Therefore, it is necessary to solve a system of six equations. This implies that we need six sample points on the triangle instead of three. Therefore, we can sample the intensities at the midpoints on edges of the triangle.

Let us denote the six color intensities needed as $I_1, I_2, I_3, I_{12}, I_{13}, I_{23}$ correspondingly for vertices of the triangle and the midpoints of the edges (Fig. 2.14).

The system of six equations become:

$$\begin{cases} I_1 = F, \\ I_2 = Ax_1{}^2 + By_1{}^2 + Cx_1y_1 + Dx_1 + Ey_1 + F, \\ I_3 = Ax_2{}^2 + By_2{}^2 + Cx_2y_2 + Dx_2 + Ey_2 + F, \\ I_{12} = A\dfrac{x_1{}^2}{4} + B\dfrac{y_1{}^2}{4} + C\dfrac{x_1y_1}{4} + D\dfrac{x_1}{2} + E\dfrac{y_1}{2} + F, \\ I_{13} = A\dfrac{x_2{}^2}{4} + B\dfrac{y_2{}^2}{4} + C\dfrac{x_2y_2}{4} + D\dfrac{x_2}{2} + E\dfrac{y_{21}}{2} + F, \\ I_{23} = A\dfrac{(x_1+x_2)^2}{4} + B\dfrac{(y_1+y_2)^2}{4} + C\dfrac{(x_1+x_2)(y_1+y_2)}{4} + D\dfrac{(x_1+x_2)}{2} + E\dfrac{(y_1+y_2)}{2} + F. \end{cases} \tag{2.23}$$

The solution according to Abbas et al. (Hill 2002) is:

$$F = I_1,\ E = \frac{C_3x_2 - C_2x_3}{x_2y_3 - y_2x_3},\ D = \frac{C_2y_3 - C_3y_2}{x_2y_3 - y_2x_3},\ C = \frac{2C_{12} - Ax_2^2 - Bx_2y_2}{y_2^2},$$

$$B = \frac{(4C_{13}y_2 - C_{23}y_3)D_{23} - (4C_{12}y_3 - C_{23}y_2)D_{32}}{E_{32}D_{23} - E_{32}D_{32}},$$

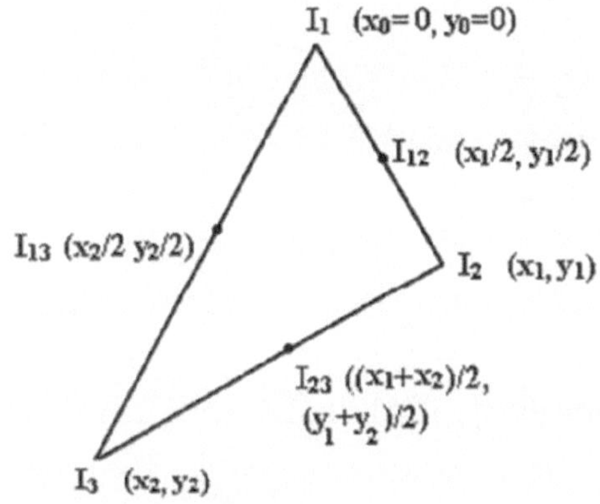

Figure 2.14 Values of color intensities at the sample points of the triangle.

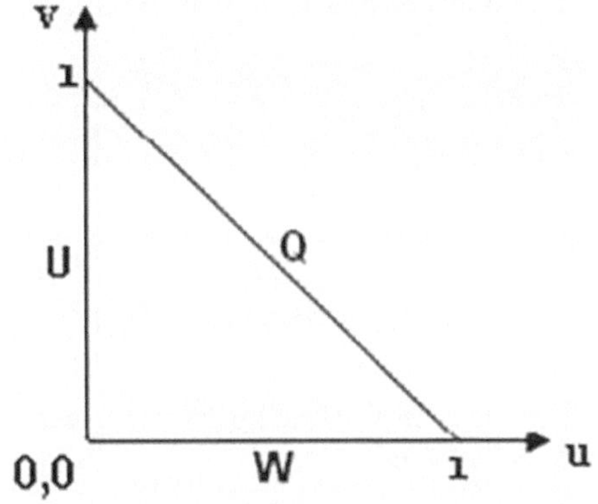

Figure 2.15 Orthonormalized triangle.

$$A = \frac{(4C_{12}y_3 - C_{23}y_3)E_{32} - (4C_{13}y_2 - C_{23}y_3)E_{23}}{E_{32}D_{23} - E_{32}D_{32}},$$

where:

$$C_2 = 4I_{12} - 3I_1 - I_2, C_{12} = I_1 + I_2 - 2I_{12}, C_3 = 4I_{13} - 3I_1 - I_3,$$
$$C_{13} = I_1 + I_3 - 2I_{13}, C_{23} = 4I_1 - 4I_{12} - 4I_{13} + 4I_{23},$$
$$D_{23} = (2x_2^2 y_3 - 2x_2 y_2 x_3),\ D_{32} = 2y_2 x_3^2 - 2x_2 x_3 y_3,$$
$$E_{23} = x_2 y_2 y_3 - y_2^2 x_3,\ E_{32} = y_2 x_3 y_3 - x_2 y_3^2.$$

It is calculated (Hill 2002), that it is necessary to execute 25 additions, 51 multiplications and 5 divisions to determine the unknowns A, B, C, D, E, F.

The obtained solution is rather complex and computationally expensive. It is possible to simplify the problem essentially by defining the problem over an orthonormalized triangle (Hast et al. 2003) (Fig. 2.15) and transforming the obtained results to the initial triangle.

For the orthonormalized triangle we use the following equation:

$$I = au^2 + bv^2 + cuv + du + ev + f. \tag{2.24}$$

Let us write down the system of equations (2.24) in matrix form for the orthonormalized triangle, considering the new variables.

$$\begin{bmatrix} I_1 \\ I_2 \\ I_3 \\ I_{12} \\ I_{13} \\ I_{23} \end{bmatrix} = \begin{bmatrix} 0 & 0 & 0 & 0 & 0 & 1 \\ 1 & 0 & 0 & 1 & 0 & 1 \\ 0 & 1 & 0 & 0 & 1 & 1 \\ \frac{1}{2} & 0 & 0 & \frac{1}{2} & 0 & 1 \\ 0 & \frac{1}{2} & 0 & 0 & \frac{1}{2} & 1 \\ \frac{1}{4} & \frac{1}{4} & \frac{1}{4} & \frac{1}{2} & \frac{1}{2} & 1 \end{bmatrix} \cdot \begin{bmatrix} a \\ b \\ c \\ d \\ e \\ f \end{bmatrix}. \tag{2.25}$$

The solution becomes (Hast et al. 2003):

$$\begin{bmatrix} a \\ b \\ c \\ d \\ e \\ f \end{bmatrix} = \begin{bmatrix} 2(I_1 + I_2 - 2I_{12}) \\ 2(I_3 - I_1 - 2I_{13}) \\ 4(I_1 + I_{23} - I_{13} - I_{12}) \\ I_2 - I_1 - a \\ I_3 - I_1 - b \\ I_1 \end{bmatrix}. \tag{2.26}$$

For the points of the initial triangle and the normalized triangle the following transformation can be used:

$$u = x\alpha_u + y\beta_u,$$
$$v = x\alpha_v + y\beta_v,$$

where:

$$\alpha_u = y_2\omega, \beta_u = -x_2\omega, \alpha_v = -y_1\omega, \beta_u = x_1\omega, \omega = 1/x_1y_2 - x_2y_1.$$

Let us substitute the last equations in the equation (2.24) and equate corresponding factors in (2.22) and (2.24), then we will obtain (Hast et al. 2003):

$$\begin{aligned} A &= a\alpha_u^2 + b\alpha_v^2 + c\alpha_u\alpha_v, \\ B &= a\beta_u^2 + b\beta_u^2 + c\beta_u\beta_v, \\ C &= 2a\alpha_u\beta_u + 2b\alpha_v\beta_v + c(\alpha_u\beta_v + \alpha_v\beta_u), \\ D &= d\alpha_u + ea\alpha_v, \\ E &= d\beta_u + e\beta_v, \\ F &= f. \end{aligned}$$

This solution will be fast and simple. However, it can still be simplified further as shown in (Hast et al. 2003). The normalization of the vectors at the mid edges is approximated using the first step of the Newton-Raphson as shown by Wynn (Foley et al. 1996):

$$N_{norm} = \frac{\vec{N}}{2}(3 - \vec{N}\vec{N}).$$

Applying the given formula for the vector $\vec{N}_{1/2} = \frac{\vec{N}_i + \vec{N}_j}{2}$, , we receive the following formula for the near-normalized value of the sum of two vectors (Hast et al. 2003):

$$(\vec{N}_i + \vec{N}_j)_{norm} = (\vec{N}_i + \vec{N}_j)\frac{5 - \vec{N}_i\vec{N}_j}{8}. \tag{2.27}$$

The formula is quite simple, however it has rather high relative approximation error when the angle between the vectors involved increases over 45° and comes closer to 90°. Let us find a formula for a better approximation for these cases.

For the vector $\vec{N}_{1/2}$, obtained by addition of the vectors $\vec{N}_i$ and $\vec{N}_j$, which are located at two vertices of the triangle, it is possible to rewrite the normalization:

$$\vec{N}_{1/2} = (\vec{N}_i + \vec{N}_j)_{norm} = \frac{\vec{N}_i + \vec{N}_j}{\sqrt{(\vec{N}_i + \vec{N}_j)^2}} = \frac{\vec{N}_i + \vec{N}_j}{\sqrt{(\vec{N}_i)^2 + (\vec{N}_j)^2 + 2\vec{N}_i\vec{N}_j}}$$

As the normal vectors $\vec{N}_i, \vec{N}_j$ are normalized, $\vec{N}_i^2 = \vec{N}_j^2 = 1$, their scalar product is equal to the cosine of the angle between them, i.e. $\vec{N}_i\vec{N}_j = \cos\psi$. Considering these facts, the following formula for the normalized value of the sum of two vectors can be obtained:

$$\vec{N}_{1/2} = \frac{\vec{N}_i + \vec{N}_j}{\sqrt{2(1+\cos\psi)}}.$$

After expansion $\frac{1}{\sqrt{2(1+\cos\psi)}}$ in a Chebyshev series and having limited it by three terms, we obtain the following formula:

$$\frac{1}{\sqrt{2(1+\cos\psi)}} \approx (0{,}103\cos^2\psi - 0{,}306\cos\psi + 0{,}705).$$

Thus:

$$\vec{N}_{1/2} \approx (\vec{N}_i + \vec{N}_j)(0{,}103\cos^2\psi - 0{,}306\cos\psi + 0{,}705). \tag{2.28}$$

In the Figure 2.16 it has shown the relative error of approximating the vector $\vec{N}_{1/2}$, using the two mentioned formulas (2.27) and (2.28).

Using formula (2.27) (solid curve) as Figure 2.16 shows, the maximum of relative error approximation does not exceed 0,36%, while using formula (2.26) (dotted curve) reaches a maximum of 11,64%.

Main disadvantage of the presented approaches consists in fact that the color intensities are calculated for midpoints of the triangle edges. In this way, there might be higher intensity values along the edges that are not taken into consideration. It is more accurate to determine the color intensities in those points of an edge where color intensities have their maximum values. In this way, the generated shading surface will more truly follow the true shading curve for the color intensities of the three-dimensional object.

Let us denote the normal vectors as $\vec{N}_0, \vec{N}_1, \vec{N}_2$ at the vertices $(x_0, y_0), (x_1, y_1), (x_2, y_2)$ of the triangle.

In many computer graphics applications, where speed is crucial, it is often assumed that the viewer and the light source are placed at infinity (Hern et al. 2011). This implies that the vector $\vec{L}$ in the direction at the light source is constant for all points on the triangle. It was proved (Kautz et al. 2000) that in this case, the maximum value of the color intensities occurs on the edges of the triangle at:

$$t_1 = \frac{\cos\gamma\cos\varphi - \cos\beta}{(\cos\varphi - 1)(\cos\beta + \cos\gamma)},$$
$$t_2 = \frac{\cos\gamma\cos\phi - \cos\lambda}{(\cos\phi - 1)(\cos\lambda + \cos\gamma)},$$
$$t_3 = \frac{\cos\beta\cos\vartheta - \cos\lambda}{(\cos\vartheta - 1)(\cos\lambda + \cos\beta)}$$

The angles between vectors in question are shown in Figure 2.17.

The variables t_1, t_2, t_3 are parametric values in the interval from 0 to 1. To establish the correspondence between the points of the edges of the actual triangle and the orthonormalized triangle, it is necessary to keep a proportional ratio of the point position relative to the vertices of that edge. Parameter t_3 varies from 0 to 1 and determines this ratio for the point on the edge BC, where the maximum value of intensity takes place (Figure 2.16).

This point divides the edge into two segments. This ratio should also be kept for edge Q of the orthonormal triangle.

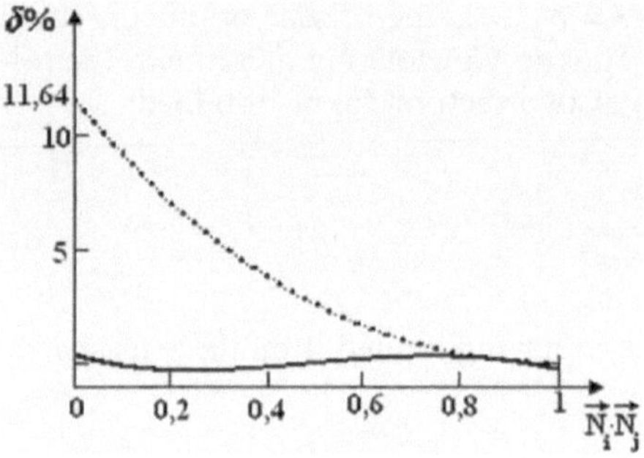

Figure 2.16 The relatives errors of the two approximations of the true normalized vector depending on the scalar product of N_i and N_j.

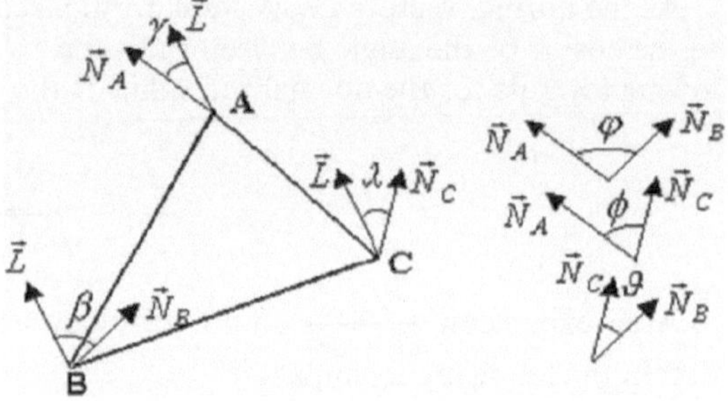

Figure 2.17 Normal vectors of the ABC triangle.

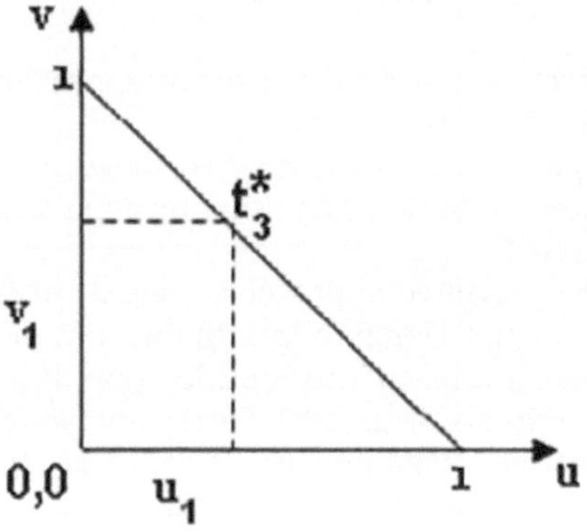

Figure 2.18 Position of point on the hypotenuse of the orthonormal triangele.

If parameter t_3^* on the edge Q corresponds to the parameter t_3, then the condition $\frac{t_3}{1} = \frac{t_3^*}{\sqrt{2}}$ should be satisfied, where $\sqrt{2}$ is the length of edge Q. Figure 2.18 shows that:

$$u_1 = t_3^* \sin 45^0 = t_3\sqrt{2}\frac{\sqrt{2}}{2} = t_3,\ v_1 = 1 - t_3^* \cos 45^0 = 1 - t_3.$$

If t_1 has a correspondence on edge V, t_2 on edge W, and t_3 on edge Q, then $I_{12\max}, I_{13\max}, I_{23\max}$ are maximum values of the intensity on the edges W, V, Q, respectively. Now we have the following equation for an orthonormal triangle:

$$\begin{matrix} I_1 \\ I_2 \\ I_3 \\ I_{12\max} \\ I_{13\max} \\ I_{23\max} \end{matrix} = \begin{bmatrix} 0 & 0 & 0 & 0 & 0 & 1 \\ 1 & 0 & 0 & 1 & 0 & 1 \\ 0 & 1 & 0 & 0 & 1 & 1 \\ t_1^2 & 0 & 0 & t_1 & 0 & 1 \\ 0 & t_2^2 & 0 & 0 & t_2 & 1 \\ u_1^2 & v_1^2 & u_1 v_1 & u_1 & v_1 & 1 \end{bmatrix} \cdot \begin{bmatrix} a \\ b \\ c \\ d \\ e \\ f \end{bmatrix}.$$

The solution is:

$$\begin{bmatrix} a \\ b \\ c \\ d \\ e \\ f \end{bmatrix} = \begin{bmatrix} \dfrac{(I_1 - I_2)t_1 + I_{12} - I_1}{t_1(t_1 - 1)} \\ \dfrac{(I_1 - I_3)t_2 + I_{13} - I_1}{t_2(t_1 - 1)} \\ \dfrac{I_{23} - au_1^2 - bv_1^2 - du_1 - ev_1 - I_1}{u_1 v_1} \\ \dfrac{(I_2 - I_1)t_1^2 + I_1 - I_{12}}{t_1(t_1 - 1)} \\ \dfrac{(I_3 - I_1)t_2^2 + I_1 - I_{13}}{t_2(t_2 - 1)} \\ I_1 \end{bmatrix}.$$

Let us simplify the solution by finding $b + e$, $a + d$.

$$b + e = \frac{(I_1 - I_3)t_2 + I_{13} - I_1}{t_2(t_2 - 1)} + \frac{(I_3 - I_1)t_2{}^2 + I_1 - I_{13}}{t_2(t_2 - 1)} = I_3 - I_1,$$

$$a + d = \frac{(I_1 - I_2)t_1 + I_{12} - I_1}{t_1(t_1 - 1)} + \frac{(I_2 - I_1)t_1^2 + I_1 - I_{12}}{t_1(t_1 - 1)} = I_2 - I_1.$$

The obtained equations show that $e = I_3 - I_1 - b$, $d = I_2 - I_1 - a$. Considering that $u_1 = t_3$, $v_1 = 1 - t_3$, it is possible to obtain more simple expression for c.

$$c = \frac{(a+b)t_3^2 + (a + b + I_2 - I_3)t_3 + I_3 - I_{23}}{t_3(1 - t_3)}.$$

Taking into consideration the simplifications, it is now possible to write the equations as:

$$\begin{bmatrix} a \\ b \\ c \\ d \\ e \\ f \end{bmatrix} = \begin{bmatrix} \dfrac{(I_1 - I_2)t_1 + I_{12} - I_1}{t_1(t_1 - 1)} \\ \dfrac{(I_1 - I_3)t_2 + I_{13} - I_1}{t_2(t_1 - 1)} \\ \dfrac{(a+b)t_3^2 + (a + b + I_2 - I_3)t_3 + I_3 - I_{23}}{t_3(1 - t_3)} \\ I_2 - I_1 - a \\ I_3 - I_1 - b \\ I_1 \end{bmatrix}.$$

The computational analysis has shown that under the condition that the color intensities $I_1, I_2, I_3, I_{12}, I_{13}, I_{23}$ are known it is necessary to perform 34 multiplications, 28 additions and 4 divisions for calculation of the coefficients A, B, C, D, E, F when using the orthonormal triangle. The number of operations can be compared to the approach by (Abbas et al. 2001). Obviously, the proposed approach is computationally less expensive. Furthermore, it should be noted that thanks to the usage of the orthonormalized triangle it is feasible to compute the intensity in the point where it has its maximum along the edge.

The previous formulation by (Abbas et al. 2001) yields much more complicated expressions using the maximum point instead of the midpoint along the edge. The cost analysis has shown that the proposed approach for scanline-fill reduces the time for shading about 8–9 times compared to the Phong method. Sometimes the intensity at the edges is almost the same as the intensities at the vertices, so that the difference is neglected. When the difference in intensities is smaller than a preset threshold, then the computation of the maximum value of color intensity on an edge of a triangle is unnecessary. In this case, it is sufficient to compute the intensity at the midpoint of the edge.

For this case the calculation of the unknown coefficients becomes simpler. So, for example, when the difference of color intensities on the edge Q is smaller than the threshold value, then:

$$c = 4(I_{23} - I_1) - a - b - 2(d + e).$$

When this occurs for two edges, for example, U and Q, then:

$$c = 4(I_{23} - I_{12}) + b - 2e,$$

$$\mathrm{a} = 2(I_2 + I_1 - 2I_{12}),$$

$$\mathrm{d} = 4\mathrm{I}_{12} - \mathrm{I}_2 - 3\mathrm{I}_1.$$

The proposed approach is a little bit more computationally expensive than the mid edge approach proposed in (Hast et al. 2003), but the advantage of the approach proposed herein is that the shading produced will follow more closely the true shading since it will take extremes into account. The mid edge approach will filter out these extremes unless they happen to lie on the mid edge or in the end points, i.e. the vertices.

7 CONCLUSIONS

A new Bidirectional Reflectance Distribution Functions (BRDF) for reproduction of specular characteristics of the surfaces have been proposed and explored in this chapter. The main feature of the new BRDF is lower computational complexity. They have simple hardware implement in systems of computer graphics. BRDFs have been developed by using approximation by polynomial of the third degree, logarithmic and new cosine functions.

BRDF approximation using polynomial of the third degree has the least power among all proposed ones. It can be used in computer graphic for conceptual design, as well as in the means of forming dynamic images.

BRDF approximation using the logarithmic function can be used for hardware implementation because it is possible to set the $\log_2(\cos\gamma)$ function in tabular form and approximate 2^x function. The usage of the new BRDF provides formation of visually identical images compared with the Phong and Schlick functions.

New cosine-power functions provide high precision of specular color component for both the epicenter and for the blooming zone. The function has much smaller degree in comparison with Blinn (Phong 1975) function. Proposed BRDF has a simple hardware implementation, which makes it effective in the construction of high-performance special means. Highly accurate color reproduction ensures this function to use for full range of specular factors both in software and hardware implementations.

A method for accelerated computation and determination of color intensities for shading of three-dimensional graphics objects is proposed. The main idea of this method consists in the generation of a second order surface using six sample points of a triangle, three of which determine color intensity in vertices, and three where the maximum values of color intensities on edges occurs. Using these points realism of the shading increases, as the maximum color intensity along edges of a triangle is considered. The offered approach allows an increase in speed of rasterization about 8–9 times compared with a classical implementation of the Phong method, with a Normalized Mean Square Error (NMSE), which does not exceed 0,00015, and that is acceptable for realistic graphics.

REFERENCES

Abbas A.M., Szirmay-Kalos L., Szijarto G., Horvath T., Foris T. 2001: Quadratic Interpolation in Hardware Rendering, Spring Conference of Computer Graphics.

Foley J.D., van Dam A., Feiner S.K. and Hughes J.F. 1996: Computer Graphics; Principles and Practice. Addison Wesley. Chpt. 16, pp. 800–807.

Gouraud H. 1971: Continuous Shading of Curved Surfaces. IEEE Transactions on Computers, Vol. c-20, No 6, June 1971.

Hast A., Barrera T., Bengtsson E. 2003: Fast Specular Highlights by modifying the Phong-Blinn Model. International Conference on Computer Graphics and Interactive Techniques.

Hearn D.D, Baker M.P., Warren Carithers W. 2011: Computer Graphics with Open GL, 4th Edition,| Pearson.

Hill F. 2002: OpenGL. Computer Graphics Programming for Professionals. Piter.

Kautz J., McCool M. 2000: Approximation of glossy reflection with pre-filtered environment maps. Proceeding graphics interface—Technical report. pp. 119–126.

Levoy M., Hanrahan P. 1996: Light Field Rendering. SIGGRAPH 96, pp. 31–42.

Lyon R.F. 1993: Phong Shading Reformulation for Hardware Renderer Simplification. Apple Technical Report No. 43.

Phong B. T. 1975: Illumination for Computer Generated Pictures. Communications of the ACM, Vol. 18, No 6, June 1975.

Rogers D. 2001: Mathematical Basics of Computer Graphics. Moscow, Mir.

Romanuyk O. 2005: Methods for Specular Color Component Accelerate Calculation. Edited by O. Romanuyk, A. Chernij: IEEE Workshop on Intelligent Data Acquisition and Advanced Computing systems; Technology and Applications. Sofia, pp. 615–619.

Romanyuk A., Hast A., Lyashenko Y. 2008: The Methods of Fast Shading, 9th Conference of Development and Application Systems, Suceava, Romania.

Romanyuk A. 2006: Efficient Methods of 3D Objects Shading. Monography. Edited by A.N. Romanyuk, A.V. Chorniy. Vinnitsa: Universum-Vinnitsa.

Romanyuk S.O., Pavlov S.V., Melnyk O.V. 2007: New method to control intensity for antialiasing. In S.O. Romanyuk, S.V. Pavlov, O.V. Melnyk: Control and Communications (SIBCON), International Siberian Conference. 21–23 May, pp. 1–4.

CHAPTER 3

Modified method of parallel-hierarchical network teaching based on population coding

L.I. Timchenko
State University of Transport Economy and Technologies, Kyiv, Ukraine

M. Zlepko
Vinnytsia National Technical University, Vinnitsa, Ukraine

A. Smolarz & K. Gromaszek
Lublin University of Technology, Lublin, Poland

B. Suleimenov
K.I. Satpaev Kazakh National Research Technical University, Almaty, Kazakhstan

A. Kalizhanova
Al-Farabi Kazakh National University, Almaty, Kazakhstan

1 INTRODUCTION

Absence of time-consuming operations indicates a sufficient simplicity of the computational procedure that realises the parallel hierarchical transformation, and makes it an efficient method for use in various applied areas requiring a combination of a high level of parallelism and a compact form of data representation.

A general algorithm of fast recognition of laser beam spots (LBS) images can be developed based on the proposed method of parallel-hierarchical transformation for processing dynamic images (Fig. 3.1).

This algorithm envisages a call to subroutine NetForm, a subprogram serving to construct network structures for images. A detailed description of the subroutine is shown as an algorithm (Fig. 3.2).

This subroutine performs input of the initial information to the PH network. After that, G-transformation of information takes place at all levels of the PH network.

2 THE G-TRANSFORMATION

The G-transformation is performed in the following way. The vector of the incoming image is sent to the PH network input (to input elements of first level branches of the network). A mathematical model of the parallel decomposition of the set $\mu=\{a_i\}, i=\overline{1,n}$ (Timchenko et al. 2011), used in each branch of the PH network, looks as follows:

$$\sum_{i=1}^{n} a_i = \sum_{j^*=1}^{P} \left(n - \sum_{k=0}^{j^*-1} n_k \right) \left(a^{j^*} - a^{j^*-1} \right),$$

where $a_i \neq 0$, P is the dimensionality of this set (a number of set elements) or the dimensionality of the PH network branch at its every level, a^z, $z=\overline{1,P}$ are elements of subsets consisting

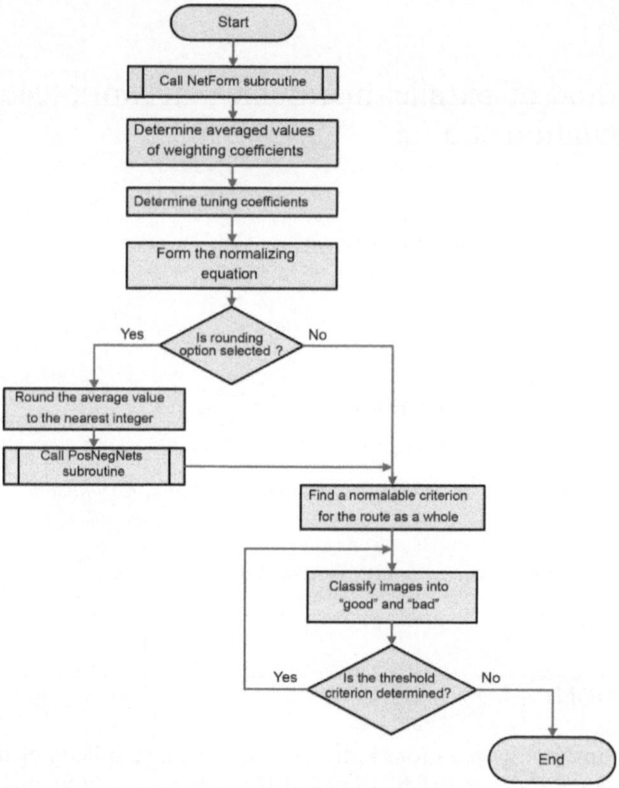

Figure 3.1 A general algorithm of laser beam spots image recognition.

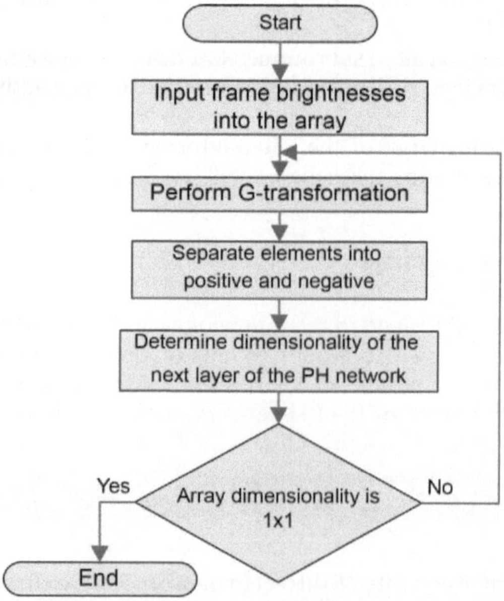

Figure 3.2 A subroutine algorithm of the creation of image network structure.

of equal elements, n_z is the number of elements in the kth subset (i.e. the order of number a_i), a^{j^*} is the 1st element of the set $\{a^z\}$, selected at the j^*-th step, $j^* = \overline{1,P}, a^0 = 0,\ n_0 = 0$.

When a structure of two networks is constructed, the average values of weighting coefficients and tuning coefficients (2) are being determined. Based on the calculated tuning coefficients, a normalising equation (6) is being formed.

If an average value $\overline{a}_i^t$ is rounded up to the nearest integer, the subroutine *PosNegNets* is called. It is a subprogram that forms two connected PH networks for processing positive and negative difference components. A formation algorithm of the two networks is similar to the formation algorithms of the network structure for images.

After that, a normalising criterion for the route as a whole is being found with further classification of images into "good" and "bad" according to the ratio.

If the threshold criterion is determined, the classification is conducted again.

Let us develop a preliminary processing algorithm of route fragments (Fig. 3.3)

An image of the laser route fragment arriving to the system input undergoes the following preliminary processing:

1. Determine maximum fragment brightness to form n border lines;
2. Having selected a necessary number of boundaries, find their geometrical centres and average parameters for the whole frame;
3. Form tunnel boundaries using a trained sample and averaged frame parameters;
4. Check if calculated frame parameters are included into the tunnel. Based on this verification, frame image classification is performed. If an image was classified as "bad", image parameters are corrected, included into the taught sample, and an additional training of the system is performed.

The developed application is intended to process and classify laser beam spots images.

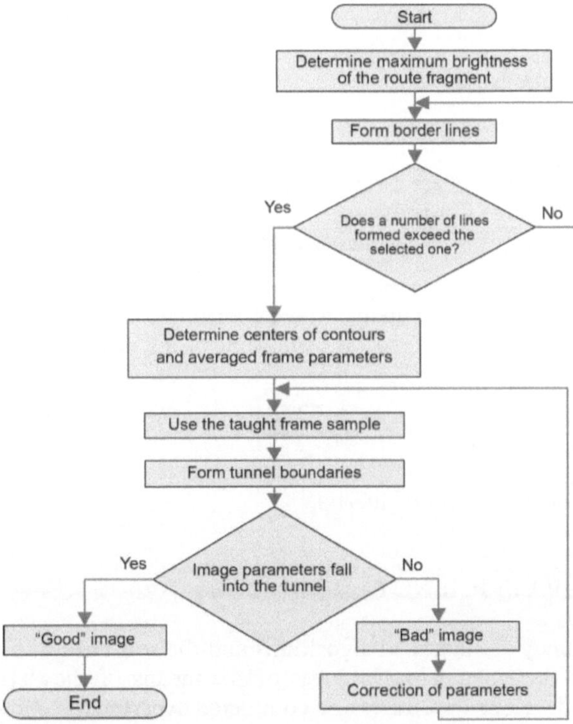

Figure 3.3 A preliminary processing algorithm of route fragments.

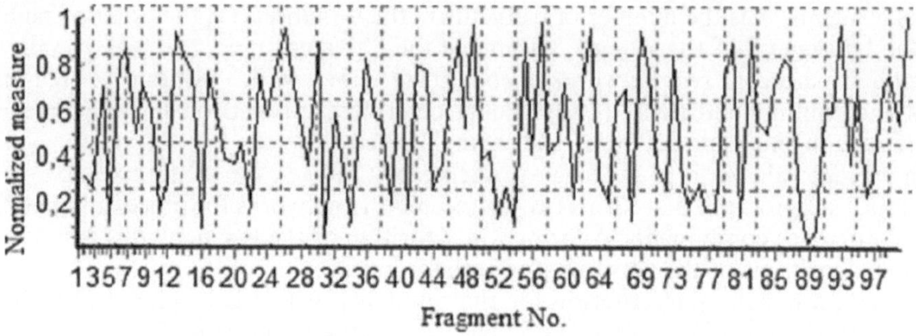

Figure 3.4 Screen form of the PH network application for fast recognition of laser beam spot images.

The software window (Fig. 3.4) represents a form divided into two parts: the left part contains a processing panel of the reference frame of the laser beam spots images route, and the right one—that of the current frame of the laser beam spots images route.

3 INFORMATION ABOUT THE FRAME PARAMETERS

Information about the frame parameters is exhibited in the upper part:

- frame width, pixels;
- frame height, pixels;
- information about the route containing the frame;
- frame file name;
- number of frames in the route.

The bottom part contains tabs:

- construction of the network graph, which can be obtained and saved as a PH network graph file;
- route fragment processing, where a route fragment can be processed;
- image comparison, where laser beam spot images are compared and classified;
- determination of energy centres, where laser beam spot energy centres are determined and the PH network is trained.

An energy centre is a point in the image, where coordinates (x,y) of a two-dimensional signal with a specific nonlinear density meet a given value of $f(x,y)$, and are expressed as follows:

$$x_{ec} = \frac{1}{M}\sum_{x=0}^{N-1}\sum_{y=0}^{N-1} w\big(f(x,y)\big)\cdot x, y_{ec} = \frac{1}{M}\sum_{x=0}^{N-1}\sum_{y=0}^{N-1} w\big(f(x,y)\big)\cdot y, M = \sum_{x=0}^{N-1}\sum_{y=0}^{N-1} w\big(f(x,y)\big)$$

where M is the first order moment of inertia.

4 ESTIMATION OF EFFICIENCY

To estimate the efficiency of suggested algorithms and the soft hardware developed on their basis, let us describe the technical advantages of the means of the PH transformation as demonstrated by the developed products and conducted experiments. A comparative characterisation is shown in Table 3.1.

Table 3.1 Comparative characterisation of the means of the parallel-hierarchical transformation.

Parameter	Indices			
	Known soft hardware (imitational modelling based on MLP and RBF networks).	Known soft hardware (imitational modelling based on neural-like network technology)	Known soft hardware (CPU, PH transformation method based on the Q-decomposition)	Proposed soft hardware (GPU, method of the PH network training based on the normalising equation)
Average size of good route fragments (%)	70	74	50	18
Average value of correct recognition (%)	92	92,5	84,8	94
Accuracy of the energy centre determination, decomposition elements	1,5	1,5	1,2	0,01
Average recognition time of network processing (s)	–	–	8,4	1,52
Average time of preliminary processing of route fragments (s)	–	–	3,32	0,6

The use of neural-like network technologies for classification of extended laser route images is analysed in (Timchenko et al. 2011). The computer modelling revealed 92.5% correctly recognised images, including 74% "good" images and 60% "bad" images. In (Timchenko et al. 2011), a recognition system was modelled on the basis of the MLP neural-like network and RBF-based neural-like network. Recognition of a sample that included 140 laser route spot objects by the RBF-based neural-like network modelled in the Statistica Neural Networks 4.0 yielded 92% correctly recognised images. Comparing the results of (Timchenko et al. 2011, Timchenko et al. 2013) and those studied in this article tells us about the potential of the latter.

Therefore, the suggested method, algorithms and soft hardware permit to measure energy centre coordinates of laser route fragment images based on the normalising equation with an accuracy of no more than 0.01 decomposition elements, thus exceeding known methods (e.g. those based on determination of the gravity centre using the method of moment characteristics (Timchenko et al. 2011, Timchenko et al. 2013, Timchenko et al. 2014) by the accuracy of 1.5 times on average, which is reflected in Table 3.1. The time necessary for preliminary and network processing of the laser route fragment images decreases as well.

Four routes, each containing 100 frames, were used in experimental research of the parallel-hierarchical transformation for fast recognition of laser beam spot images. Using the normalising equation, let us determine the normalised measures for Route 1 (Fig. 3.5).

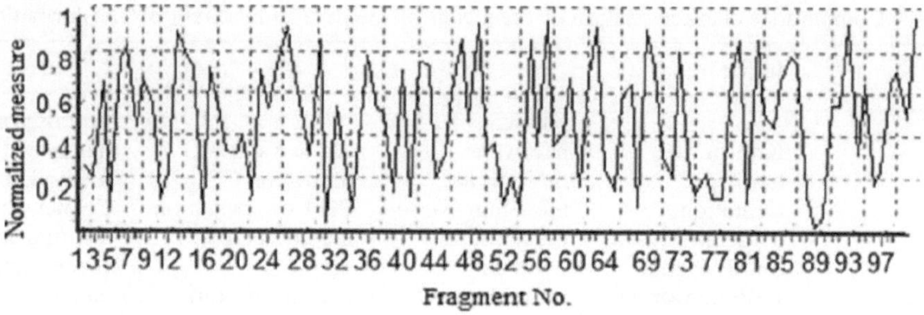

Figure 3.5 Determination of the normalised measure for further classification of Route 1 fragments.

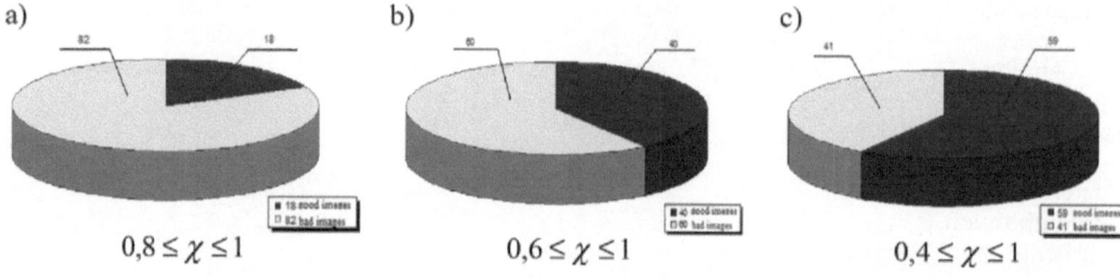

Figure 3.6 Classification of Route 1 fragments (with the respective threshold criterion).

Using inequations, let us classify images (Fig. 3.6a).

As can be seen, the portion of "good" images is 18%. As a rule, in real conditions, positions of energy centres cannot be determined absolutely accurately, therefore less tight limits should be set for the threshold criterion using relation (Figure 3.6b and 3.6c) An average portion of "good" images in this case is 40% and 59% respectively. Then the PH network is trained for repeated processing of "bad" route fragments.

In physical modelling of the method of PH transformation and determination of extended laser route image coordinates using the graphic adapter Radeon X1300, processing of a single image takes about 0.6 s. Radeon X1300 is a basic solution in the ATI Radeon family of graphic adapters based on the graphic processor RV515 with the main characteristics of 4 pixel pipelines, 4 texture units and 2 vertex pipelines.

An approach of flow programming is suggested to program the GPU. This approach includes splitting a program into relatively small stages (core programs) that process data flow elements. Core programs go into shaders, and data flows go into textures in the GPU. A shader is a program performed in the GPU and processing the data flow. "Data flow" means information about the coordinates of polygon vertices, each vertex illumination, normal mapping, texture coordinates and so on, that permanently arrives in blocks to the shader program. A video processor receives outgoing information for all three vertices of the polygon. Having data on the three vertices, the GPU goes through all the pixels of a single polygon, while gradually changing (interpolating) vertex values from one vertex to another. A shader length is a memory space of the shader program. Considering that data arriving to the shader are random for the programmer, in a sense that the order in which the data will be sent to the shader is not preset, the shader program does not have any statistical or general variables; there is nothing similar to files or information storage between calls. Otherwise, the shader program is similar to a regular C program: there are input, output and time variables, standard functions, structures, arrays, cycles and conditional operators.

Image processing takes place in the GPU with cores realised at all elements covered by the initial region. The only obvious way to calculate a scalar of the input vector is to represent 1×1 initial elements and use a core that is read in all values from the input texture. This approach has several drawbacks. First, only one of the parallel elementary processors would be busy. Second, that would probably exceed the maximum memory size, including the memory of the shader and static instruction of calculation for some hardware. That is why we will perform a parallel operation of reduction based on global methods of communication on parallel computers.

5 EXPERIMENT

At the high level, GPU-based parallel calculation is a correction of sizes of the input and output texture and of index elements. For the presented vector M of the length M, the output of the first step is M/2 with texture M/2. For each of its elements, coordinates for input texture are corrected in such a way that they correspond to disconnected 2×2 subregions. Then the values in those subregions are compared. This is repeated recursively until the 2×2 texture is reduced finally to the 1×1 "scalar" texture through a logarithmic series of repetitions.

Next series of images finalise the first step of the 8×8 algorithm reduction of the input texture (Fig. 3.7). The left image demonstrates the input texture. Initial elements are marked in green (Fig. 3.7a). The right image is a result of the first round of reduction. Each initial element contains a local transfer maximum of the 2×2 subregion in the input texture. This relation, in addition, is distinguished in the second line of images (Fig. 3.7b). Next, let us determine the coordinates of energy centres of a fragment of Route 1 (Fig. 3.8). A diagram of changes in the energy centre coordinates of fragments of Route 1 is shown in Figure 3.9.

a)

47	2	3	57	5	12	7	8
10	20	6	13	14	15	16	17
19	11	21	22	23	68	25	26
38	29	64	31	32	33	35	34
37	28	39	49	53	42	41	52
46	1	48	40	61	51	44	43
55	71	4	58	69	62	50	60
30	65	66	67	24	59	70	56

47	57	15	17
38	64	68	35
46	49	61	52
71	67	69	70

b)

47	2	3	57	5	12	7	8
10	20	6	13	14	15	16	17
19	11	21	22	23	68	25	26
38	29	64	31	32	33	35	34
37	28	39	49	53	42	41	52
46	1	48	40	61	51	44	43
55	71	4	58	69	62	50	60
30	65	66	67	24	59	70	56

47	57	15	17
38	64	68	35
46	49	61	52
71	67	69	70

Figure 3.7 A diagram of pixel processing using the Radeon X1300 graphic adapter.

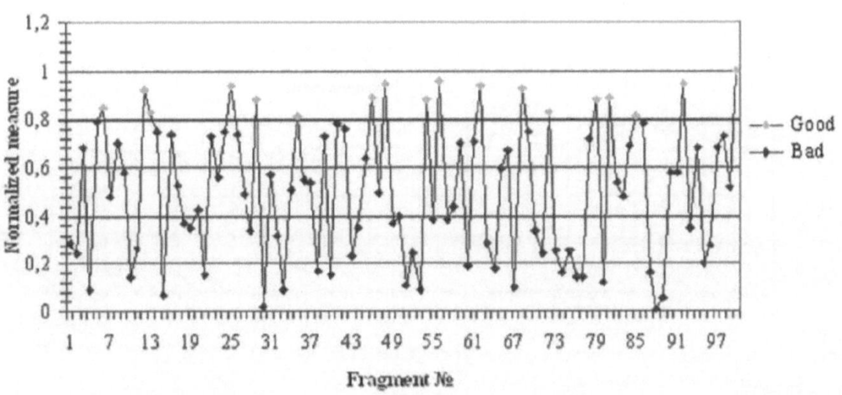

Figure 3.8 A diagram of formation of "good" and "bad" images in Route 1.

After the PH network training, a portion of "good" images was 83% (as compared to 18%). The graphic interpretation of determination of energy centre coordinates after the PH network training is demonstrated in Figure 3.10.

After the PH network training, a portion of "good" images of Route 2 was 76% (12% before training) (Fig. 3.11 versus Fig. 3.12).

After the PH network training, a portion of "good" images of fragments of Route 3 was 65% (15% before training) (Fig. 3.13 versus Fig. 3.14).

Finally, after the PH network training, a portion of "good" images of route 4 reached 83% as compared to 17% before training (Fig. 3.15 versus Fig. 3.16).

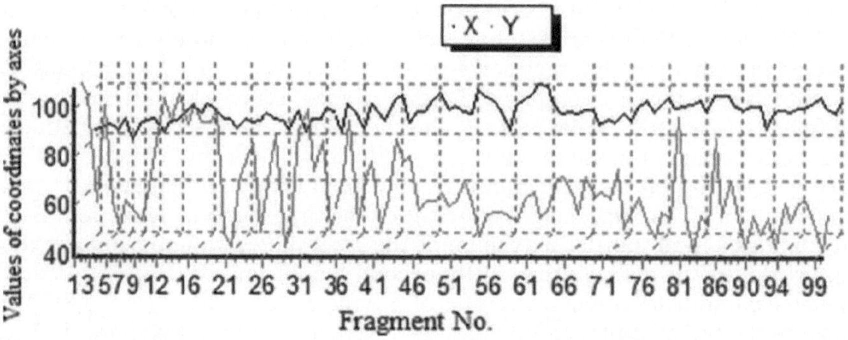

Figure 3.9 Determination of coordinates of energy centers of Route 1 fragments.

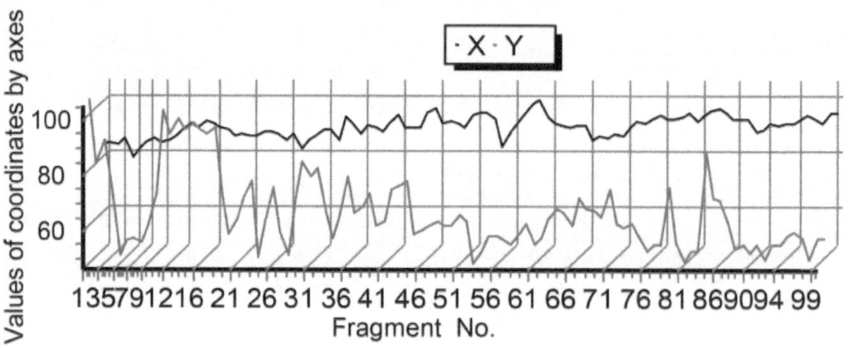

Figure 3.10 Determination of energy centre coordinates of fragments of Route 1 after the PH network training.

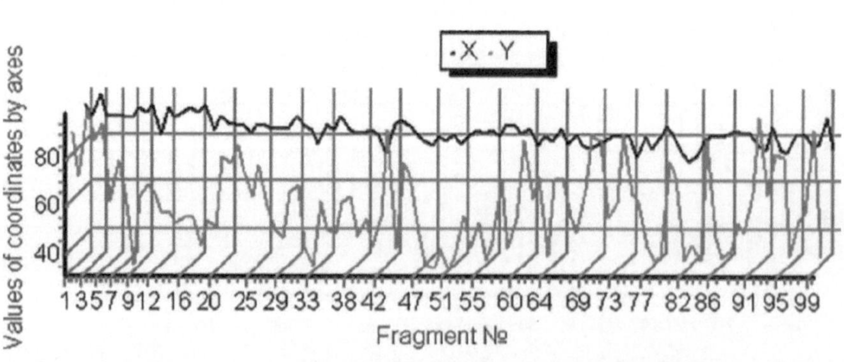

Figure 3.11 Determination of energy centre coordinates of fragments of Route 2.

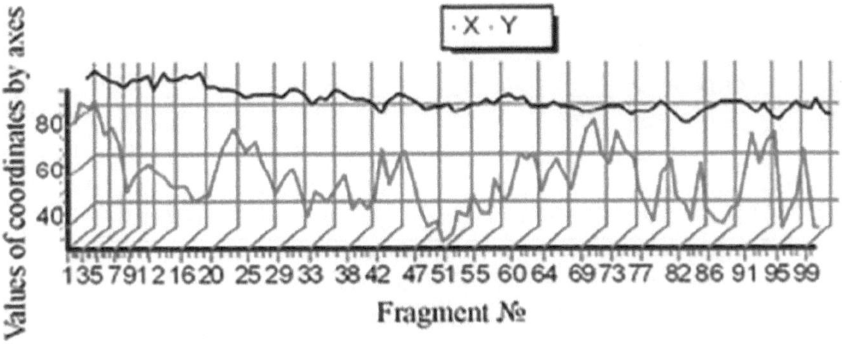

Figure 3.12 Determination of energy centre coordinates of fragments of Route 2 after the PH network training.

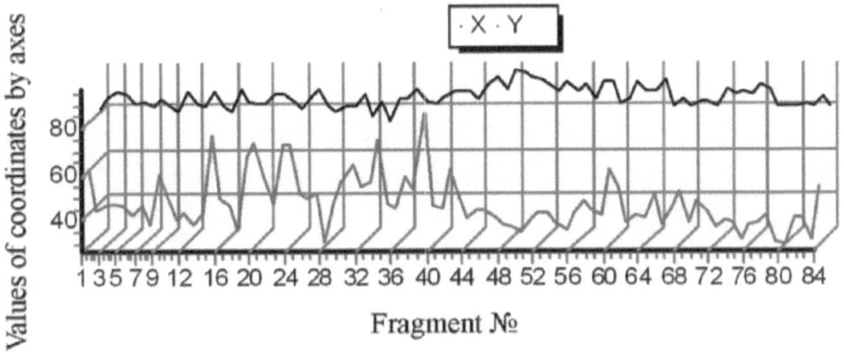

Figure 3.13 Determination of energy centre coordinates of fragments of Route 3.

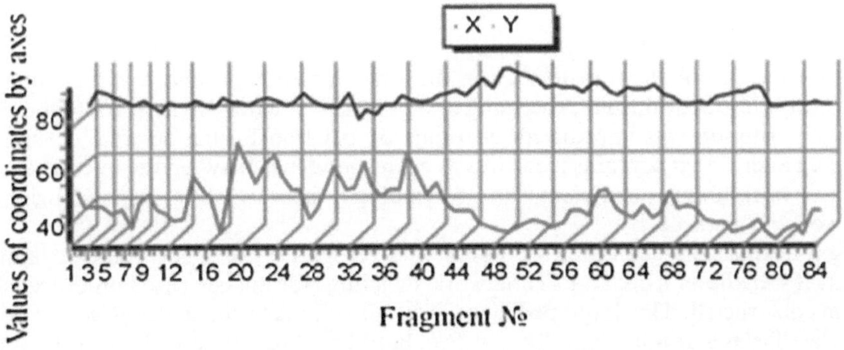

Figure 3.14 Determination of energy centre coordinates of fragments of Route 3 after the PH network training.

The work deals with an important problem of improved efficiency of dynamic image recognition. The analysis of modern trends in the development of fast recognition technologies for dynamic images, as well as the analysis of the PH transformation development, allows to classify the suggested parallel-hierarchical approach as a neural-like method of transformation with a network of direct propagation and the space-time organisation of connections.

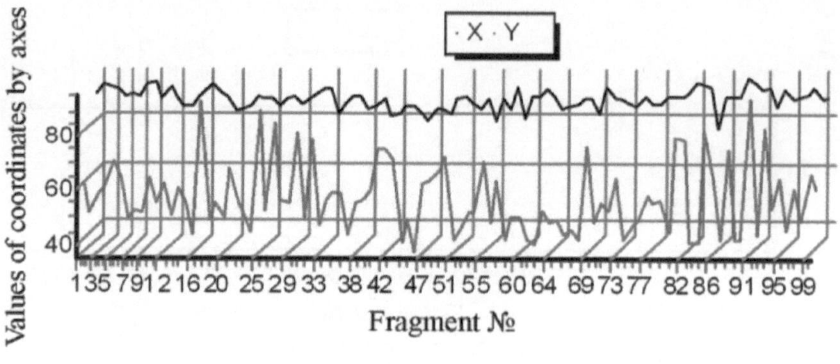

Figure 3.15 Determination of energy centre coordinates of fragments of Route 4.

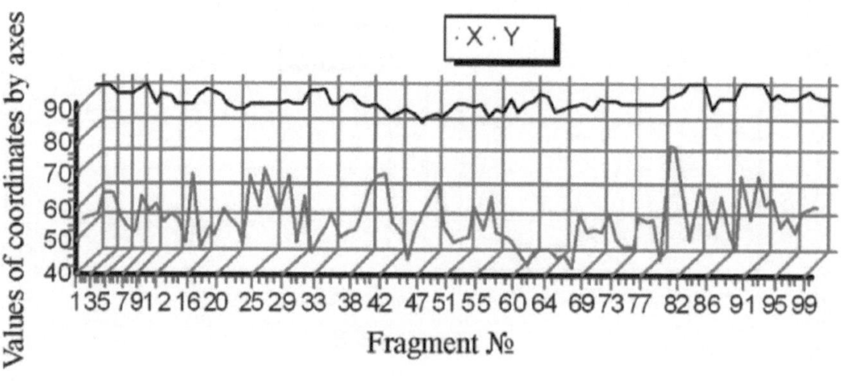

Figure 3.16 Determination of energy centre coordinates of fragments of route 4 after the PH network training.

The authors think that efficiency of computational structures can be increased by applying a developed method of PH transformation with the formation of a normalising equation.

For quality classification and processing of a sequence of extended laser route spot images, a threshold criterion was introduced. Methods of PH transformation were developed: by introducing a set A that contains measures of correspondence between the reference and current PH network tuning coefficients, and by finding a measure of correspondence between two networks as a whole.

Using a normalising equation, processing and recognition of algorithms for laser beam spot images were developed, and PH network structures for images based on G-transformation were constructed. The developed algorithms allow to determine energy centre positions and to classify laser route image frames. Peculiarities of real-time realisation of the algorithm of the developed method for route fragments are discussed, and a choice of means for software development is explained. On the basis of the developed algorithms, software was created for modelling a neural-like parallel-hierarchical network, which was used for image classification and fast processing.

Experimental methods to study the processing of laser beam spot image fragments were developed, which allow to verify the adequacy of the proposed algorithms and to obtain results of fast processing and classification of laser beam spot image fragments.

In the conducted experiments, an average portion of "good" route fragments was 17%, as compared to 50% in (Timchenko et al. 2011). However, after the training, it increased to 79.25%

(as compared to 65% (Timchenko et al. 2013)). It was also established that an average rate of correct recognition was 94% (84.8% (Timchenko et al. 2013)), and the accuracy of energy centre determination was no more than 0.01 decomposition elements (as compared to 1.2 decomposition elements (Kim & Wunsch 2003)), which is reflected in Table 3.1. This is, on average, 1.5 times higher than the accuracy of the known methods, for instance in comparison to gravity centre determination using a method of moment characteristics. Physical modelling of the PH transformation method for fast image recognition using the Radeon X1300 graphic adapter demonstrates that the processing of one image requires approximately 0.6 s (3.32 s (Timchenko et al. 2013)), and network processing requires 1.52 s (8.4 s (Timchenko et al. 2013)).

From recent achievements in the sphere of neurobiological research it is known that for coding within the frame of such an approach the information is presented by the population of active neurons (Haykin 1999, Timchenko et al. 2011). This important property was demonstrated in the experiments performed by Sparks, analysing how the brain of a monkey controls the motion of its eyes. The conclusion was made that the needed motion is coded by a population of the cells, each of which presents a motion different from others. The motion performed by the eye corresponds to the average of all the motions, coded by the active cells. As Yaung and Yamane showed in the experiments with the cerebral cortex of a monkey, population coding is valid not only for the motion of eyes but also for features of the face.

In accordance with the idea of population coding, the currently recognised image must be compared with a certain average representation of the reference pattern—average by all current patterns (in other words, by all the teaching sample) on the basis of averaging the PH network parameters.

Let us use the general idea of population coding (Timchenko et al. 2013) and construct a model of any finite operation conducted by all current operations, i.e. a finite operation consisting of a sequence of current operations. For instance, a finite operation in the form of a visual saccade consists of a sequence of current micro-saccades. At the branch level of the neural network, this finite operation with the realisation of population coding meets the averaged parameters of this network (Timchenko et al. 2013). For the PH network, both a number of elements in the branch of each level, which are determined on the basis of the model, and the values of the element itself may be taken as averaged parameters. In this case the currently recognised pattern will be reflected by the current PH network and compared with the reference PH network with averaged parameters (the PH network with averaged parameters forms a reference network of the reference pattern).

Having denoted the average value of the random element of the first level as $\overline{a}^1_{i,j}$, the second level as $\overline{a}^2_{i,j}$, the third level as $\overline{a}^3_{i,j}$, etc., the kth last level as $\overline{a}^k_{i,j}$, and the average number of elements of the first level as $N_{\overline{a}^1_{i,j}}$, the second level as $N_{\overline{a}^2_{i,j}}$, the third level as $N_{\overline{a}^3_{i,j}}$, etc., and the kth level as $N_{\overline{a}^k_{i,j}}$, one can form a PH network with averaged parameters according to the idea of population coding. The average number of certain layer elements is calculated according to the formula:

$$\overline{a}^k_{i,j} = \frac{\sum_k a^k_{i,j}}{N_{\overline{a}^k_{i,j}}}.$$

The structure of the PH network with averaged parameters thus synthesised is shown in Figure 3.17.

A current pattern or a tested pattern prepared by the parallel-hierarchical network with current parameters $a^1_{i,j}, a^2_{i,j}, a^3_{i,j}, \ldots, a^k_{i,j}$ and a respective number of elements in branches of each level $N_{a^1_{i,j}}, N_{a^2_{i,j}}, N_{a^3_{i,j}}, \ldots, N_{a^k_{i,j}}$ is being compared with the reference pattern prepared by the parallel-hierarchical network with averaged parameters $\overline{a}^1_{i,j}, \overline{a}^2_{i,j}, \overline{a}^3_{i,j}, \cdots, \overline{a}^k_{i,j}$ and an average number of elements in branches of the respective level $N_{\overline{a}^1_{i,j}}, N_{\overline{a}^2_{i,j}}, N_{\overline{a}^3_{i,j}}, \cdots, N_{\overline{a}^k_{i,j}}$ Current parallel-hierarchical network parameters $a^1_{i,j}, a^2_{i,j}, a^3_{i,j}, \ldots, a^k_{i,j}$ are calculated in network branches.

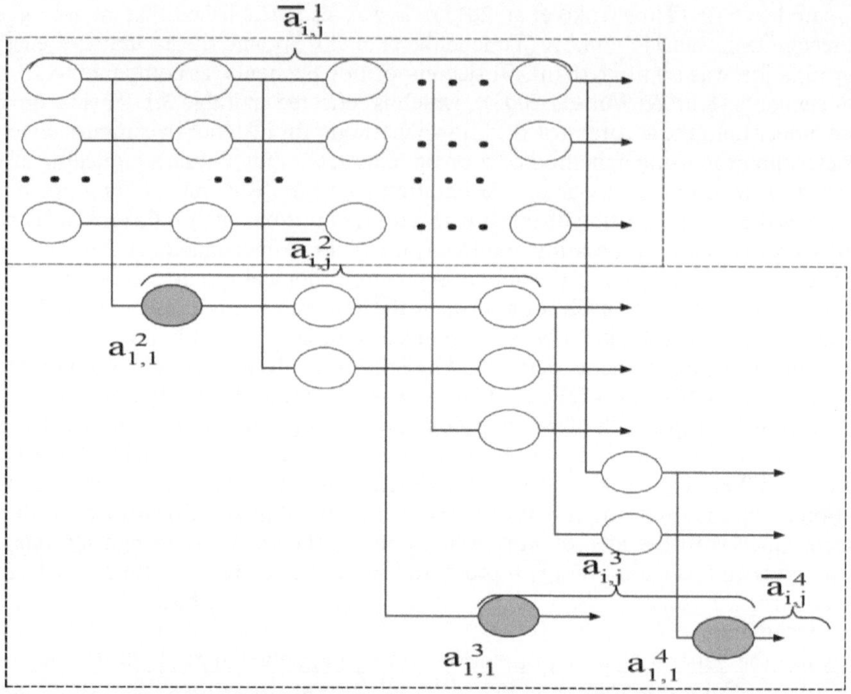

Figure 3.17 Structure of the parallel-hierarchical network with averaged parameters.

A current pattern or a tested pattern prepared by the parallel-hierarchical network with current parameters $a^1_{i,j}, a^2_{i,j}, a^3_{i,j}, \ldots, a^k_{i,j}$ and a respective number of elements in branches of each level $N_{a^1_{i,j}}, N_{a^2_{i,j}}, N_{a^3_{i,j}}, \cdots, N_{a^k_{i,j}}$ is being compared with the reference pattern prepared by the parallel-hierarchical network with averaged parameters $\bar{a}^1_{i,j}, \bar{a}^2_{i,j}, \bar{a}^3_{i,j}, \ldots, \bar{a}^k_{i,j}$ and an average number of elements in branches of the respective level $N_{\bar{a}^1_{i,j}}, N_{\bar{a}^2_{i,j}}, N_{\bar{a}^3_{i,j}}, \cdots, N_{\bar{a}^k_{i,j}}$. Current parallel-hierarchical network parameters $a^1_{i,j}, a^2_{i,j}, a^3_{i,j}, \ldots, a^k_{i,j}$ are calculated in network branches.

Using an adaptive threshold transformation with a computed threshold based on a formula for boundary preparation of the parallel-hierarchical network elements for each level as described in (Timchenko et al. 2013), and on the basis of the three-level coding, it is possible to represent averaged parameters $\bar{a}^1_{i,j}, \bar{a}^2_{i,j}, \bar{a}^3_{i,j}, \ldots, \bar{a}^k_{i,j}$ with their ternary labels (–1, 0, +1). Then arrays of difference of the element with an average brightness value of decomposition elements of the pattern (or of its fragment) are determined.

For a random averaged parameter, a ternary level transition may be presented by three types of labels: zero label $a^0_{i,j}$, positive $a^1_{i,j}$, and negative $a^{-1}_{i,j}$. In this case a parallel-hierarchical network with numerical counts is transformed into a parallel-hierarchical network with counts $a^0_{i,j}, a^1_{i,j}, a^{-1}_{i,j}$ (Timchenko et al. 2011). This ternary transformation procedure may be described in the following form:

$$R_{i,j} = a^k_{i,j} - \bar{a}^k_{i,j}.$$

To prepare a pattern, the resulting difference is compared with the computed threshold δ, i.e.

$$a^{(\ )}_{i,j} = \begin{cases} 1, & \text{if } R_{i,j} > \delta \\ -1, & \text{if } R_{i,j} < -\delta. \\ 0, & \text{if } |R_{i,j}| \le \delta \end{cases} \tag{3.1}$$

The threshold δ is calculated from the condition:

$$N_t^{(1)} \cdot N_t^{(-1)} \cdot N_t^{(0)} = \text{Max}, \tag{3.2}$$

When condition (3.2) is satisfied, the relation $N_t^{(1)} \approx N_t^{(-1)} \approx N_t^{(0)}$ will be true.

In contrast to the threshold transfer function of a neuron for the known neural networks (Haykin 1999), when a parallel-hierarchical network is realised for the threshold function (3.1), a threshold is not set as a certain constant, but is a function of a number of positive, negative and zero preparations, and is calculated by (3.2).

Therefore, the threshold adaptive transformation ensures that when forming ternary labels, current and averaged image elements are not compared at the level of noise signals, or with zero, in (3.1). Instead, for each image its own threshold δ is calculated that would be adapted to a particular image, thus increasing noise immunity of the transformation.

Such a transformation simplifies the correlation comparison procedure of current and reference parallel-hierarchical network counts, because it is performed on simple labels (0, +1, −1) instead of halftone counts.

In order to form reference images, training within a sample should be conducted. For this purpose, it is necessary to perform averaging in branches of each level, i.e. to form averaged elements $\bar{a}_{i,j}^1, \bar{a}_{i,j}^2, \bar{a}_{i,j}^3, \ldots, \bar{a}_{i,j}^k$ and then move to ternary labels $a_{i,j}^0, a_{i,j}^1, a_{i,j}^{-1}$. Having completed the manipulations described above, it is possible to form a parallel-hierarchical network with reference parameters for current images. After that a correlation coefficient of the parallel-hierarchical network with current parameters can be found. (Under the parallel-hierarchical network with current parameters we understand a PH network with current values of its elements $a_{i,j}^1, a_{i,j}^2, a_{i,j}^3, \ldots, a_{i,j}^k$ with a transfer to ternary labels $a_{i,j}^0, a_{i,j}^1, a_{i,j}^{-1}$ and a current number of elements in the branch of each level $N_{a_{i,j}^1}, N_{a_{i,j}^2}, N_{a_{i,j}^3}, \cdots, N_{a_{i,j}^k}$).

To analyse the data when their sequence is important, time series are used. In this method, coordinates of energy centres of laser beam spot images are used as estimates of interest.

That is, for a random average parameter such a transition can be presented by three kinds of preparations: $a_{i,j}^o, a_{i,j}^1$ and $a_{i,j}^{-1}$. In this case, a parallel-hierarchical network with numerical counts will be transformed into a PH network with binarised counts $a_{i,j}^o, a_{i,j}^1$ and $a_{i,j}^{-1}$. As a result, the comparison procedure of binarised counts of current and reference PH networks is considerably simplified.

For the formation of referenced image, for instance of a biomedical image of the norm and images with pathologies, it is necessary to carry out their teaching within the limits of the teaching sample.

For this purpose it is necessary, during each teaching stage, to make an average by the element of the branch of each level, i.e. from average elements $\bar{a}_{i,j}^1, \bar{a}_{i,j}^2, \bar{a}_{i,j}^3, \ldots, \bar{a}_{i,j}^k$ further passing to the binarised preparations $a_{i,j}^0, a_{i,j}^1, a_{i,j}^{-1}$. Having performed the above-mentioned actions, PH networks can be formed with reference parameters for the images of the form and images with various pathologies.

Having realised parallel-hierarchical networks with reference parameters for normal images and images with various pathologies, a comparison with the parallel-hierarchical network can be made, using current parameters. By the PH network with current parameters we imply the parallel-hierarchical network with current values of its elements $a_{i,j}^1, a_{i,j}^2, a_{i,j}^3, \ldots, a_{i,j}^k$ with the transition to the binarised preparations $a_{i,j}^0, a_{i,j}^1, a_{i,j}^{-1}$ and the current number of elements in the branches of each level $N_{a_{i,j}^1}, N_{a_{i,j}^2}, N_{a_{i,j}^3}, \ldots, N_{a_{i,j}^k}$. The comparison procedure of the parallel-hierarchical network with reference parameters and the PH network with current parameters comprises their topographic superposition and calculation of the number of coincidences of the same binarised elements.

Two binarised PH networks coincide if all the counts of each preparation similarly located in the network are pairwise equal. In case of detergency dimensionalities of the compared parallel-hierarchical networks it is necessary to introduce in its branches additional codes with coding of the fourth state. For evaluation of the result of binarised parallel-hierarchical networks we will introduce a quantitative index, characterising their degree of coincidence (3.3)

$$R(c_e,c_n)=\Sigma(a_{i,j}^{1(\cdots)})_e \cap (a_{i,j}^{1(\cdots)})_n+\cdots+\Sigma(a_{i,j}^{k(\cdots)})_e \cap (a_{i,j}^{k(\cdots)})_n, \tag{3.3}$$

where $c_e = f_e(a_{i,j}^1, a_{i,j}^2, \cdots, a_{i,j}^k)$ is the networking function of a reference image, $c_n = f_n(a_{i,j}^1, a_{i,j}^2, \cdots, a_{i,j}^k)$ is the networking function of the current image and $a_{i,j}^{k(\cdots)} \in \{ a_{i,j}^{k(0)}, a_{i,j}^{k(1)}, a_{i,j}^{k(-1)} \}$, and $\cap$ denotes a coincidence of similar binarised preparations, when they are compared. Components (3.3) equal unit only in the case, when similar preparations coincide, i.e.:

$$(a_{i,j}^{k(\cdots)})_e \cap (a_{i,j}^{k(\cdots)})_n = \begin{cases} 1, \text{ if } (\cdots)=(\cdots) \\ 0, \text{ else} \end{cases}$$

The total number of the elements in the reference PH network is calculated in the following manner

$$N_e = N_{a_{i,j}^1} + N_{a_{i,j}^2} + \ldots + N_{a_{i,j}^{k-1}} + N_{a_{i,j}^k}$$

Normalised degree of binarised preparations comparison is calculated in the following way:

$$\Re = \frac{R(c_e,c_n)}{N_e}$$

We suggest the following example of binarised preparations comparison at the second level for two PH networks (Fig. 3.18).

Let us calculate for this example (Fig. 3.18) the degree of coincidence $R(c_e,c_n)$ and the normalised degree of comparison R for the second level of the current and reference PH networks.

$$R(c_e,c_n)=(1)+(1+1)+(1+1)+(1+1+1)+(1+1+1+1)+(1+1+1+1)=16.$$

The total number of elements in the reference PH network at the second level is $N_e = 21$. The normalised degree of comparison R while comparing the binarised counts of the current and reference PH networks for their other levels will be the following:

$$\Re = \frac{R(c_e,c_n)}{N_e} = \frac{16}{21} \approx 0{,}762$$

It is obvious that the normalised measure of comparison of two PH networks is defined within the following limits

$$0 \le \Re \le 1.$$

a)	b)
1	1
0 −1	0 −1
−1 0 1	0 0 1
0 1 0 1	0 1 0 −1
1 −1 0 0 −1	1 −1 1 0 −1
0 1 0 1 −1 1	0 1 0 0 −1 0

Figure 3.18 Example of the comparison of binarised preparations at the second level of: a) the reference PH network, and b) the current PH network.

6 CONCLUSIONS

An important factor is that the normalised measure of comparison can be calculated not only separately for each two levels, but also in common for two PH networks. This improves the probability of the recognition of results formation. Thus, for network teaching, we suggest applying the idea of population coding in an artificial neural network and its similarity to natural neural networks, to represent the current image by the current PH network with current parameters and transform it on the basis of generalised content preparation into a binarised preparation, with further comparison on the basis of the normalised measure of comparison with the reference PH network of a reference pattern having average parameters, elements of which are binarised preparations. Unlike the known structures of artificial neural networks, where non-normalised (absolute) similarity criteria are used for comparison, in the considered method of teaching a normalised criterion is used. A normalised measure of comparison is suggested not only for separate calculations for each of the two levels, but also for joint calculations for each level of PH networks. This improves the accuracy of the recognition of results formation.

REFERENCES

Haykin S. 1999. *Neural Networks*. New Jersey: Prentice Hall.

Kim, S. & Wunsch, D.C. 2003. A GPU based parallel hierarchical fuzzy ART clustering. *Proc IJCNN*: 2778–2782.

Timchenko, L.I., Melnikov, V.V., and Kokryatskaya, N.I. 2011. Method of parallel-hierarchic organization of network for proceeding of image. *Cybernetic and System Analysis* 47(1):140–151.

Timchenko, L.I., Kokryatskaya, N.I. and Shpakovych V.V. 2013. Modeling of a method of parallel hierarchical transformation for fast recognition of dynamic images. *EURASIP Journal on Advances in Signal Processing* 2013:87.

Timchenko, L., Kutayev, Y., Cheporniuk, S., Kokriatskaya, N., Yarovyy, A. and Denysova, A. 2014. A new approach to detection of noise-distorted signals based on the method of S-preparation. *Journal of IET Image Processing* 8(11): 627–638.

CHAPTER 4

Methods and systems of 2D polarization multi-matrix tomography of birefringent biological tissues and fluids

S.V. Pavlov & N.I. Zabolotna
Vinnytsia National Technical University, Vinnytsia, Ukraine

T. Małecka-Massalska & Z. Omiotek
Lublin University of Technology, Lublin, Poland

A. Burlibay & N.A. Orshubekov
Kazakh University of Railways and Communications, Almaty, Kazakhstan

1 INTRODUCTION

Creation of a new class of intelligent optic-electronic devices and systems for the control of the parameters of structure inhomogeneity of biological tissues with high information content, accuracy and wide functional possibilities is an important problem. Solution of which promotes the increase of the efficiency of medical diagnostics and treatment, thus promoting the improvement of nations health. In recent decade, optic methods of formation of biological objects layered images have been widely used in biomedical diagnostics. Optic medical diagnostics uses various spectral and laser methods, including spectrophotometry of near-IR band, fluorescent laser spectrometry, optic coherent and diffusion tomography, confocal spectroscopy, opto-acoustic tomography, photon correlation spectroscopy, Doppler tissue imaging and speckle-monitoring of biological flows (Shuliang et al. 2002, de Boer et al. 2002, Bickel et al. 1985, Sikora 2007).

It is determined that the field of optic radiation, scattered by biological layers is, objectively, multidimensional and multiparametric carrier of the information about their structure. In this sense, all multidimensional set of optic radiation parameters becomes the carrier of the information ("information print") regarding morphological, biochemical, optic-anisotropic etc., structure of biological objects (Pierce et al. 2004).

Proceeding from above-mentioned, construction of new systems of optic diagnostics becomes an important and urgent problem. These systems enable: maximally use the information content of experimental measurements; reproduce the distribution of the parameters of biological layers' structure; provide multiparametric objective complex mathematical analysis of the information, obtained in the process of experiments.

One of the promising directions for the solution of this problem is the development of modern polarization-sensitive optic coherent tomography, using the methods of laser polarimetry (Shuliang et al. 2002, de Boer et al. 2002, Pierce et al. 2004). Such tomography are based on measurement of Mueller's matrices of the investigative samples (Bickel et al. 1985, Angelsky 2005).

Measurement of Mueller's matrices of light scattering layers enables to obtain the complete information regarding polarizing properties of biological object.

Introduction of two-component amorphous-crystal model of biological tissues become the basis for the establishment of the relations between the distributions of Mueller's matrix elements set with the distributions of orientations and birefringent ability of biological tissues layers. Thus, criteria of muscular dystrophy diagnosis, precancerous state of connective tissues, collagenases, etc. were formulated (Shuliang et al. 2002, de Boer et al. 2002,

Pierce et al. 2004). Numerous world known as scientific-research institutions and companies develop and manufacture systems of biological objects polarimetry. The world well known leaders in this area are Axometrics, Texas A&M University, John Hopkins University, University of Toledo (USA), Perkin Elmer, M. Chernyshevskiy Saratov State University, Scientific-Research Centre of Unique Instrumentation of the Russian Academy of Sciences (Russia), Stepanov Institute of Physics of National Academy of Sciences of Byelorussia and Yuriy Fedkovych Chernivtsi National University. Potential possibilities in the sphere of construction of high information multiparametric system of laser polarimetry of biological layers provides the concept, suggested in (Bickel et al. 1985, Angelsky 2005). This concept relies on creation of the system of complex 2D Mueller-matrix tomography, that comprises the methods of Mueller-matrix mapping of biological layers (direct problems of 2D Mueller-matrix tomography) and methods of polarization-phase reconstruction of optic anisotropy structure parameters of biological (inverse problem of Mueller-matrix tomography).

With the introduction of objective complex analysis, based on the set of statistic, correlation and spectral moments of the 1st–4th orders (Ushenko et al. 2004).

In the given research, the set of experimental methods of 2D Mueller-matrix, orientation— and phase tomography of the histological sections of biological tissues and films on biological liquids, realized by the above-mentioned system. Its complex application forms the basis of multistage algorithm of polarization reproduction of the parameters of linear birefringence of multilayer biological tissues.

2 MATERIALS AND METHODS OF 2D POLARIZATION MUELLER-MATRIX TOMOGRAPHY

2.1 *General characteristic of direct and inverse problems of 2D Mueller-matrix tomography of biological tissues*

For the analysis of the information, obtained within the limits of laser polarimetry of biological tissues and liquids (coordinate distribution of azimuths and polarization ellipticity, Mueller matrices elements) we use the following model approach (de Boer et al. 2002, Pierce et al. 2004):

1. All the variety of human Biological Tissues (BT) may by presented in the form of four basic types – connective, muscular, epithelial and nervous tissues.
2. Morphologic structure of any type of BT is considered in the form of two-component amorphic-crystalline structure.
3. Crystalline component or extra-cellular matrix is architectonic grid that consists of coaxial cylindrical protein (collagen, myosin and elastin) fibrils.
4. From optic point of view, protein fibrils possess the properties of uniaxial birefringent crystals.
5. Interaction of laser radiation with BT is considered in approximation of single-time scattering, when attenuation coefficient of its layer corresponds the condition $\tau \leq 0{,}1$.

It is known (de Boer et al. 2002, Pierce et al. 2004), that anisotropic component each of these layers is formed by the grids of protein fibrils. They are characterized by Mueller-matrix operator of optically uniaxial birefringent crystal:

$$\{Z\}_j = \begin{Vmatrix} 1 & 0 & 0 & 0 \\ 0 & z_{22} & z_{23} & z_{24} \\ 0 & z_{32} & z_{33} & z_{34} \\ 0 & z_{42} & z_{43} & z_{44} \end{Vmatrix}, \qquad (4.1)$$

where:

$$z_{ik}(\rho,\delta)=\begin{cases} z_{22}=\cos^2 2\rho+\sin^2 2\rho\ \cos\delta; \\ z_{23;32}=\cos 2\rho\ \sin 2\rho\ (1-\cos\delta); \\ z_{33}=\sin^2 2\rho+\cos^2 2\rho\ \cos\delta; \\ z_{34;43}=\pm\cos 2\rho\ \sin\delta; \\ z_{24;42}=\pm\sin 2\rho\ \sin\delta; \\ z_{44}=\cos\delta. \end{cases} \tag{4.2}$$

Here ρ is the detection of optic axis, determined by the direction of birefringent fibril placement; $\delta=2\pi/\lambda\cdot\Delta n\cdot d$ is the phase shift introduced between orthogonal components of the amplitude of laser wave length λ that passes across fibril with linear dimension of geometrical cross-section d and birefringence index Δn.

The term direct problems of 2D Mueller-matrix tomography means complex of experimental steps for measurement of coordinate distributions of the set of Mueller-matrices elements (Mueller-matrix images) with further analytic (statistic, correlation, fractal) algorithmic analysis of obtained data arrays to define the criteria (interconnections) of diagnostics, differentiation and classification of parametric of anisotropy of phase-inhomogeneous biological layers. The groups of Mueller-matrix images of biological layers are the object of the research: "orientation" Mueller-matrix images z_{22}, z_{33}, that carry information mostly regarding the directions of the axes of biological crystal structure; "phase" Mueller-matrix images, z_{44}, that carry information regarding phase shifts between orthogonal components of laser wave, amplitude, stipulated by birefringence of biological crystals; "orientation-phase" Mueller-matrix images z_{42}, z_{43}, z_{24}, z_{34}, z_{23}, z_{32} that simultaneously characterize simultaneously orientations of optical axes and phase shifts of biological crystals.

Problems of 2D Mueller-matrix tomography – it is complex of experimental steps aimed at revealing orientation-phase structure (ρ,δ) of polycrystalline network of biologic layers, that are created in the form of "orientation" tomograms (2D distribution of the directions of birefringent fibrils axes $\rho(x, y)$) and phase tomograms (2D distribution of phase shifts $\delta(x, y)$).

2.2 *Architecture of the system of automated laser polarimetry for the solution of direct and inverse problems of Mueller-matrix tomography of biological tissues*

In (Ushenko et al. 2011) the architecture (Fig. 4.1) of the system that realized functions for the solution of direct and inverse problems of Mueller-matrix tomography was demonstrated, correspondingly:

- "direct" 2D Mueller-matrix mapping of multilayered BT with the formation the series of "orientation", "orientation-phase", "phase" tomograms and determination of the set of objective parameters that characterize them;
- polarization reproduction of Mueller-matrix images of fractional layers of two-component real biological structure with determination of the set of object parameters, that characterize them.

Main structural blocks of the system (see Fig. 4.1) are laser 1 (semi-conductor or helium-neon laser) with the wavelength $\lambda=0.638$ μm, that radiates the beam, that passes across the collimator 2, which forms broader beam of rays, to the block of polarization radiation 3. This block must form: series of probing beams with necessary azimuths of polarization by means of rotating the bandwidth of linear polarizer 5_1, within the limits of $0° \leq \theta \leq 180°$ while removing from propagation way filtered radiation of quarter-wave plate 4_2; if quarter-wave 4_2 is available during the organization of probing laser beam with "right circulation" polarization.

Thus, laser beam, formed by block 3, probes object 6 and by means of projecting block 7, angular aperture of which is matched with the indicatrix of laser beam diffusion, forms the

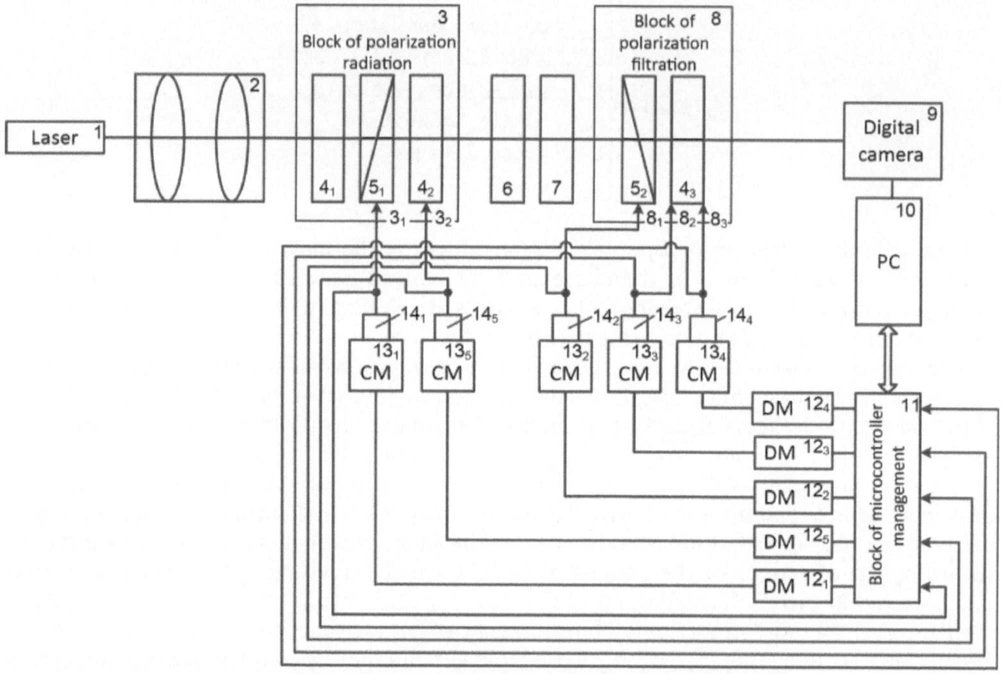

Figure 4.1 Architecture of the system of 2D Mueller-matrix tomography and complex analysis of the obtained images of orientation-phase structure of biological tissues.

images of optic-anisotropic layer of the object. These images are filtrated by the block of polarization filtration 8, in the phase of digital photosensitive camera 9. Block of polarization filtration 8 consists of linear polarizer 5_2, with the rotation of transmission plane at necessary angles (for instance 0°; 90°; 45°; 135° or other preset angle). The quarter-wave plate 4_3; its optic axis can be oriented under the angle +45° relatively linear polarizer 5_2 (mode of right circulation "⊗") and under the angle –45° polarizer 5_2 (mode of left circulation "⊕").

When multifunctional polarization filter-analyzer 8 is used, coordinate distributions of the values of polarization-filtered intensities of laser images of optic-anisotropic layer 6 are measured, which across frames separator of video camera 9 are transmitted to the computer 10 and are stored there.

Control of the position of the above-mentioned polarization elements is realized by means of special microcontroller block 11. For organization of the exchange between basic program of the computer 10 and block 11 command-line mode is used. A main function of the block 11 is the control of the turns and positioning of the motors 13_1–13_5 by the means of motor drivers 12_1–12_5. Rotating devices of moving polarization elements of the circuit are equipped with position sensors 14_1–14_{14} (opto-pairs), by means of which the feedback with block of microcontroller management (Fig. 4.1) is organized.

Determining a feature of the given system of Mueller-matrix tomography is the possibility to perform programmable complex analysis of measured orientation-phase images of biological tissue structures, based on application of complex statistic, correlation and fractal approaches. Complex approach to the obtained orientation-phase structure images of biological layers, initiated in (Zabolotna 2011, Angelsky et al. 2007, Zabolotna et al. 2014), was developed and applied for the first time to inverse problem of Mueller-matrix tomography.

2.3 *Methods of analysis of Mueller-matrix images of orientation-phase structure of biological layers*

2.3.1 *Statistical approach*

As the basic analytical tool for estimation of 2D distributions of Mueller-matrix images $z_{ik}(X,Y)$, statistic moments of the first (M_1), second (M_2), third (M_3) and fourth (M_4) orders were used. They were calculated by the following algorithms (Zabolotna 2011, Angelsky et al. 2007, Zabolotna et al. 2014).

$$
\begin{aligned}
M_1 &= \frac{1}{N}\sum_{j=1}^{N}\left(\left|z_{ik}\right|\right)_j; \\
M_2 &= \sqrt{\frac{1}{N}\sum_{j=1}^{N}\left(z_{ik}^2\right)_j}; \\
M_3 &= \frac{1}{M_2^3}\frac{1}{N}\sum_{j=1}^{N}\left(z_{ik}^3\right)_j; \\
M_4 &= \frac{1}{M_2^4}\frac{1}{N}\sum_{j=1}^{N}\left(z_{ik}^4\right)_j,
\end{aligned}
\tag{4.3}
$$

where $N = 800 \times 600$ is the number of digitalization elements, determined by several pixels of photo-sensitive area of CCD camera.

2.3.2 *Correlation approach*

Statistical approach does not take into consideration coordinate inhomogeneity or homogeneity of the distribution, i.e., the same histograms may have different by structure two 2D arrays. To reveal such situations the method of autocorrelation is used. For instance, two identical distributions of 2D array of Mueller-matrix image $z_{ik}(X,Y)$ are formed and linearly bias one relatively another. At each step of bias the set of correlation or coordinated that are overlapped, is determined. Dependence of such correlation on the step of bias is described by autocorrelation function (Zabolotna 2011, Angelsky et al. 2007, Zabolotna et al. 2014).

$$
\mathrm{K}(\Delta x,\Delta y) = \lim_{\substack{x\to 0\\ y\to 0}} \frac{1}{X_0 Y_0}\int_0^x\int_0^y \left[z(x,y)\right]\left[z(X-\Delta x, Y-\Delta y)\right] dxdy, \tag{4.4}
$$

where $(\Delta x,\Delta y)$ – "steps", at which coordinates (X, Y) change.

For quantitative estimation of autocorrelation dependences structure, we will calculate the set of their statistic moments of the first, second, thirds and fourth orders (relation 4.3), further they will be called correlation moments Q_1–Q_4.

2.3.3 *Fractal approach*

Fractal analysis of MMI elements $z_{ik}(X,Y)$ is performed in the following succession of actions (Zabolotna 2011, Angelsky et al. 2007, Zabolotna et al. 2013):

- autocorrelation functions $\mathrm{K}(\Delta x,\Delta y)$ were computed and corresponding spectra of power $PSD(z_{ik})$ of coordinate distributions of Mueller matrix elements $z_{ik}(X,Y)$ were found;
- log-log dependences of power spectra $\lg PSD(z_{ik}) - \log(\nu)$ of distributions $z_{ik}(X,Y)$ were determined;
- dependences $\lg PSD(z_{ik}) - \log(\nu)$ were linearly approximated applying the method of least squares into curves $\Phi(z_{ik})$, for direct sections of which slopes η_i were determined and values of fractal dimensionalities of set values z_{ik} were calculated by the relation:

$$
D(z_{ik}) = 3 - tg\,\eta_i. \tag{4.5}
$$

Classification of self-similarity of coordinate distributions of matrix elements $z_{ik}(X, Y)$ was carried out in accordance with such criteria:

- MMI $z_{ik}(X,Y)$ – are fractal on condition of linear character of the dependence $\Phi(z_{ik})(\eta = \text{const})$ for 2-3 decades of dimensions' d crystal grid elements;
- MMI $z_{ik}(X,Y)$ – are stochastic on condition of the presence of slopes $\Phi(z_{ik})$;
- MMI $z_{ik}(X,Y)$ – are random on condition of the absence of stable slopes $\Phi(z_{ik})$ in the whole interval of dimensions d.

For objective evaluation of the values of logic dependences of MMI power spectra we will apply statistic moments of the 1st–4th orders (relation (4.3)), which further we will call spectral moments W_i that characterize average, dispersion, asymmetry and excess of above-mentioned logarithmic dependences.

2.4 *Experimental technique of measurement and complex analysis of "orientation", "phase", "orientation-phase" Mueller-matrix images of biological layers*

Elements of Mueller matrix of biological layer are determined by the algorithm, realized in the above-mentioned system of 2D laser polarimetry. We irradiate the biological layer 6 by laser beams of light of four various types of polarization with the azimuths α polarization "0°", "90°", "45°" and ellipticity β "right circulation ⊗", formed by the block 3. For each type of polarization of probing beam, six coordinate distributions of the intensity of anisotropic layer laser beam are measured by means of polarization filtration carried out by block 8 ("0°", "90°", "45°", "135°" "right circulation" and "left circulation").

The set of 24 images is obtained, based on these images we define, by turns, coordinate distributions of 4 parameters of the Stokes vector for the series of corresponding probing laser images with the azimuth α and ellipticity β by the relation:

$$\begin{cases} S_1^{\alpha,\beta} = I(0) + I(90) \\ S_2^{\alpha,\beta} = I(0) - I(90) \\ S_3^{\alpha,\beta} = I(45) - I(135) \\ S_4^{\alpha,\beta} = I(\otimes) - I(\oplus) \end{cases} \tag{4.6}$$

On the base of this relation, elements of Mueller matrix are formed by the relations (Shuliang et al. 2002).

$$\begin{array}{lll} z_{11} = 0,5(S_1^0 + S_1^{90}); & z_{21} = 0,5(S_2^0 + S_2^{90}); & z_{31} = 0,5(S_3^0 + S_3^{90}); \\ z_{12} = 0,5(S_1^0 - S_1^{90}); & z_{22} = 0,5(S_2^0 - S_2^{90}); & z_{32} = 0,5(S_3^0 - S_3^{90}); \\ z_{13} = S_1^{45} - z_{11}; & z_{23} = S_2^{45} - z_{21}; & z_{33} = S_3^{45} - z_{31}; \\ z_{14} = S_1^{\otimes} - z_{11}; & z_{24} = S_2^{\otimes} - z_{21}; & z_{34} = S_3^{\otimes} - z_{31}; \\ z_{41} = 0,5(S_4^0 + S_4^{90}); & & \\ z_{42} = 0,5(S_4^0 - S_4^{90}); & & \\ z_{43} = S_4^{45} - z_{41}; & & \\ z_{44} = S_4^{\otimes} - z_{41}. & & \end{array} \tag{4.7}$$

Further application of complex statistic, correlation and fractal analysis of 2D Mueller-matrix images enables to enlarge functional possibilities of the systems of registration of classic, polarizing, phase and stokes polarimetric micro images of biological layers and obtain new and exhaustive information data regarding of (Fig. 4.2):

- statistic moments of the degrees of distribution;
- correlation similarity of distributions $f_{ik}(m \times n)$ and quantitative characteristics (correlation moments) of autocorrelation coordination;

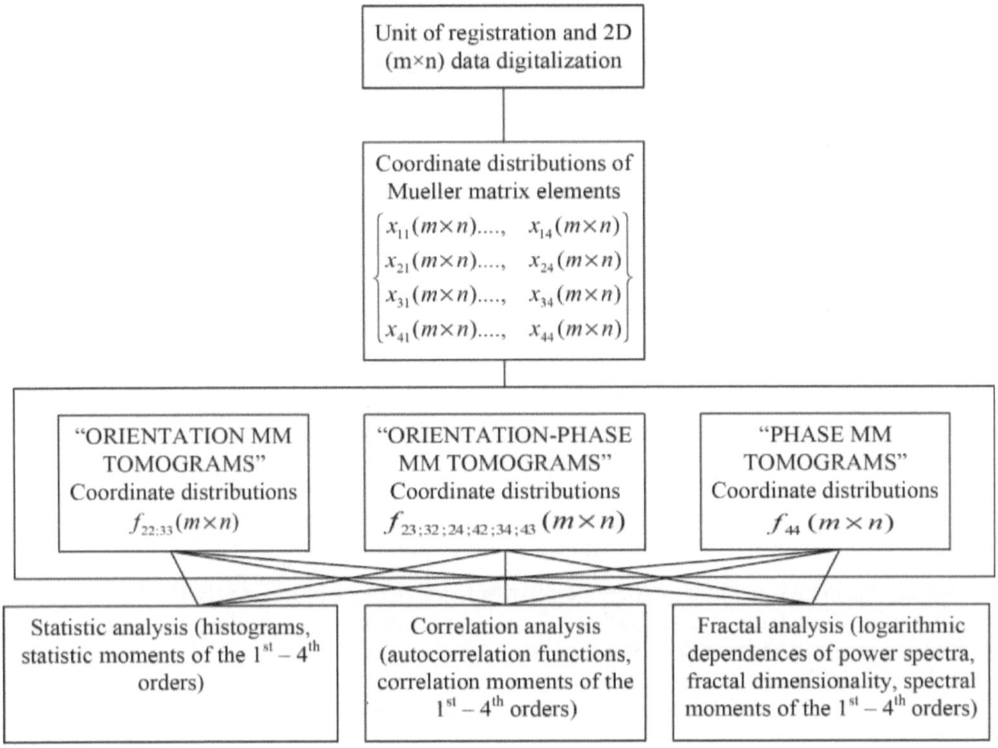

Figure 4.2 Formation of Mueller-matrix image elements and their complex analysis.

– scale self-similarity, fractal dimensionality and quantitative characteristics (fractal dimensionality, spectral moments) of space-frequency distribution $f_{ik}(m \times n)$.

2.5 *Mueller-matrix "orientation" and "phase" tomography of biological layers*

Because of theoretical studies, it is established that the geometry of fibrillar architectonics of biological tissues has hierarchical filamentous construction. That is discrete by its structure and is characterized be scale repetends in the range of three decades of optic dimensions (Pierce et al. 2004). On the base of this model concepts regarding the processes of interaction of polarization radiation with such geometrical structures are analytically developed and experimentally verified. According to these concepts fibrillar elements of the architectonics of biological tissues possess properties of uniaxial crystals. Directions of optic axes are determined by the angles of fibrils stacking in the layer of biological tissue (ρ) and the value of the anisotropy of their substance – by the value of birefringence index (Δn).

Within the frame of a single scattering there exists definite connection between the values of Mueller-matrix and values of orientation (ρ) and phase (δ) parameters of fibrillar grid of architectonic network (Pierce et al. 2004).

Further widening of functional possibilities of the considered architecture of the system, shown in Fig. 4.2 is reached by means of realization of the methods aimed at the solution of inverse problem of Mueller-matrix tomography (reproduction of the parameters of coordinate distribution of directions $\rho(m \times n)$ of optic axes of birefringent polycrystal network of biological tissue layers and coordinate distributions of phase shifts $\delta(m \times n)$) by means of analytical calculations by the formulas.

The established algorithm of optic axis of uniaxial birefringent crystal direction, described in (Ushenko et al. 2004), allows to carry out the calculation by the formula:

$$\rho(jk) = 0,5\text{arctg}\left[\frac{z_{34;43}(jk)}{z_{24;42}(jk)}\right]. \tag{4.8}$$

The obtained 2D distributions $\rho(m \times n)$ will be called Mueller-matrix "orientation tomograms" of birefringent network of anisotropic layer.

On the base of the algorithm, described in (Shuliang et al. 2002, Ushenko et al. 2004) the possibility of determination in explicit form the coordinate distributions of phase shifts $\delta(m \times n)$, that emerge between orthogonal components of laser wave amplitude at the expense of birefringent tissues layers by experimentally measured Mueller-matrix "phase" $z_{ik}(m \times n)$ maps.

$$\delta(jk) = 0,5\,\text{arccos}\left[z_{44}(ik)\right] \tag{4.9}$$

The obtained 2D distributions $\delta(m \times n)$ will be called Mueller-matrix "phase tomograms" of birefringent network of anisotropic layer.

Further application of complex statistic, correlation and fractal analysis of discrete 2D arrays $\rho(m \times n)$, $\delta(m \times n)$, enables to widen functional possibilities of the systems of Mueller-matrix mapping of biological layers and obtain data about:

- statistic moments of higher orders of distributions $\delta(m \times n)$ and $\rho(m \times n)$;
- correlation similarity of distributions $\delta(m \times n)$ and $\rho(m \times n)$ as well as quantitative characteristics of autocorrelation coordination;
- scale self similarity fractal dimensionality and quantitative characteristics of space-frequency structure of distributions $\delta(m \times n)$ and $\rho(m \times n)$.

However, the considered methods are methods of indirect measurement of the parameters of optical structure of biological layers that possess corresponding errors. It is possible to reduce these errors, developing the methods of direct (without using calculations of Mueller matrices) experimental orientation and phase tomography of polycristal networks of biological layers.

2.6 *Experimental Mueller-matrix tomography of the two-layer structure "muscular tissue- dermis of the skin" and complex analysis of the obtained images*

Two-layer structure, formed by overlapping of two optically thin histological cuts is taken as the objects of experimental study: muscular biological tissue (MT) and dermis of the skin (DS). Samples of such tissues are characterized by the following optic-geometric parameters:

- Dermis of the skin (DS): (absorption coefficient μ_a = 2.2 cm^{-1}, scattering coefficient μ_s = 185 cm^{-1}, anisotropy coefficient g = 0.82, geometric thickness L = 30 μm);
- Muscular tissue (MT) (μ_a = 2 cm^{-1}, μ_s = 215 cm^{-1}, g = 0.96, L = 30 μm).

Applying experimental technique of Mueller matrix elements measurements, realized in the system presented in Fig. 4.1, Mueller matrices of muscular tissue histological cuts (see Fig. 4.3) (Zabolotna et al. 2014), dermis of the skin (Fig. 4.4, a) (Zabolotna et al. 2014), two-layered structure "muscular tissue-dermis of the skin" (Fig. 4.4, b) (Zabolotna et al. 2014), autocorrelation functions and power spectra of corresponding distributions $z_{ik}(m \times n)$ as well as the set of their statistic $M_{i=1;2;3;4}$, correlation $Q_{2;4}$ and spectral $J_{i=1;2;3;4}$ statistic moments (Tables 4.1–4.3) were obtained, that is described in the research (Zabolotna et al. 2014).

2.6.1 *Muscular tissue*

Statistic moments M_i, that describe coordinate distributions of Mueller-matrix images, have individual values. The most sensitive (the range of value change) to phase or orientation mechanisms of laser radiation parameters change by birefringent grid of myosin fibrils the 3rd and 4th statistic moments.

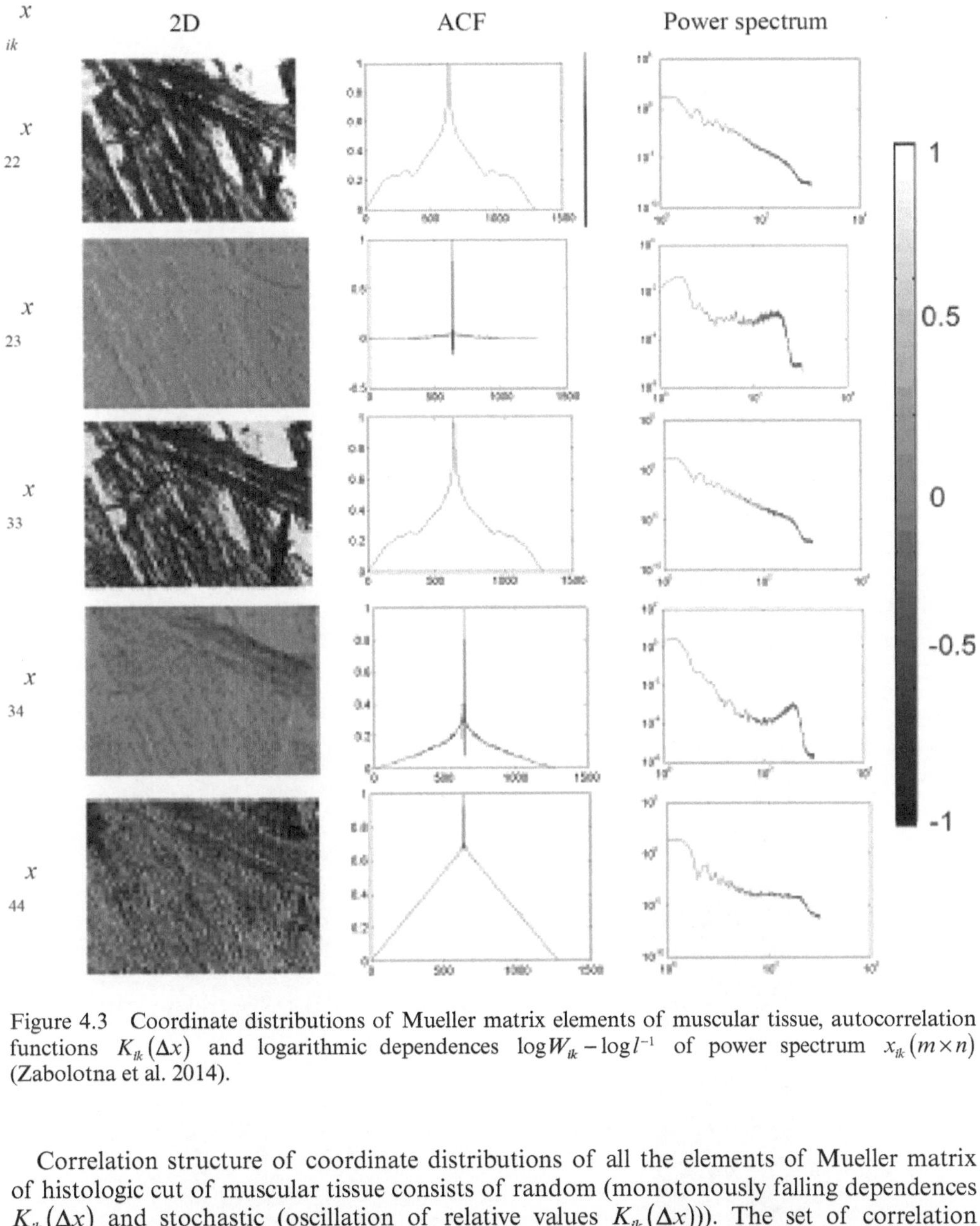

Figure 4.3 Coordinate distributions of Mueller matrix elements of muscular tissue, autocorrelation functions $K_{ik}(\Delta x)$ and logarithmic dependences $\log W_{ik} - \log l^{-1}$ of power spectrum $x_{ik}(m \times n)$ (Zabolotna et al. 2014).

Correlation structure of coordinate distributions of all the elements of Mueller matrix of histologic cut of muscular tissue consists of random (monotonously falling dependences $K_{ik}(\Delta x)$ and stochastic (oscillation of relative values $K_{ik}(\Delta x)$)). The set of correlation moments $Q_{i=2;4}$ distinctly depends on peculiarities of correlation matching of coordinate structure of matrix elements $x_{ik}(m \times n)$ distributions. Thus, the greater half-width $L \uparrow$ of autocorrelation functions of diagonal elements $x_{22;33;44}(m \times n)$ the higher the values of $Q_2 \uparrow$ are. And vice versa, the greater correlation discoordination $L \downarrow$ of non-diagonal matrix elements $x_{23;32;34;43;24;42}(m \times n)$ distributions, the higher values of correlation moments of the 4th $Q_4 \uparrow$ order are. Such changes are accompanied by extremely great dynamic range of correlation moments change – from 5 to 10 times (Table 4.1).

Spectra of power (Log – log dependences of power spectra) of Mueller matrix images of diagonal elements $f_{ik}(X,Y)$ are characterized by two slopes of approximating curve. For coordinate distributions of non-diagonal matrix elements $x_{ik;i \neq k}(m \times n)$ values corresponding dependences are transformed in curves.

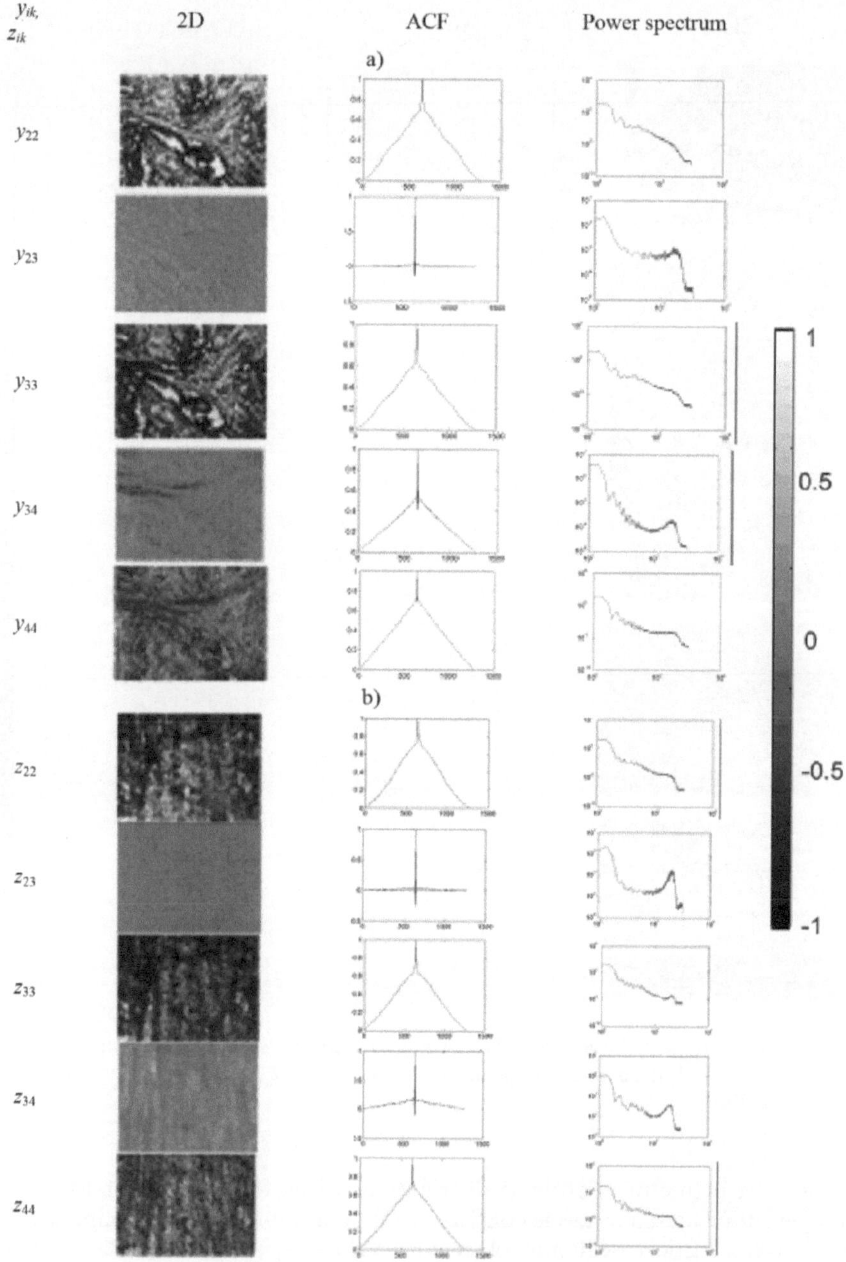

Figure 4.4 Coordinate distributions of Mueller matrix elements, autocorrelation functions and logarithmic dependences of power spectra, a) dermis of the skin tissue, b) two-layered structure "muscular tissue – dermis of the skin" (Zabolotna et al. 2014).

High diagnostic sensitivity of the 2nd spectral moment to change of self similarity of Mueller matrix elements $x_{ik}(m \times n)$ coordinate distributions of muscle tissue – differences between the values of spectral moment J_2, calculated for diagonal and non-diagonal matrix elements are within the limits of 3–4 times (Table 4.1).

Table 4.1 Statistic M_i, correlation Q_i and spectral j_i moments of coordinate distributions $y_{ik}(m \times n)$ of Mueller matrix elements of the layer of muscular tissue (Zabolotna et al. 2014).

x_{ik}	x_{22}	x_{23}	x_{24}	x_{33}	x_{34}	x_{44}
M_1	0,29	0,02	0,09	0,33	0,1	0,23
M_2	0,08	0,03	0,05	0,09	0,05	0,06
M_3	0,45	0,38	0,39	0,43	0,71	0,23
M_4	5,51	1,73	3,79	1,19	6,84	1,05
Q_2	0,16	0,019	0,011	0,18	0,09	0,12
Q_4	0,99	5,71	6,18	1,17	3,85	1,87
J_1	0,51	0,18	0,23	0,55	0,26	0,62
J_2	0,17	0,57	0,66	0,19	0,44	0,29
J_3	0,06	0,86	0,91	0,08	0,59	0,11
J_4	0,13	1,54	1,75	0,16	0,77	0,28

Table 4.2 Statistic M_i, correlation Q_i and spectral j_i moments of coordinate distributions $y_{ik}(m \times n)$ of Mueller matrix elements of the layer of dermis of the skin tissue (Zabolotna et al. 2014).

y_{ik}	y_{22}	y_{23}	y_{24}	y_{33}	y_{34}	y_{44}
M_1	0,39	0,01	0,01	0,34	0,21	0,37
M_2	0,07	0,02	0,04	0,08	0,04	0,06
M_3	0,17	0,03	0,13	0,52	0,77	0,22
M_4	7,51	4,61	5,08	3,33	1,11	1,78
Q_2	0,21	0,001	0,0013	0,22	0,12	0,18
Q_4	0,78	4,87	5,51	0,89	1,48	1,18
J_1	0,62	0,24	0,32	0,67	0,37	0,68
J_2	0,14	0,53	0,61	0,15	0,41	0,23
J_3	0,09	0,78	0,97	0,012	0,65	0,18
J_4	0,42	2,05	2,34	0,33	0,84	0,53

Table 4.3 Statistic M_i, correlation Q_i and spectral j_i moments of coordinate distributions $z_{ik}(m \times n)$ of Mueller matrix elements of two-layer tissue "muscular tissue-dermis of the skin" (Zabolotna et al. 2014).

z_{ik}	z_{22}	z_{23}	z_{24}	z_{33}	z_{34}	z_{44}
M_1	0,31	0,03	0,05	0,25	0,11	0,38
M_2	0,04	0,04	0,04	0,04	0,06	0,06
M_3	0,49	0,44	0,53	0,42	0,33	0,33
M_4	2,12	1,79	0,89	2,32	0,36	0,48
Q_2	0,19	0,031	0,025	0,21	0,11	0,15
Q_4	0,83	3,97	4,31	0,87	2,48	1,26
J_1	0,48	0,15	0,2	0,51	0,22	0,53
J_2	0,19	0,54	0,61	0,17	0,39	0,23
J_3	0,06	0,82	0,78	0,07	0,52	0,1
J_4	0,11	1,15	1,27	0,13	0,68	0,22

2.6.2 *Dermis of the skin*

Statistic moments $M_{(i)}$, that describe coordinate distributions of Mueller matrix elements of dermal layer, are characterized by greater values of average $M_{(1)}$ and excess $M_{(4)}$ of diagonal elements $y_{ik;i=k}(m \times n)$ as compared with analogous statistic parameters of Mueller-matrix images of MT layer. Accordingly, autocorrelation functions $K_{ik}(\Delta x)$, experimentally measured coordinate distributions of Mueller matrix elements of skin dermis layer, are characterized by greater half-width weakly expressed oscillations.

Quantitative statistic M_i, correlation Q_i; and spectral J_i moments, that characterize distributions $y_{ik}(m\times n)$ and dependences $K_{ik}(\Delta x)$ and $\log W(x_{ik}) - \log l^{-1}$ of histological cut of DS possess individual values (Table 4.2), different from the analogous parameters, determined for MT (Table 4.1).

Two-layered "MT – DS" biological tissue. Values of statistic $M_{z_{ik}}^{j=1,2,3,4}$ correlation $Q_{z_{ik}}^{j=2,3,4}$ and spectral $J_{z_{ik}}^{j=1,2,3,4}$ moments of all Mueller matrix images $z_{ik}(m\times n)$ of the given biological object (Table 4.3) have intermediate values between corresponding quantitative parameters (Table 4.1 and Table 4.2) of coordinate distributions of Mueller matrix elements of partial layers of MT $(x_{ik}(m\times n))$ and DS $(y_{ik}(m\times n))$.

Approximating curves log-log dependences of power spectra of Mueller matrix images of diagonal elements possess two characteristic slopes that correspond to the slope of such dependence for MT.

Thus, the relations between statistic, correlation and fractal parameters of two-layered biological tissue and its partial layers are established, this fact was used as the basis for the development of new methods of Mueller-polarimetry of complex biological structures.

2.7 *Method and system of polarization reproduction of Mueller-matrix images of partial layers of two-layered biological structure*

The process of probing of two-layered biological structure in model notion is relation of the structure (Fig. 4.5) that consists of subsurface and internal (shielded) layers, radiation, that is described by certain input relatively to biological structure the Stokes vector S_0. Each layer is characterized by its values of Mueller matrix relatively $\{X\}$ and $\{Y\}$. When radiation passes across the structure, output Stokes vector S^* is formed, which is determined from the known expression:

$$S^* = \{X\}\cdot\{Y\}\cdot S_0 \tag{4.10}$$

The idea of the method of polarization reproduction (reconstruction) of Mueller-matrix images of internal (shielded) layers of biological tissues is the variation of polarization state $(\alpha_0;\beta_0)$ of laser beam that probes biological tissue (z_{ik}) and monitors changes of Stokes vector parameters $S_{i=1:2:3:4}(X,Y)$ in points (X,Y) of its polarization-inhomogeneous $(\alpha(X,Y);\beta(X,Y))$ image (Angelsky et al. 2005, Dubolazov et al. 2013, Ushenko et al. 2013).

Analysis of expressions of Mueller matrix elements (relation 4.2) shows, that at certain values of optic axis ρ orientation and phase shift δ of biological crystal, they take "extreme values", which, from physical point of view correspond to the formation of linearly or circularly polarized wave, that radiate the grid of biological crystals of external layer $y_{ik}(\rho,\delta)$ of biological tissue (Angelsky et al. 2005, Dubolazov et al. 2013, Ushenko et al. 2013).

From physical point of view this can be interpreted as uncertainty of correlation connections between manifestations polarization properties of organic crystals in various points of architectonic grid of biological tissue, i.e., uncertain or singular mechanisms are the processes of S_0 Stokes vector transformation of probing biostructure beam into S^* (first case of "uncertainty" of Mueller matrix elements) (Pierce et al. 2004).

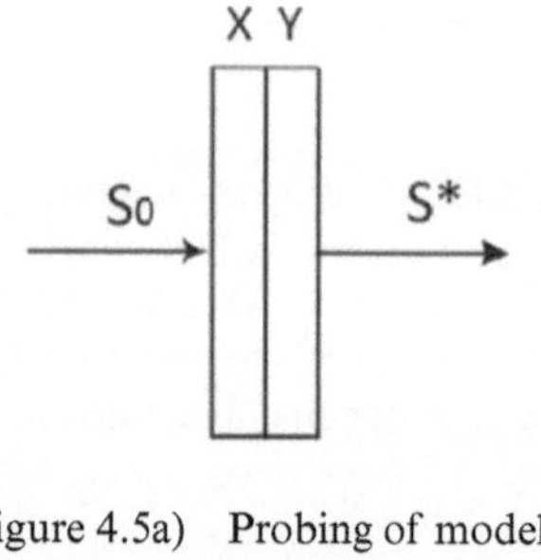

Figure 4.5a) Probing of model.

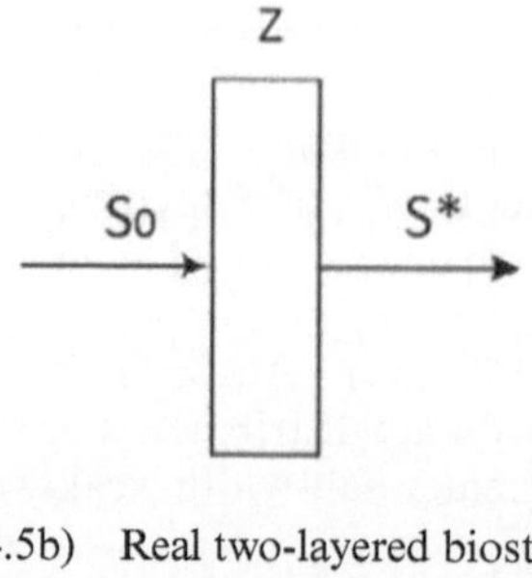

Figure 4.5b) Real two-layered biostructure.

Analysis of the information regarding the conditions of formation of singular values of Mueller matrix elements of biological tissues (Pierce et al. 2004) enables to determine:

- Complete set of points ($\delta = \pm\pi/2$), in the image of biological object, coordinate position of which correspond the conditions $z_{44} = z_{22} = z_{33} = 0$.
- Complete set of "S"- points ($\delta = 0$) of polarization image with arbitrary azimuths ($0 \le \rho \le \pi$), to which conditions $z_{22} = z_{33} = 1$ correspond.

Besides, the selection of various types of polarization singularities of biological tissue ("right" and "left"-rotation singular points) is possible. Table 4.4 illustrates in details the connection of singular values of Mueller matrix elements set with polarization singularities of biological tissues images (Pierce et al. 2004).

In case of linear polarized radiation $\left(x_{ik}(\delta = 0), x_{ik}(\delta = \pi)\right)$ elements z_{ik} of Mueller matrix of two-layered biological structure are described by the expressions (Dubolazov et al. 2013, Ushenko et al. 2013):

$$S_x = \begin{pmatrix} 1 \\ \cos(2\alpha_x) \\ \sin(2\alpha_x) \\ 0 \end{pmatrix} \Leftrightarrow z_{ik}(s_x) = \begin{cases} z_{22} = y_{22};\ z_{23} = y_{23};\ z_{32} = y_{32};\ z_{33} = y_{33}; \\ z_{34} = y_{34};\ z_{43} = y_{43};\ z_{24} = y_{24};\ z_{42} = y_{42}; \\ z_{44} = y_{44}. \end{cases} \qquad (4.11)$$

In other case $\left(x_{ik}(\delta = \pm 0{,}5\pi)\right)$ the following transformation of matrix elements z_{ik} of multi-layered biological object occurs (Dubolazov et al. 2013, Ushenko et al. 2013):

$$S_x^{\otimes} = \begin{pmatrix} 1 \\ 0 \\ 0 \\ 1 \end{pmatrix} \Leftrightarrow z_{ik}(S_x^{\otimes}) = \begin{cases} z_{22} = y_{23} + y_{24};\ z_{23} = y_{23} + y_{24}; \\ z_{32} = y_{33} + y_{34};\ z_{33} = y_{32} + y_{34}; \\ z_{34} = y_{32} + y_{33};\ z_{43} = y_{42} + y_{44}; \\ z_{24} = y_{22} + y_{23};\ z_{42} = y_{43} + y_{44}; \\ z_{44} = y_{42} + y_{43}. \end{cases} \qquad (4.12)$$

Table 4.4 Relations of characteristic values of Mueller matrix elements of biological tissues and their polarization-inhomogeneous images.

f_{ik}		Linear polarization ($\delta = 0$, $\delta = \pi$)	Circular polarization ($\delta = +\pi/2$)
f_{22}	0	–	+ ($\rho = +\pi/4$)
	1	+ ($\delta = 0$)	–
	–1	+ ($\delta = \pi$)	–
$f_{23} = f_{32}$	0	+ ($\delta = \pm\pi/4$)	–
	1	–	+ ($\rho = +\pi/4$)
	–1	–	+ ($\rho = +\pi/4$)
$f_{24} = -f_{42}$	0	+ ($\rho = 0,\pi$)	–
	1	–	+ ($\rho = +\pi/4$)
	–1	–	+ ($\rho = -\pi/4$)
f_{33}	0	–	+ ($\rho = 0$)
	1	+ ($\delta = 0$)	–
	–1	+ ($\delta = \pi$)	–
$f_{34} = -f_{43}$	0	+ ($\delta = \pm\pi/4$)	–
	1	–	+ ($\rho = 0$)
	–1	–	+ ($\rho = +\pi/4$)
f_{44}	0	–	+ ($\rho = 0 \div \pi$)
	1	+ ($\delta = 0$)	–
	–1	+ ($\delta = \pi$)	–

In other words, there exists certain state of polarization (linear or circular) of laser radiation, converted by the grid of biological crystals of subsurface layer, at which measurement of Mueller matrix elements becomes simpler, that allows to use them for the reproduction of oriental-phase structure of subsurface layer of BT.

Realization of the method occurs in automated system shown in Fig. 4.1 without any changes in its structure, by means of corresponding principle of automated control of structure elements. By means of complete rotation $(0 \le \vartheta \le \pi)$ of polarization plane of laser beam, formed by unit 3, probing two-layered biological tissue 6 and measurement (in each pixel of photosensitive platform of digital camera 9) of Stokes vector parameters set $S_{i=1;2;3;4}(r)$ for each value ϑ on condition (Dubolazov et al. 2013):

$$S_2^2(\vartheta^*) + S_3^2(\vartheta^*) + S_4^2(\vartheta^*) \to 1, \tag{4.13}$$

we obtain the following algorithms of polarization reproduction of orientation $(\rho(m \times n))$ and phase $(\delta(m \times n))$ parameters of biological objects grids of the subsurface layer crystals of optic anisotropic object (Dubolazov et al. 2013):

$$\begin{cases} \rho_x = 0,25\pi + \vartheta^*, \\ \rho_y = 0,5\, arctg\left(\dfrac{S_3(\vartheta^*)}{S_2(\vartheta^*)}\right). \end{cases} \tag{4.14}$$

$$\begin{cases} \delta_x = \arccos\left(\dfrac{-a_2 \pm \sqrt{a_2^2 - 4a_1a_3}}{2a_1}\right), \\ \delta_y = \arccos\left[S_4(\vartheta^*)\right], \end{cases} \tag{4.15}$$

where:

$$\begin{aligned} a_1 &= \cos\delta_y, \\ a_2 &= \sin^2\delta_y \cos^2 2(\rho_x - \rho_y) - 2\cos^2\delta_y, \\ a_3 &= \cos^2\delta_y - \sin^2\delta_y \cos^2 2(\rho_x - \rho_y). \end{aligned} \tag{4.16}$$

Thus, widening of functional possibilities of the system (Fig. 4.1) at the expense of the method polarization reproduction of "shielded" externally layers of biologic tissues is reached by means of organization of polarization feedback for determination of optimal state of probing laser beam polarization $(\alpha_0^*(\vartheta); \beta_0^*(\vartheta))$.

This feedback is realizes algorithmically applying computer program, that produces corresponding sign, realization of which leads to certain arrangement of polarization elements of unit 3 by means of commands of the unit microcontroller 11 and the set of step motors, their drivers and position sensor, connected with it.

2.8 *Polarization reproduction of Mueller-matrix images of partial layers of two-component biological structure "muscular tissue-dermis of the skin"*

Optic-thin (attenuation ratio $\tau \le 0,1$) histologic cryocuts of muscular tissue (MT) and Dermis of the Skin (DS) were used as the objects of experimental research. Three groups of Mueller-matrix images of biological layers serve as the object of the research. Fig. 4.6–Fig. 4.9 show the comparative series of experimentally measured and polarizationally reproduced Mueller-matrix images of various types of elements as well as their autocorrelation functions $K_x(\Delta X)$; $K_y(\Delta X)$ and Log-log dependences of power spectra W_x; W_y (Dubolazov et al. 2013, Ushenko et al. 2013).

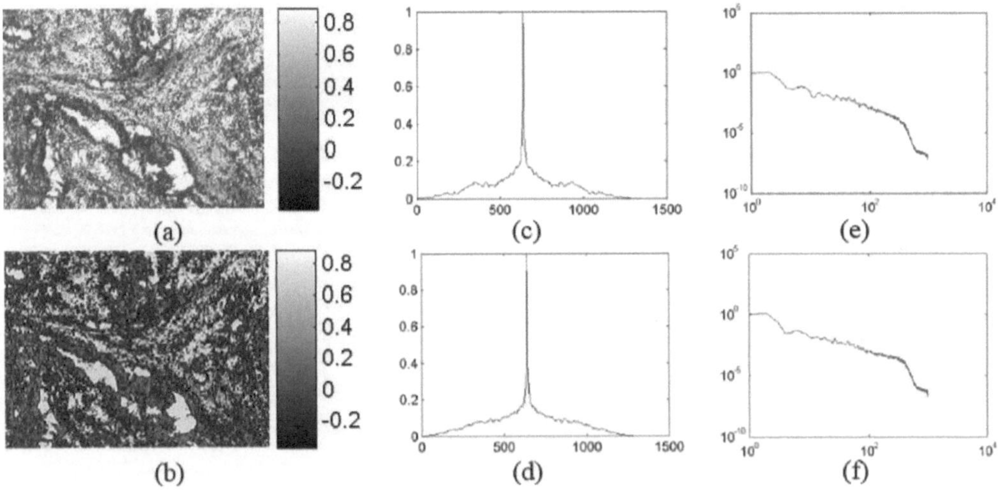

Figure 4.6 Experimental and polarizationally reproduced parameters for dermis of the skin, case 1.

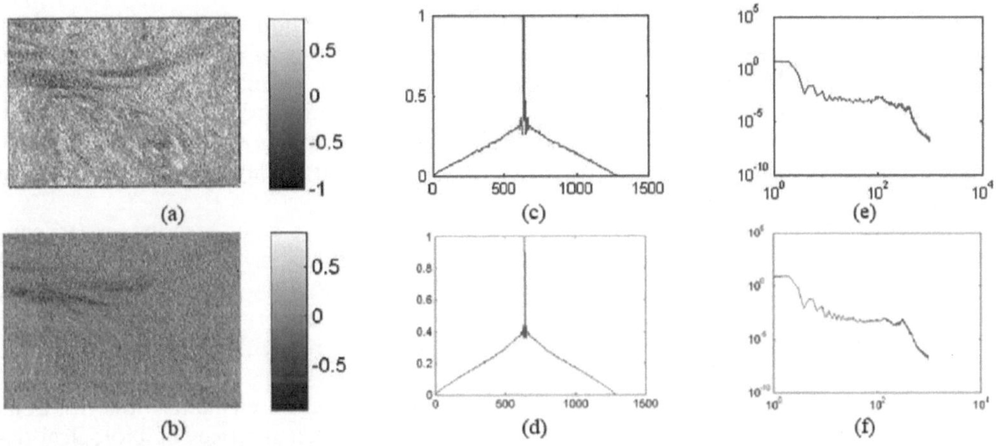

Figure 4.7 Experimental and polarizationally reproduced parameters for dermis of the skin, case 2.

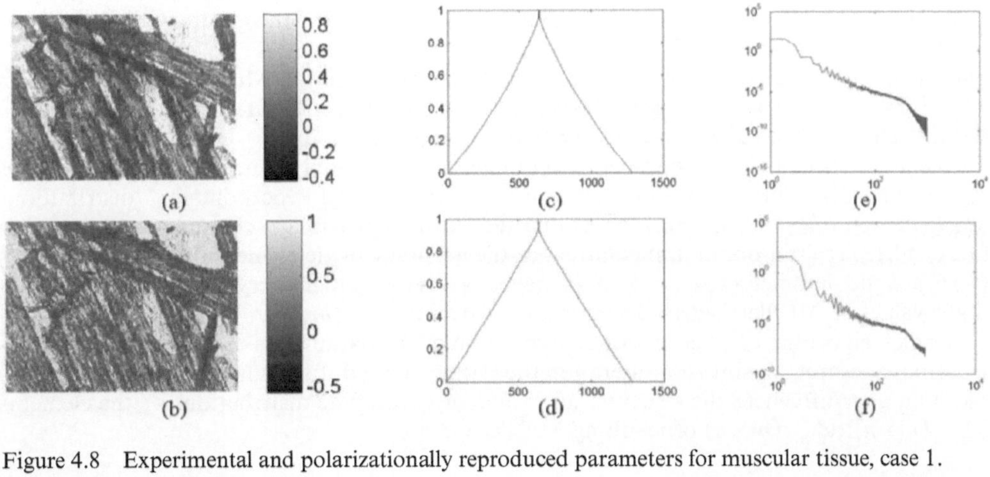

Figure 4.8 Experimental and polarizationally reproduced parameters for muscular tissue, case 1.

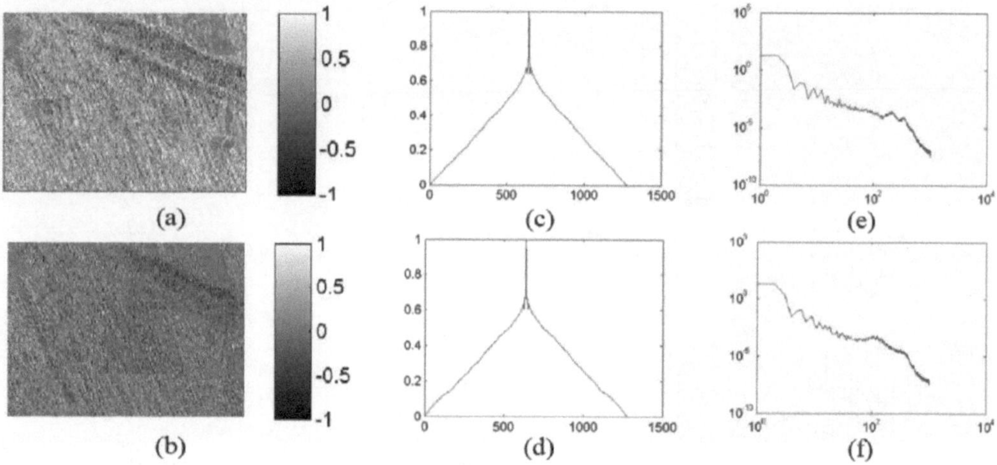

Figure 4.9 Experimental and polarizationally reproduced parameters for muscular tissue, case 2.

The comparative analysis of the data obtained by the method of polarization reconstruction with the results of direct Mueller-matrix tomography of two-layered biological layers revealed the following fact. Coordinate distributions of polarizationally reproduced elements $x^*_{ik}(m\times n)$; $y^*_{ik}(m\times n)$ Mueller matrix of skin dermis and muscular tissue have overall similar but more "blurred" topological structure as compared with experimentally determined Mueller-matrix images $x_{ik}(m\times n)$; $y_{ik}(m\times n)$ partial layers of real biological tissues.

Discrepancies in the values of statistic moments $M_{i=1;2;3;4}$, that describe experimentally measured and polarizationally reproduced distributions $x_{ik}(m\times n)$; $y_{ik}(m\times n)$ $x^*_{ik}(m\times n)$; $y^*_{ik}(m\times n)$, reach 10%–15% for average $\left(M^{(1)}_{ik}\right)$; 20% - 30% for dispersion $\left(M^{(2)}_{ik}\right)$; 30% - 40% for asymmetry $\left(M^{(3)}_{ik}\right)$ and excess $\left(M^{(4)}_{ik}\right)$ (Table 4.5 and Table 4.6).

Differences between the set of correlation models $Q_{i=2;3;4}$ are within the limits from 15% ($Q_{i=2}$) to 35% ($Q_{i=4}$).

Log-log dependences of power spectra of diagonal elements distributions $x_{ik}(m\times n)$; $y_{ik}(m\times n)$ and $x^*_{ik;i=k}(m\times n)$; $y^*_{ik;i=k}(m\times n)$ of Mueller matrices of biological tissues partial layers are characterized by broken approximating lines within the limits of the whole range of space frequencies l^{-1}. Polarizationally reproduced values of slopes are greater than experimental data of laser polarization by 2^0–5^0. Quantitatively values of the set of spectral moments $J_{i=1;2;3;4}$ differ within the limits from 15% ($J_{i=1;2}$) to 30% ($J_{i=3;4}$).

The obtained data, regarding the statistic $M_{i=1;2;3;4}$ correlation $Q_{i=2;3;4}$ and fractal $J_{i=1;2;3;4}$ parameters of polarizationally reproduced 2D distributions of Mueller matrix elements $x^*_{ik;i=k}(m\times n)$; $y^*_{ik;i=k}(m\times n)$ of partial layers of real biological structure "muscular tissue-skin dermis" allow to state diagnostic efficiency of the given method.

Available discrepancies between experimentally-measured Mueller matrices images $x_{ik}(m\times n)$; $y_{ik}(m\times n)$ and polarizationally reproduced coordinate distributions $x^*_{ik;i=k}(m\times n)$; $y^*_{ik;i=k}(m\times n)$ may be connected with approximate character of condition (4.11)–(4.13) realization, that may influence the accuracy of determination (relation (4.14)–(4.16)) of the parameters $\rho_x,\rho_y,\delta_x,\delta_y$ of partial grids of biological crystals and, correspondingly, values of Mueller matrix elements $x^*_{ik;i=k}(m\times n)$; $y^*_{ik;i=k}(m\times n)$.

Besides, algorithm of polarization reproduction of the parameters of biologic tissue architectonics does not take into consideration the ratio of light diffusion in the width of the samples that also influences the structure and value of coordinate distributions of the elements $x^*_{ik;i=k}(m\times n)$; $y^*_{ik;i=k}(m\times n)$ of resulting Mueller matrix.

Table 4.5 Statistic M_i, correlation Q_i and spectral J_i moments of coordinate distributions of experimentally measured $x_{ik}(m \times n)$ and polarizationally – reproduced $x^*_{ik}(m \times n)$ Mueller matrix elements of muscular tissue layer.

x_{ik}	x_{22}	x^*_{22}	x_{24}	x^*_{24}	x_{44}	x^*_{44}
M_1	0,29	0,32	0,09	0,07	0,23	0,17
M_2	0,08	0,07	0,05	0,06	0,06	0,04
M_3	0,45	0,36	0,39	0,44	0,23	0,32
M_4	5,51	4,69	3,79	5,08	1,05	1,41
Q_2	0,16	0,17	0,11	0,15	0,12	0,09
Q_4	0,99	1,12	6,18	7,85	1,87	2,27
J_1	0,51	0,54	0,66	0,71	0,62	0,69
J_2	0,17	0,14	0,23	0,29	0,29	0,33
J_3	0,06	0,09	0,91	1,28	0,11	0,09
J_4	0,13	0,16	1,75	2.37	0,28	0,21

Table 4.6 Statistic M_i, correlation Q_i and spectral J_i moments of coordinate distributions of experimentally measured and polarizationally – reproduced $y^*_{ik}(m \times n)$ Mueller matrix elements of muscular tissue layer.

y_{ik}	y_{22}	y^*_{22}	y_{24}	y^*_{24}	y_{44}	y^*_{44}
M_1	0,39	0,33	0,01	0,015	0,37	0,29
M_2	0,07	0,09	0,04	0,03	0,06	0,08
M_3	0,17	0,13	0,13	0,19	0,22	0,17
M_4	7,51	5,89	5,08	6,18	1,78	1,46
Q_2	0,21	0,25	0,015	0,018	0,18	0,22
Q_4	0,78	0,97	5,51	6,94	1,18	1,65
J_1	0,62	0,64	0,61	0,66	0,68	0,71
J_2	0,14	0,16	0,32	0.35	0,23	0,28
J_3	0,09	0,12	0,97	1,21	0,18	0,24
J_4	0,42	0,56	2,34	2,87	0,53	0,62

3 METROLOGICAL CHARACTERISTICS OF MEASUREMENT ERRORS DISTRIBUTIONS IN THE SYSTEM OF MUELLER-MATRIX MAPPING OF BIOLOGICAL LAYERS

Analysis of metrological errors of the systems of 2D Mueller-matrix mapping is an urgent problem in the process of creation of similar diagnostic systems. In (Zabolotna, Pavlov et al. 2014) the known technique of theoretical integral and individual errors evaluation of Mueller-matrix elements values measurement in the system of Mueller-matrix mapping based on conditioning ratio of characteristic matrix of the system was used. It is shown that the above-mentioned errors may be stipulated by the error of the azimuth of polarizer transmission plane, error of the phase shift of quarter-wave retarder, error of phase plate fast axis establishment random noise, caused by instability of the intensity of laser source radiation. Experimental evaluation of measurement errors of matrix reference elements on the experimental installation of Mueller matrix mapping system allowed to determine the value of experimental integral absolute error within the limits of 3.2% to 8.7%, which is a satisfactory result (Zabolotna, Pavlov, Ushenko et al. 2014).

Thus, in (Zabolotna, Pavlov et al. 2014, Zabolotna, Pavlov, Ushenko et al. 2014) classic analysis of “single-channel” errors of Mueller matrix parameters measurement were applied. The traditional phenomenological approach, is described in details in (Zabolotna et al. 2015).

Actual problem is the problem of analysis of the errors of "2D" measurement of Mueller matrix elements within the limits of statistic, correlation and fractal approaches to the analysis of the obtained data.

For investigation of the characteristics of the errors of Mueller matrices measurements by means of the developed system we select 5% of glucose. The solution in distilled water, which is optically anisotropic layer with circular birefringence, for which Mueller matrix is known.

Determination of statistic, correlation and fractal characteristics of coordinate distributions of the measured coordinate distribution errors of Mueller matrix elements is based on the following principles:

- statistic ("one-dimensional" within the limits of local pixel) – calculation of statistic moments of the first and second orders, which characterize the coordinate distributions of the values of relative errors of Mueller matrix determination, presented in (Zabolotna, Pavlov et al. 2014):

$$S_0 \frac{|\Delta(S_{0,*})|}{|(S_{0,*})|^{\mathrm{T}}} = \frac{|(S_{0,*})|^{\mathrm{E}} - |(S_{0,*})|^{\mathrm{T}}}{|(S_{0,*})|^{\mathrm{T}}}, \qquad \frac{|\Delta z_{ik}|}{|z_{ik}|^{\mathrm{T}}} = \frac{|z_{ik}|^{\mathrm{E}} - |z_{ik}|^{\mathrm{T}}}{|z_{ik}|^{\mathrm{T}}}, \tag{4.17}$$

here T – means theoretical values; E – experimental values.

- statistic ("two-dimensional" within the limits of the set of pixels) – calculation of statistic moments of the 1st–4th orders which characterize the coordinate distributions of the values of the elements of theoretically $\left(M^T_{i=1;2;3;4}(z_{ik})\right)$ known and experimentally $\left(M^E_{i=1;2;3;4}(z_{ik} \pm \Delta z_{ik})\right)$ measured Mueller matrix:

$$\begin{aligned} M_1^T &= \frac{1}{N}\sum_{j=1}^{N}\left(|z_{ik}|\right)_j, \\ M_2^T &= \sqrt{\frac{1}{N}\sum_{j=1}^{N}\left(|z_{ik}|\right)_j^2}, \\ M_3^T &= \frac{1}{\left(M_2^T\right)^3}\frac{1}{N}\sum_{j=1}^{N}\left(|z_{ik}|\right)_j^3, \\ M_4^T &= \frac{1}{\left(M_2^T\right)^4}\frac{1}{N}\sum_{j=1}^{N}\left(|z_{ik}|\right)_j^4, \end{aligned} \tag{4.18}$$

$$\begin{aligned} M_1^E &= \left(M_1^T \pm \Delta M_1\right) = \frac{1}{N}\sum_{j=1}^{N}\left(|z_{ik}| \pm |\Delta z_{ik}|\right)_j, \\ M_2^E &= \left(M_2^T \pm \Delta M_2\right) = \sqrt{\frac{1}{N}\sum_{j=1}^{N}\left(|z_{ik}| \pm |\Delta z_{ik}|\right)_j^2}, \\ M_3^E &= \left(M_3^T \pm \Delta M_3\right) = \frac{1}{\left(M_2^E\right)^3}\frac{1}{N}\sum_{j=1}^{N}\left(|z_{ik}| \pm |\Delta z_{ik}|\right)_j^3, \\ M_4^E &= \left(M_4^T \pm \Delta M_4\right) = \frac{1}{\left(M_2^E\right)^4}\frac{1}{N}\sum_{j=1}^{N}\left(|z_{ik}| \pm |\Delta z_{ik}|\right)_j^4, \end{aligned} \tag{4.19}$$

$$\frac{\Delta M_{i=1;2;3;4}|\Delta z_{ik}|}{M_{i=1;2;3;4}|z_{ik}|^{\mathrm{T}}} = \frac{M_{i=1;2;3;4}|z_{ik}|^{\mathrm{E}} - M_{i=1;2;3;4}|z_{ik}|^{\mathrm{T}}}{M_{i=1;2;3;4}|z_{ik}|^{\mathrm{T}}} \tag{4.20}$$

Correlation – calculations of averaged within the limits of all raw $(1, \ldots, k)$ autocorrelation function of Mueller matrix values of elements distribution (Zabolotna, Pavlov, Ushenko et al. 2014):

$$\bar{K}(\Delta m) = \sum_{j=1}^{n} \frac{K_j(\Delta m)}{n} \tag{4.21}$$

For evaluation of linearity of autocorrelation dependences of ($S_0(m \times n)$, $S_*(m \times n)$, $Z_{ik}(m \times n)$) distributions linearly coefficient ξ, described in (Zabolotna, Pavlov 2014) as:

$$\xi(\Delta m, S_0, S_*, z_{ik}) = 1 - \frac{\Pi^E(\Delta m, S_0, S_*, z_{ik})}{\Pi^T(\Delta m, S_0, S_*, z_{ik})} = 1 - 2\int_1^m \bar{K}(\Delta m, S_0, S_*, z_{ik})\, dm \tag{4.22}$$

Here Π^E - is the area, under experimentally determined function, Π^T - is the area under theoretically determined function;

- correlation ***moments of the 1st–4th orders***

For evaluation of the error values of correlation moments of the 1st–4th orders the relation will be as follows:

$$\delta Q_{i=1;2;3;4} = \frac{\Delta Q_{i=1;2;3;4}(\bar{K}|\Delta z_{ik}|)}{Q_{i=1;2;3;4}(\bar{K}|\Delta z_{ik}|)^T} = \frac{Q_{i=1;2;3;4}(\bar{K}|\Delta z_{ik}|)^E - Q_{i=1;2;3;4}(\bar{K}|\Delta z_{ik}|)^T}{Q_{i=1;2;3;4}(\bar{K}|\Delta z_{ik}|)^T} \tag{4.23}$$

- fractal – calculations of logarithmic dependences of power spectra distributions of Mueller matrix elements values.

For evaluation of self-similarity degree of $(S_0(m \times n), S_*(m \times n), z_{ik}(m \times n))$ distributions fractality coefficient μ was introduced in accordance with the statements described in (Zabolotna, Pavlov, Ushenko et al. 2014):

$$\mu = 1 - \frac{\eta_{max} - \eta_{min}}{\eta_{max} + \eta_{min}} \tag{4.24}$$

Here η_{max} and η_{min} – are maximal and minimal values of the slope of approximating curve $\Phi(\eta)$ to logarithmic dependence of power spectra of values Mueller matrix elements distribution.

- spectral ***moments of the 1st–4th orders***

For evaluation of the errors of spectral moments of the 1st–4th orders value the following relation will be introduced

$$\delta W_{i=1;2;3;4} = \frac{\Delta W_{i=1;2;3;4}(J|\Delta z_{ik}|)}{W_{i=1;2;3;4}(J|\Delta z_{ik}|)^T} = \frac{W_{i=1;2;3;4}(J|\Delta z_{ik}|)^E - W_{i=1;2;3;4}(J|\Delta z_{ik}|)^T}{W_{i=1;2;3;4}(J|\Delta z_{ik}|)^T} \tag{4.25}$$

Here $J|\Delta z_{ik}|$ – are logarithmic dependences of power spectra distributions of Mueller matrix element values.

The results of measurements of Mueller matrix elements values of 5% glucose solution in distilled water in flat-parallel dish 20 mm of thickness.

From theoretical point of view turn of polarization plan occurs linearly polarized with azimuth $\alpha_0 = 0°$. The laser radiation, that already passed across such layer, remains flat-polarized, but with different azimuth $\alpha = \theta = 10°$. In other words, the given process is characterized by the following Mueller matrix of circular birefringence:

$$\{Z\}=\begin{Vmatrix}1 & 0 & 0 & 0\\ 0 & \cos\theta & \sin\theta & 0\\ 0 & -\sin\theta & \cos\theta & 0\\ 0 & 0 & 0 & 0\end{Vmatrix}=\begin{Vmatrix}1 & 0 & 0 & 0\\ 0 & 0{,}984 & 0{,}174 & 0\\ 0 & -0{,}174 & 0{,}984 & 0\\ 0 & 0 & 0 & 0\end{Vmatrix} \tag{4.26}$$

Quantitative parameters that characterize coordinate distributions of the values of Mueller matrix elements of glucose solution and the degree of their coordinate and scale self-similar homogeneity, are given in Table 4.7 and Table 4.8.

From the data, given above, it is seen the value of integral (within the limits of $m \times n$) absolute errors Δq of elements $z_{i=1\div3,k=1\div3}$ measurements in within the limits of 0,03–0,04, and elements $z_{i=4,k=1\div4}$, $z_{i=1\div4,k=4}$ – 0,06–0,08.

In the limits of digital camera pixel set high level of coordinate $(0{,}019 \leq \xi \leq 0{,}029)$ scale self-similar $(0{,}97 \leq \mu \leq 0{,}905)$ homogeneity of 2D distributions registration of Mueller matrix elements of optically active layer of glucose solution is realized.

Analysis of Table 4.8 values allowed to reveal:

- range of errors change of statistic moments values of the 1st–4th orders, that characterize coordinate distributions of "orientation", "orientation-phase" and "phase" elements of Mueller matrix are within such limits:

$$\begin{cases} 0{,}058 \leq \Delta M_1 \leq 0{,}07; \\ 0{,}064 \leq \Delta M_2 \leq 0{,}073; \\ 0{,}072 \leq \Delta M_3 \leq 0{,}08; \\ 0{,}079 \leq \Delta M_4 \leq 0{,}085; \end{cases}$$

Table 4.7 Objective parameters, that characterize distributions errors Δz_{ik}.

Parameters	z_{11}	z_{12}	z_{13}	z_{14}	z_{21}	z_{22}	z_{23}	z_{24}
$\overline{\Delta z}_{ik}$	0,051	0,063	0,075	0,089	0,067	0,049	0,063	0,094
Δz_{ik}	0,019	0,021	0,023	0,025	0,022	0,15	0,021	0,026
ξ	0,019	0,0205	0,022	0,025	0,02	0,021	0,022	0,026
μ	0,97	0,95	0,94	0,92	0,96	0,97	0,95	0,93
Parameters	z_{31}	z_{32}	z_{33}	z_{44}	z_{41}	z_{42}	z_{43}	z_{44}
$\overline{\Delta z}_{ik}$	0,042	0,048	0,053	0,094	0,081	0,092	0,096	0,098
Δz_{ik}	0,014	0,015	0,016	0,027	0,022	0,024	0,025	0,026
ξ	0,021	0,022	0,023	0,026	0,025	0,026	0,028	0,029
μ	0,96	0,95	0,94	0,92	0,93	0,92	0,925	0,905

Table 4.8 Parameters, characterizing the errors of the value of statistic $M_{i=1;2;3;3}$ correlation $Q_{i=1;2;3;3}$ and spectral $W_{i=1;2;3;3}$ moments.

Parameter	δM_1	δM_2	δM_3	δM_4	δQ_2	δQ_3	δQ_4	δW_1	δW_2	δW_3	δW_4
z_{33}	0,058	0,064	0,072	0,079	0,031	0,035	0,037	0,091	0,11	0,124	0,141
z_{34}	0,065	0,067	0,076	0,083	0,037	0,047	0,051	0,11	0,135	0,154	0,174
z_{44}	0,07	0,073	0,08	0,085	0,044	0,05	0,054	0,142	0,153	0,165	0,186

– range of errors change of spectral moments values of the 2nd–4th orders, that characterize coordinate distributions of "orientation", "orientation-phase" and "phase" elements of Mueller matrix are within the limits:

$$\begin{cases} 0{,}031 \le \Delta Q_2 \le 0{,}044; \\ 0{,}035 \le \Delta Q_3 \le 0{,}05; \\ 0{,}037 \le \Delta Q_4 \le 0{,}054; \end{cases}$$

– range of errors change of spectral moments values of the 1st–4th orders, that characterize coordinate distributions of "orientation", "orientation-phase" and "phase" elements of Mueller matrix are within the limits:

$$\begin{cases} 0{,}091 \le \Delta W_1 \le 0{,}142; \\ 0{,}11 \le \Delta W_2 \le 0{,}153; \\ 0{,}124 \le \Delta W_3 \le 0{,}165; \\ 0{,}141 \le \Delta W_4 \le 0{,}186. \end{cases}$$

Experimental evaluation of measurement errors of Mueller matrix elements in the system of Mueller-matrix mapping of biological optically inhomogeneous layers with theoretically known Mueller matrix with circular birefringent is realized.

For the first time on the base of statistic, correlation and fractal approaches to the description of 2D distribution values and the range of error changes of statistic, correlation and spectral moment values are determined. They characterize coordinate distributions of orientation, "orientation-phase" and "phase" Mueller matrix images of optic-anisotropic layer.

4 DIAGNOSTIC POSSIBILITIES OF ORIENTATION AND PHASE MUELLER-MATRIX TOMOGRAPHY OF POLYCRYSTAL NETWORKS OF BLOOD PLASMA

In many cases study of optically-anisotropic structure not of biological tissues but of biological fluids, such as blood, urine, bile, etc. is more accessible. That is why, further development of new approaches to the analysis of vector structure of laser radiation fields, transformed not only optically-anisotropic layers of biological tissues by also films of biological fluids, in particular polycrystal networks proteins is very important.

In (Angelsky et al. 2010, Ushenko, Boychuk et al. 2013) diagnostic possibilities of static and fractal analysis of Mueller matrix and polarization images of blood plasma of the human being in case of cardiac insufficiency (ischemia), acute inflammatory processes (acute colitis), oncologic changes of mammary gland were proved. Determination of diagnostic possibilities of other methods of blood plasma laser polarimetry, particularly orientation and phase Mueller matrix tomography within the limits of statistic, correlation and fractal analysis of the obtained tomograms is still actual.

In (Ushenko, Boychuk et al. 2013) scenarios of formation and complex analysis of the structure of orientation and phase Mueller matrix tomogram of blood plasma films for determination of objective criteria of human physiologic state diagnostic are presented.

As the object of experimental research blood plasma smears (optically thin structure with attenuation factor of $\tau = 0{,}07$) of a healthy man and sick person suffering from carcinoma of the stomach, were used. Smear is prepared by means of drying at the temperature of 20–22°C for 24 hours. During this period the complete evaporation of water and crystallization of protein (albumin-globulin) structures occurs.

Experimental research was carried out by means of multifunctional system, shown in Fig. 4.1 in Mueller-matrix "orientation" and "phase" tomography modes.

The statement of protein networks of biological tissues is the base of modeling of blood plasma optic properties (Angelsky, Pishak et al. 2007, Angelsky et al. 2010, Ushenko, Boychuk et al. 2013)):

- the film of human blood plasma is considered in the form of two-component amorphic-crystalline structure;
- crystalline component is formed by the set (network) of albumin and globalin crystals;
- optically-liquid crystals of amino acids possess properties of optically uniaxial birefringent crystals, that are characterized by Mueller matrix operator, described by relation (4.1).

Thus, for description of optical properties of human layer blood plasma it is necessary to possess information regarding the coordinate distributions of the two groups of parameters ρ and δ, which characterize crystallized amino acids of albumin and globulin. On the base of the given information we will consider the process of laser radiation transformation by the monolayer of partial crystals of blood plasma amino acids.

Analytically orientation-phase structure of such monolayer or flat polycrystalline network can be presented in the form of two 2D arrays, called orientation tomogram of the form (4.27) and phase tomogram of the form (4.28), respectively:

$$\rho(x,y)=\begin{pmatrix} \rho_{11} & \dots & \rho_{1y} \\ \vdots & \rho_{ik} & \vdots \\ \rho_{x1} & \dots & \rho_{xy} \end{pmatrix}, \tag{4.27}$$

$$\delta(x,y)=\begin{pmatrix} \delta_{11} & \dots & \delta_{1y} \\ \vdots & \delta_{ik} & \vdots \\ \delta_{x1} & \dots & \delta_{xy} \end{pmatrix}. \tag{4.28}$$

The established algorithm of determination of optic axis of uniaxial birefringent crystal direction enables to perform the calculation of Mueller matrix orientation tomograms of blood plasma monolayer applying the relation (4.8).

Mueller matrix phase tomograms of birefringent network of blood plasma monolayer can be obtained by means of experimentally measured Mueller-matrix "phase" maps $z_{44}(m\times n)$ from the relation (4.9).

Quantitatively distributions of orientation and phase tomograms were evaluated, applying the already known technique (Angelsky, Pishak et al. 2007), that will be given, for instance for orientation tomogram. The 2D array $\rho(m\times n)$ was scanned with the step of $1pix$ in horizontal direction $1pix; 2pix; \dots npix$. For each step ρ the number of values $N_{k=1+n}$ in limits of corresponding horizontal column $1pix; 2pix; \dots mpix$ was calculated. Thus, for each orientation tomogram $\rho^{*}(m\times n)=\text{const}$ one-dimensional coordinate dependence of the amount of values of corresponding orientation of optic axes of polycrystalline network $N^{(\rho)}(x=1\div n)\equiv N(x)$ was obtained. Further, statistic, correlation and fractal evaluation of the obtained distributions was performed by the formulas (4.6)–(4.8).

The series of Fig. 4.10–Fig. 4.11 orientation tomograms of albumin-globulin networks, coordinate $(m\times n)$, quantitative $(N(x))$, autocorrelation $(K_{ik}(\Delta x))$ and fractal $(W(Z_{ik}))$ dis-

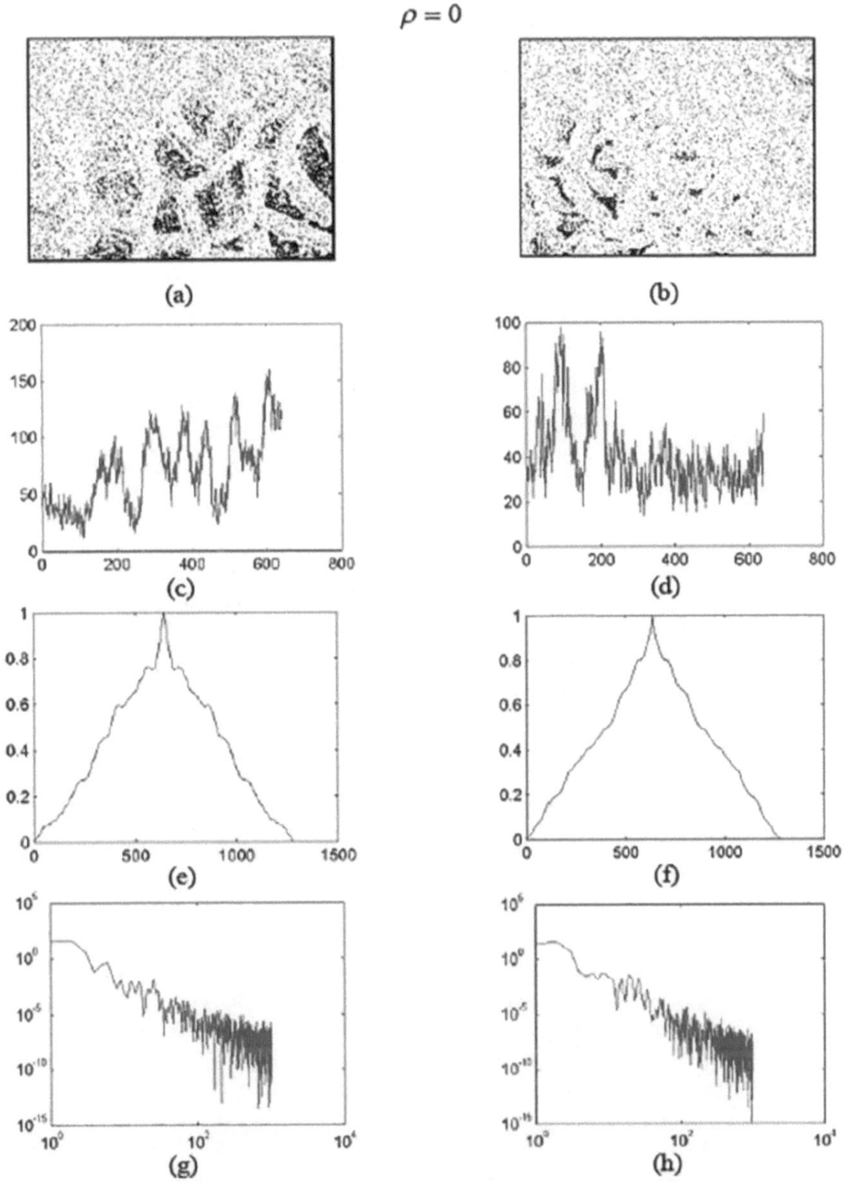

Figure 4.10 Coordinate ((a), (b)), quantitative ((c), (d)), correlation ((e), (f))) and fractal ((g), (h)) structure of direction distribution of optic axes of the crystals of healthy man blood plasma amino acids (left column) and sick person (right column) suffering from the carcinoma of the stomach.

tributions of the determined directions of optic axes of partial crystals of optic-anisotropic grid $\rho(m\times n)=0$ (Fig. 4.10), $\rho(m\times n)=0{,}25\pi$ (Fig. 4.11) of healthy man blood plasma (left column) a person suffering from carcinoma of the stomach (right column), as well as the set of their statistic $M_{i=1;2;3;4}$, correlation $Q_{2;3;4}$ and spectral $J_{i=1;2;3;4}$ of statistic moments (see Table 4.9) is shown.

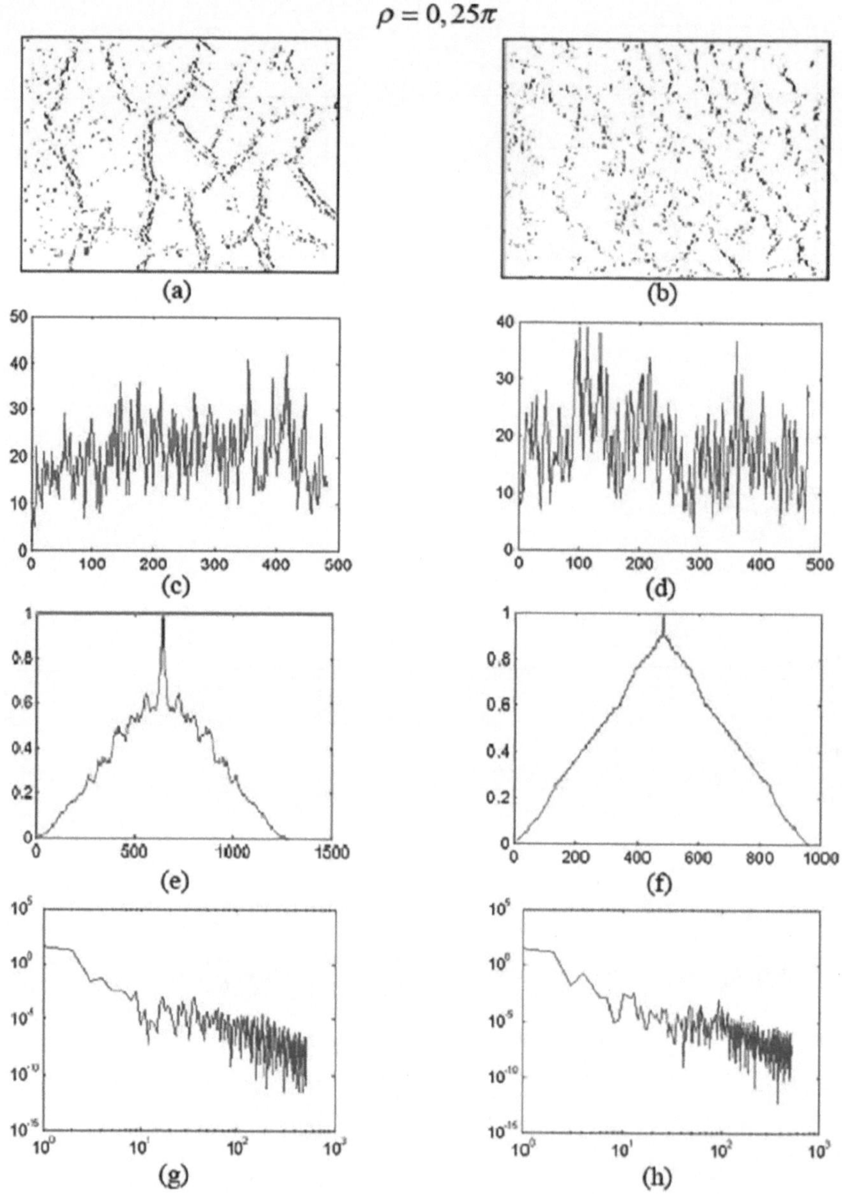

Figure 4.11 Coordinate ((a), (b)), quantitative ((c), (d)), correlation ((e), (f))) and fractal ((g), (h)) structure of direction distribution of optic axes of the crystals of healthy man blood plasma amino acids (left column) and sick person (right column) suffering from the carcinoma of the stomach.

From the analysis of the experimental data obtained the principle fact follows – availability of sufficient level of azimuth symmetry in coordinate distributions of optic axes of corresponding polycrystalline network both in blood plasma of healthy man and person suffering from carcinoma of the stomach. Comparative analysis of the set of the amount $(N(\rho = const))$ of determined directions of partial crystals distributions irrespective of specific value $\rho(m \times n) = const$ and physiological state revealed their statistic $M_i(\rho = const) \approx M_i^*(\rho = const)$, correlation $Q_i(\rho = const) \approx Q_i^*(\rho = const)$ and spectral $J_i(\rho = const) \approx J_i^*(\rho = const)$ similarity.

Quantitatively the structure of the series of orientation tomograms of optic-anisotropic network of blood plasma is illustrated by the set of statistic, correlation and spectral moments, given in Table 4.9 for three determined directions $\rho^* = 0; +0,25\pi; -0,25\pi$.

Comparative analysis of experimental data obtained indirectly determined by means of Mueller matrix orientation tomograms of blood plasma layer did not reveal enough objective differentiation criteria of polycrystal networks of various types.

Series of Fig. 4.12 and Fig. 4.13 contains directly measured phase tomograms of polycrystalline birefringent network of healthy man blood plasma (left column) and sick person, suffering from carcinoma of the stomach (right column): $\delta(m \times n) = 0$ (Fig. 4.12, a); $\delta(m \times n) = 0,1\pi$ (Fig. 4.13, a)) and static, correlation and fractal dependences (fragments (b), (c), (d), correspondingly, that characterize them (Table 4.10)).

Analysis of data, given in Table 4.10, it is seen that the method of phase tomography of birefringent structure of polycrystal network of blood plasma is highly efficient in cancer diagnostics of carcinoma of the stomach.

The reveal diagnostic efficiency of static $M_{i=1;2;3;4}$, correlation $Q_{i=2;3;4}$, and spectral $J_{i=1;2;3;4}$ parameters that characterize coordinate, correlation and self similar structure of experimentally measured determined distributions of phase shifts of polycrystalline network of healthy man blood plasma $\delta(m \times n) = 0,1\pi;\ 0,2\pi$ and sick person, suffering from carcinoma of stomach $\delta^*(m \times n) = 0,1\pi;\ 0,2\pi$:

- differences between the 2nd, 3rd and 4th statistic moments of coordinate distributions $\delta(m \times n) = 0,1\pi;\ 0,2\pi$ and $\delta^*(m \times n) = 0,1\pi;\ 0,2\pi$ are within the limits from 2 to 4 times;
- values of the 2nd, 3rd and 4th correlation moments differ 2.5–15 times;
- differences between the value of the 2nd, 3rd and 4th spectral moments reach 1.5–3 times.

Thus, it may be staled that the method of Mueller-matrix phase tomography of the coordinate distributions of birefringence amino-acids polycrystalline network of optically-thin layers of human plasma turned out to be efficient for the diagnostics of oncologic state of internal organs of the human being.

Table 4.9 Statistic M_i, correlation Q_i and spectral W_i moments of the 1st–4th orders of orientation tomograms of blood plasma crystals of amino acids.

$R_{i=1;2;3;4}$	$\rho^* = 0$		$\rho^* = +0,25\pi$		$\rho^* = -0,25\pi$	
State	Norm	Cancer	Norm	Cancer	Norm	Cancer
M_1	0,43	0,36	0,29	0,21	0,25	0,23
M_2	0,21	0,18	0,23	0,26	0,24	0,22
M_3	0,75	0,89	1,04	1,21	0,91	1,11
M_4	1,39	1,56	1,61	1,89	1,86	2,09
Q_2	0,25	0,24	0,14	0,22	0,24	0,26
Q_3	0,41	0,53	1,56	0,58	0,25	0,32
Q_4	0,86	1,11	3,32	0,83	0,13	0,18
J_1	0,69	0,64	0,56	0,59	0,58	0,62
J_2	0,17	0,21	0,28	0,24	0,27	0,31
J_3	0,09	0,11	0,71	0,59	0,51	0,45
J_4	0,14	0,18	0,53	0,68	0,42	0,39

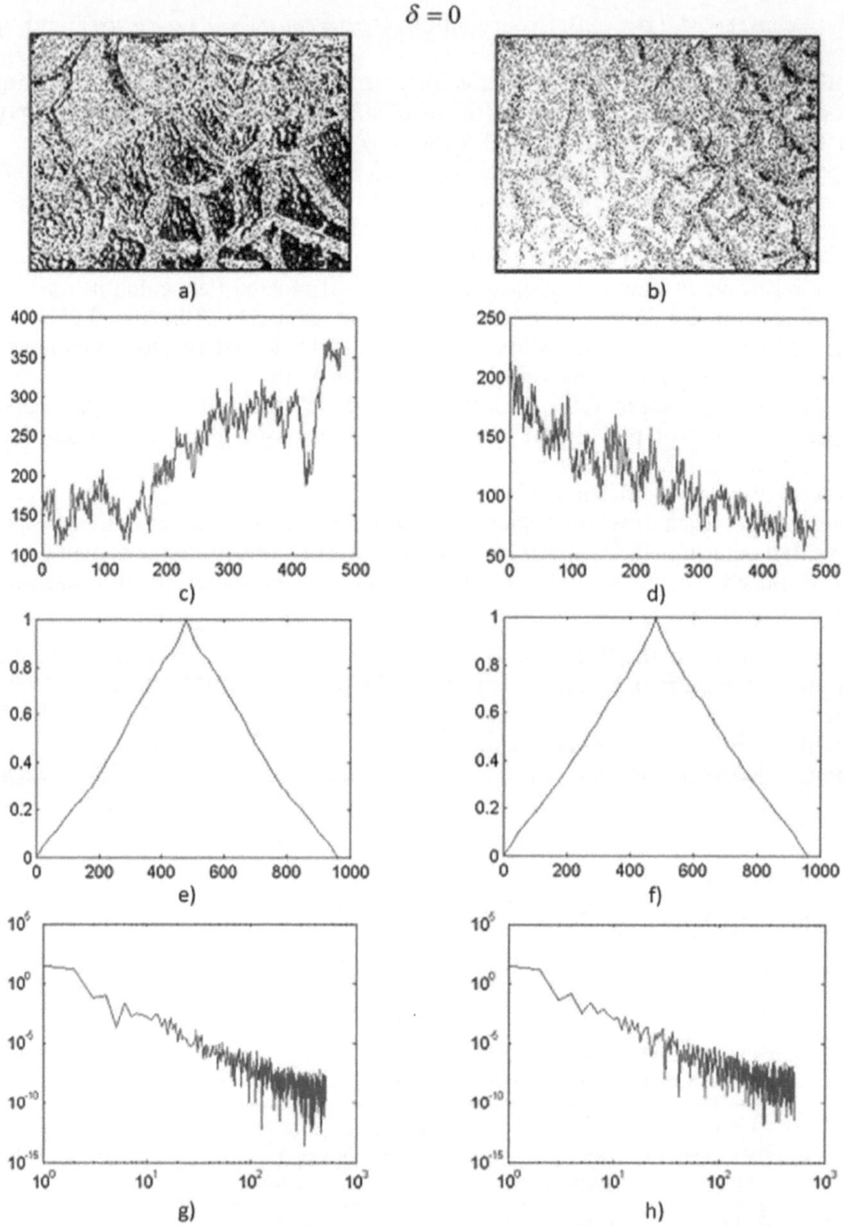

Figure 4.12 Coordinate ((a), (b)), quantitative ((c), (d)), correlation ((e), (f))) and fractal ((g), (h)) structure of determined phases level distribution $\delta = 0$ of partial crystals of blood plasma amino acids of the healthy man (left column) and sick person, suffering from the carcinoma of the stomach (right column) $\delta = 0{,}1\pi$.

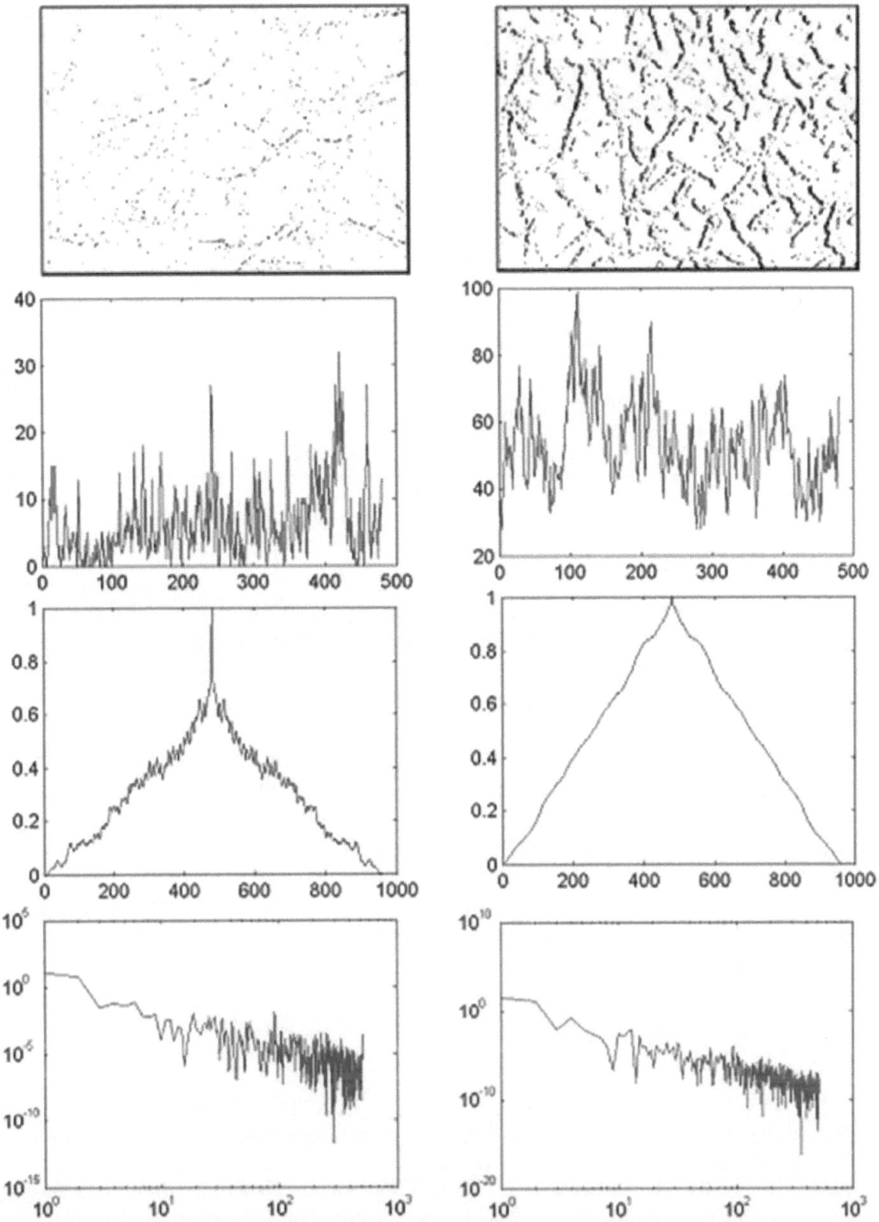

Figure 4.13 Coordinate ((a), (b)), quantitative ((c), (d)), correlation ((e), (f))) and fractal ((g), (h)) structure of determined phases level distribution of partial crystals of blood plasma amino acids of the healthy man (left column) and sick person, suffering from the carcinoma of the stomach (right column).

Table 4.10 Statistic M_i, correlation Q_i and spectral W_i moments of the 1st–4th orders of phase tomograms of the networks of blood plasma crystals of amino acids.

$R_{i=1;2;3;4}$	$\delta^* = 0$		$\delta = +0{,}1\pi$		$\delta = 0{,}2\pi$	
State	Norm	Cancer	Norm	Cancer	Norm	Cancer
M_1	0,45	0,43	0,09	0,21	0,05	0,16
M_2	0,3	0,28	0,11	0,18	0,09	0,18
M_3	0,51	0,58	1,47	0,68	3,14	0,86
M_4	0,61	0,72	2,03	0,85	4,77	1,18
Q_2	0,31	0,29	0,11	0,26	0,06	0,21
Q_3	0,09	0,1	1,17	0,31	2,81	0,53
Q_4	0,07	0,09	3,63	0,43	7,76	0,54
J_1	0,69	0,74	0,58	0,49	0,51	0,34
J_2	0,31	0,35	0,31	0,21	0,26	0,13
J_3	0,07	0,1	0,19	0,25	0,31	0,72
J_4	0,45	0,43	0,09	0,21	0,22	0,68

5 CONCLUSIONS

The methods of orientation and phase Mueller matrix tomography of blood plasma polycrystalline networks, realized on multifunctional system 2D Mueller matrix tomography, with formation and complex analysis of the structures of corresponding orientations and phase tomograms of a healthy man and a person, suffering from carcinoma of the stomach, are experimentally studied in this chapter.

Applying the method of Mueller-matrix orientation tomography of blood plasma layers' sufficient number of objective criteria of differentiation of various types of polycrystalline networks is not revealed.

Diagnostic ability of static, correlation and spectral parameters, that characterize coordinate, correlation and self similar structure of experimentally measured determined distributions of phase shifts of blood plasma crystalline network of a healthy man $\delta(m \times n) = 0{,}1\pi;\ 0{,}2\pi$ and sick person $\delta^*(m \times n) = 0{,}1\pi;\ 0{,}2\pi$, suffering from carcinoma of the stomach is revealed.

REFERENCES

Angelsky O.V., Pishak V.P., Ushenko A.G. and Ushenko Yu. A. 2007: Statistical and fractal structure of biological tissue Mueller matrix images in Optical correlation techniques and applications; Ed. by O. Angelsky. – Bellingham: SPIE Press., P. 213–266.

Angelsky O.V., Tomka Yu. Ya., Ushenko A.G., Ushenko Ye. G. and Ushenko Yu. A. 2005: Investigation of 2D Mueller matrix structure or biological tissues for pre-clinical diagnostics of their pathological states. Journal of Physics D: Applied Physics, Vol. 38, No 23, pp. 4227–4235.

Angelsky O.V., Ushenko A.G., Ushenko Y.A., Pishak V.P., Peresunko A.P. 2010: Statistical, Correlation and Topological Approaches in Diagnostics of the Structure and Physiological State of Birefringent Biological Tissues in Handbook of Photonics for Biomedical Science; Ed. by Valery V. Tuchin – London.: CRC Press., pp. 283–322.

Angelsky O.V., Ushenko A.G., Ushenko Yu. A. et al. 2007: Statistical and Fractal Structure of Biological Tissue Mueller Matrix Images, Optical Correlation Techniques and Applications, Ed. Washington: Society of Photo-Optical Instrumentation Engineers, pp. 213–266.

Bickel W.S., Bailey W.S. 1985: Stokes vectors, Mueller matrices, and polarization of scattered light, American Journal of Physics, Vol. 53, Issue 5, pp. 468–478.

de Boer J.F. and Milner T.E. 2002: Review of polarization sensitive optical coherence tomography and Stokes vector determination. J. Biomed. Opt., Vol. 7, pp. 359–371.

Dubolazov A.V., Koval G.D., Zabolotna N.I., Pavlov S.V. 2013: Fractal Structure of Optical Anisotropy Mueller Matrices Images of Biological Layers. Proc. SPIE, Vol. 9066, P.90661W.
Pierce M.C., Strasswimmer J., Park B.H., et al. 2004: Birefringence measurements in human skin using polarization-sensitive optical coherence tomography. J. Biomed. Opt. Vol. 9, pp. 287–291.
Shuliang Jiao & Lihong V. Wang 2002: Two-dimensional depth-resolved Mueller matrix of biological tissue measured with double-beam polarization-sensitive optical coherence tomography. Opt. Lett. Vol. 27, pp. 101–103.
Sikora J. 2007: Boundary Element Method for Impedance and Optical Tomography, Publishing House of the Warsaw University of Technology.
Ushenko A.G., and Pishak. V.P. 2004: Laser Polarimetry of Biological Tissue: Principles and Applications in Handbook of Coherent-Domain Optical Methods: Biomedical Diagnostics, Environmental and Material Science [ed. Valery V. Tuchin]. Kluwer Academic Publishers. Vol. 1, pp. 93–138.
Ushenko V.A., Zabolotna N.I., Pavlov S.V., Burkovets D.M., Novakovska O. Yu. 2013: Mueller matrices polarization selection of two-dimensional linear and circular birefringence images. Proc. SPIE, Vol. 9066, P. 90661X.
Ushenko Y.A., Boychuk T.M., Bachynsky V.T., Mincer O.P. 2013: Diagnostics of Structure and Physiological State of Birefringent Biological Tissues: Statistical, Correlation and Topological Approaches in Handbook of Coherent-Domain Optical Methods. New York: Springer Science+Business Media, pp. 107–148.
Ushenko Yu.A., Dubolazov O.V., Karachevtcev A.O., Zabolotna N.I. 2011: The Mueller-matrix elements characteristic values of biological tissues. Proc. SPIE. Vol. 8001, P. 80010J.
Zabolotna N.I. 2011: Principles and methods of Mueller-matrix tomography of multilayer biological tissues. Proc. SPIE 8001, International Conference on Applications of Optics and Photonics, 80010J (July 26, 2011); doi:10.1117/12.891514.
Zabolotna N.I., Pavlov S.V., Radchenko K.O., Stasenko V.A., Wójcik W., Kussambayeva N. 2015: Diagnostic efficiency of Mueller matrix polarization reconstruction system of the phase structure of liver tissue. Proc. SPIE, Vol. 9816, P. 98161E.
Zabolotna N.I., Pavlov S.V., Ushenko A.G., Karachevtsev A.O., Savich V.O., Sobko O.V., Olar O.V. 2014: System of the phase tomography of optically anisotropic polycrystalline films of biological fluids. Proc. SPIE, Vol. 9166, P. 916616.
Zabolotna N.I., Pavlov S.V., Ushenko A.G., Sobko O.V., Savich V.O. 2014: Multivariate system of polarization tomography of biological crystals birefringence networks. Proc. SPIE, Vol. 9166, P. 916615.
Zabolotna N.I., Radchenko K.O. 2014: A multifunctional automated system of 2D laser polarimetry of biological tissues. Proc. SPIE. Vol. 9205, P. 92050V.
Zabolotna N.I., Wojcik W., Pavlov S.V., Ushenko O.G., Suleimenov B. 2013: Diagnostics of pathologically changed birefringent networks by means of phase Mueller matrix tomography. Proc. of SPIE, Vol. 8698, P. 86980C.

CHAPTER 5

Subpixel edge detection and localisation based on low-frequency filtering

Y.Y. Bilynsky & P.M. Ratushny
Vinnytsia National Technical University, Vinnytsia, Ukraine

A. Kotyra & P. Kisała
Lublin University of Technology, Lublin, Poland

M. Junisbekov & E. Amirgalijev
M.Kh. Dulaty Taraz State University, Taraz, Kazakhstan

1 INTRODUCTION

Algorithms for subpixel edge localisation are becoming more popular as their goal is to provide super resolution. Many different methods for edge localisation with subpixel accuracy have been developed so far (Furman et al. 2003). In spite of numerous publications, the problem of subpixel measuring is still unsolved from the viewpoint of universal quantitative estimation. It is because any digitised image is influenced by a noise that is always present in physical measurements. A minor error in source data may actually cause a wrong decision. An object's edge in the image can be considered as a step of a gradient of one- or two-dimensional signal. Then a fragment of a real image can be approximated by an ideal gradient. The gradient is considered to be existing if the approximation standard error is lower than a certain boundary level. In the case of a one-dimensional object's edge in an image, the gradient is approximated by the following step function:

$$S(x) = \begin{cases} b, & x < x_0 \\ b+h, & x \geq x_0 \end{cases}, \tag{5.1}$$

where x = current coordinate; x_0 = coordinate of an edge point; b = function increment; h = polar coordinates of a gradient point nearest to a centre of the analysed circular area (Marr & Hildret 1980). An edge of a real object in an image can be detected both by a maximum of the 1st derivative and by zeros of the 2nd derivative (Abdou 1979, Furman et al. 2003, Rusyn 1977). Methods based on the 1st derivative enable fast and efficient localisation of edges which are nonparallel to grid axes, using gradient size and direction with the error not less than a half of an interpixel width. Methods based on zero crossing (2nd derivative) are also used for edge measuring due to their lower sensitivity to noise and potential durability. Additional numerical differentiation must be performed to determine subpixel coordinates because derivatives are very sensitive to noise. The above mentioned operations are also used for processing of low-contrast images. This can be done in two ways: the first one is data filtering by appropriate derivatives of Tychonoff filters; the second one is an interpolation of discrete data by splines and next the determination of an analytic derivative. These two procedures are equivalent, but they do not allow to eliminate the errors of image digitising (Bertero & Poggio 1988).

2 METHODS

The proposed method for edge localisation does not use a numerical differentiation but enables minimisation of the digitising error and getting the subpixel coordinates of the edge point. The method is based on finding a shared point of intersection of two boundary curves, found as a result of low-frequency filtering. The low-frequency filtering is performed by means of a Gaussian filter with specific weighting coefficients. According to this method, interpolation polynomials are built by means of k points selected from the source and filtered boundary curves. For this purpose, interpolation nodes are specified as the following vectors:

$$N = \begin{bmatrix} n-\Delta \\ n \\ n+\Delta \\ n+2\Delta \\ \dots \\ n+j\Delta \end{bmatrix}, \quad I_1 = \begin{bmatrix} l_{1,-1} \\ l_{1,0} \\ l_{1,1} \\ l_{1,2} \\ \dots \\ l_{1,j} \end{bmatrix}, \quad I_2 = \begin{bmatrix} l_{2,-1} \\ l_{2,0} \\ l_{2,1} \\ l_{2,2} \\ \dots \\ l_{2,j} \end{bmatrix}, \tag{5.2}$$

where N = coordinates vector of the boundary curve points; Δ = interpixel space; I_1 = brightness vector of the source boundary curve; I_2 = brightness vector of the filtered boundary curve; $j+2=k$ = the number of analysed pixels.

To determine the coefficients of the interpolation polynomial, matrix $N_{j,i}$ is formed on the condition that:

$$N_{j,i} = (n_j)^i = \begin{bmatrix} 1 & n-\Delta & (n-\Delta)^2 & \dots & (n-\Delta)^{j+2} \\ 1 & n & n^2 & \dots & n^{j+2} \\ 1 & n+\Delta & (n+\Delta)^2 & \dots & (n+\Delta)^{j+2} \\ \dots & \dots & \dots & \dots & \dots \\ 1 & n+j\Delta & (n+j\Delta)^2 & \dots & (n+j\Delta)^{j+2} \end{bmatrix}. \tag{5.3}$$

The polynomial coefficients are calculated by the formula:

$$a_j(N, I_1) = N_{j,i}^{-1} I_1, \tag{5.4}$$

$$b_j(N, I_2) = N_{j,i}^{-1} I_2, \tag{5.5}$$

where a_j, b_j = coefficients of the interpolation polynomials for the source and filtered boundary curves, respectively. In such a case, the boundary curves, i.e. the dependence of brightness from the pixel number, can be defined by the expressions:

$$I_1(n) = \sum_{i=0}^{j+1} a_j n^i = a_0 + a_1 n + a_2 n^2 + \dots + a_{j+1} n^{j+1} = f_1(n, l_1), \tag{5.6}$$

$$I_1(n) = \sum_{i=0}^{j+1} b_j n^i = b_0 + b_1 n + b_2 n^2 + \dots + b_{j+1} n^{j+1} = f_2(n, l_1). \tag{5.7}$$

The object's edge point is located on the intersection of two polynomial curves (5.6) and (5.7) as shown in Figure 5.1. The polynomials $I_1(n)$ and $I_2(n)$ of the boundary curves intersect in point C with the coordinates (I_C, $n+\delta$) located in the interpixel space. This coordinate with displacement δ corresponds to the edge of the image. To find the subpixel coordinate the following condition must be satisfied:

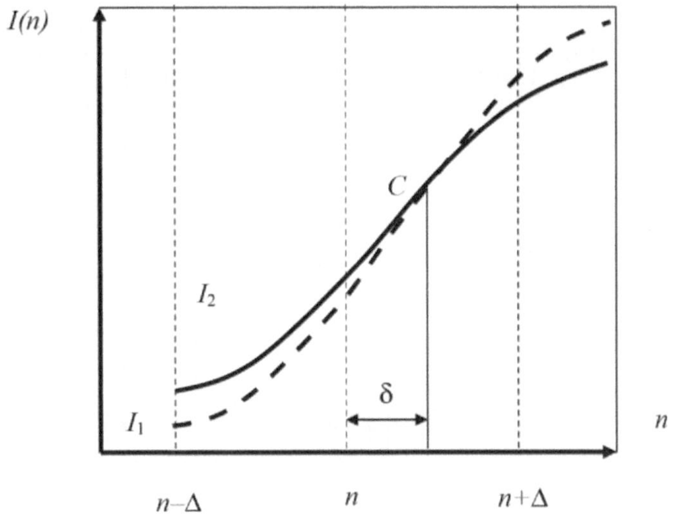

Figure 5.1 Polynomial boundary curves as a result of filtering and their shared point.

$$I_1(n+\delta) = I_2(n+\delta), \tag{5.8}$$

which makes obvious that $\delta = f(n,\ I\{I_1 = I_2\})$ is the solution of such a system:

$$\begin{cases} f_1(n, I_1) = I_C\big|_{n+\delta} \\ f_2(n, I_2) = I_C\big|_{n+\delta} \end{cases}. \tag{5.9}$$

Let us solve the system (5.9) using Newton's method for solving nonlinear equation system (Dyakonov 2001). The Jacobian matrix to be analysed is the following:

$$J(n, I) = \begin{bmatrix} \dfrac{\partial f_1(n, I_1)}{\partial n} & \dfrac{\partial f_1(n, I_1)}{\partial I} \\ \dfrac{\partial f_2(n, I_2)}{\partial n} & \dfrac{\partial f_2(n, I_2)}{\partial I} \end{bmatrix}. \tag{5.10}$$

If the Jacobian matrix is not degenerated, then the solution of the equation system (5.9) can be found from the recurrent expression:

$$(n+\delta)_i\Big|_{(n, I_C\{I_1 = I_2\})} = (n+\delta)_{i-1}\Big|_{(n, I_C\{I_1 \neq I_2\})} - J^{-1}(n, I) \times \begin{bmatrix} f_1(n, I_1) \\ f_2(n, I_2) \end{bmatrix}. \tag{5.11}$$

The process iteration is executed until the condition is satisfied:

$$\left| (n+\delta)_i\Big|_{(n, I_C\{I_1 = I_2\})} - (n+\delta)_{i-1}\Big|_{(n, I_C\{I_1 \neq I_2\})} \right| \leq \varepsilon, \tag{5.12}$$

where ε = measuring error.

A mathematical model of the discrete boundary curve for a one-dimensional space as considered in (Bilynskyy 2007) is used to calculate the coordinates of the edge point:

$$H^{**}(n)=\frac{\Delta I}{\left(I_{\max}-I_{\min}\right)}\sum_{k=0}^{K}\exp\left(-\frac{\pi\left((n-k)-0,5-\delta\right)^2\Delta I^2}{\left(I_{\max}-I_{\min}\right)^2}\right) \tag{5.13}$$

where δ = displacement of the edge of the boundary curve from the pixel center. For the research, let us use the boundary curves of different blurring degrees σ: 1; 1.25; 2 with the coordinate of the edge point $\delta = 0.1$, which correspond to a maximum difference of brightness on the curve Δ: 0.4; 0.35; 0.2 (Dyakonov 2001). For this purpose, the interpolation polynomial of the third degree will be applied, enabling the usage of four node points, in the neighborhood of which the edge is located. Let us define the vectors:

$$N=\begin{bmatrix}-1\\0\\0\\0\end{bmatrix},\quad I_1=\begin{bmatrix}0.0055\\0.1130\\0.5540\\0.9310\end{bmatrix},\quad I_2=\begin{bmatrix}0.0400\\0.2040\\0.5370\\0.8450\end{bmatrix}. \tag{5.14}$$

As a result, we get matrix $N_{4,4}$:

$$N_{4,4}=\begin{bmatrix}1&-1&1&-1\\1&0&0&0\\1&1&1&1\\1&2&4&8\end{bmatrix}. \tag{5.15}$$

The coefficients can be calculated by expressions (5.6) and (5.7) and the following polynomials will be obtained:

$$\begin{aligned}I_1(n)&=0,113+0,341n+0,167n^2-0,066n^3,\\I_2(n)&=0,204+0,281n+0,085n^2-0,032n^3.\end{aligned} \tag{5.16}$$

Based on the discrete model of the boundary curve, the subpixel coordinates were simulated. This allowed to apply a comparative analysis of the proposed and known method of zero crossing. Table 5.1 shows the subpixel coordinates of the edge point as a result of the given methods. For this purpose, the model of the boundary curve with different blurring degrees was used.

Table 5.1 Calculated values of the edge point coordinate.

Blurring degree	$\sigma = 1$ ($\Delta = 0.4$)		$\sigma = 1.25$ ($\Delta = 0.35$)		$\sigma = 2$ ($\Delta = 0.2$)	
Edge displacement δ	Interpolation crossing	Zero crossing	Interpolation crossing	Zero crossing	Interpolation crossing	Zero crossing
0	0	0	0	0	0	0
0.1	0.107	0.138	0.108	0.128	0.106	0.112
0.2	0.217	0.246	0.217	0.236	0.208	0.209
0.3	0.321	0.340	0.316	0.335	0.311	0.318
0.4	0.415	0.415	0.410	0.419	0.400	0.401
0.5	0.500	0.500	0.500	0.500	0.500	0.500
0.6	0.588	0.577	0.630	0.661	0.601	0.595
0.7	0.671	0.660	0.681	0.671	0.702	0.690
0.8	0.769	0.752	0.783	0.764	0.791	0.793
0.9	0.878	0.862	0.893	0.872	0.895	0.892

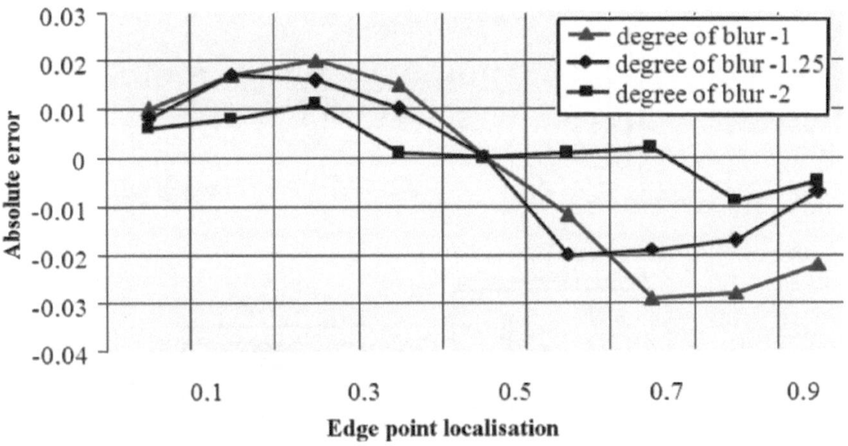

Figure 5.2 Dependence of the absolute error from the edge point localisation.

The research shows that the subpixel coordinates obtained by the proposed method for the boundary curves with a blurring degree $1 < \sigma < 2$ and the length from 5 to 20 pixels have a higher accuracy in comparison to the zero crossing method. For the boundary curves of a great length with a blurring degree $\sigma > 2$ the calculated subpixel coordinates of the edge point are practically similar. Figure 5.2 shows the dependence of the absolute error from the edge point localisation for several boundary curves with a different blurring degree. Figure 5.2 shows that the error for any boundary curve is zero when the shift of the edge point in the interpixel space is 0 or 0.5, and is nonzero in all other cases. The maximum relative error for $\sigma = 1$ is at the level of 7%.

3 EXPERIMENT

To corroborate the proposed method, a model of the imitation system was created. The model given in Figure 5.3 simulates continuous monitoring of the edge coordinates of the measured object when it changes its position.

The model consists of the digital video camera of 640×480 pixels and 8 μm interpixel space. A video camera of a low resolution has been chosen specially to get a bigger difference in measurements without and with the proposed method of edge localisation. An image of the object was projected to the 19 inch monitor of 1280×1024 pixels. To read the data from the monitor and process them further the video camera was connected to the PC via USB. The main goal of the experiment consists in finding coordinates of the object's edge point located on the monitor by capturing it by means of the video camera. At that, the position of the video camera during capturing the video is fixed. The video camera captured the image of the object from the monitor and transferred it to the computer, where a profile of the boundary curve of the object's edge was formed. At that, the object was shifted by one pixel along the *X*-axis by means of the software and an image was read repeatedly. The intensity of the object and its position were specified by the software. Thus, the coordinates of the object's edge were known on the basis of monitor pixel sizes. To preserve the same intensity, the object's edge was parallel to the matrix columns. Before measurements, a calibration of the optical system was made and dimensioning specifications of the model were determined. By measuring the metrological object of the special type with marked well-observed fixed points, a region of space was found as a result of referencing the video camera to the monitor. An optical system was considered to be isoplanatic in that region. After calibration done

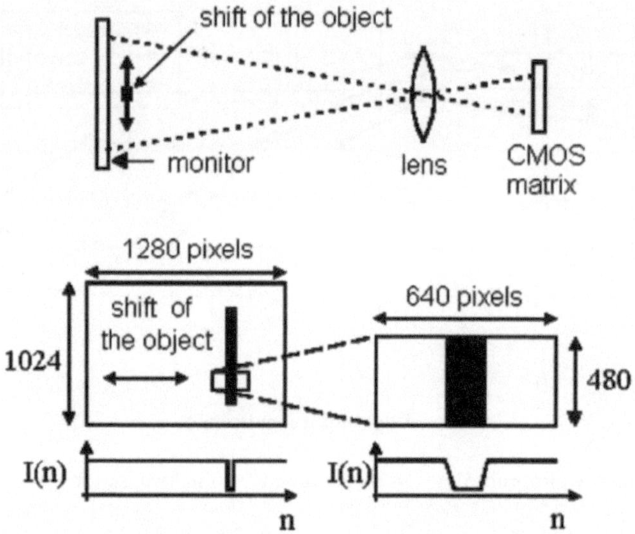

Figure 5.3 Experimental model diagram of the imitation system.

during the control procedure, the parameters of the optical system did not change. The distance between the monitor and the video camera was chosen as a ratio of the monitor pixel to the video camera pixel as 4:1. Iterative one-pixel displacement of an image on the monitor was captured by the video camera and an edge of the same line of the photo-matrix was detected. For this purpose, on the basis of the proposed method, the software for an edge point localisation of a subpixel accuracy was developed. The software made it possible to determine the edge point coordinates using known methods and the proposed low frequency filtering method. The dependence between the monitor pixels and the video camera pixels is almost linear. In order to specify the dependence parameters, the coefficients of the linear approximation were determined using the least squares method. Then, the corrected linear function was built based on the data obtained experimentally. Figure 5.4 shows the results concerning the edge position for the image formed by the video camera and the corrected position obtained using the proposed method. In Figure 5.4, M and N are coordinates, where M = the number of the monitor pixels, N = the number of the video camera pixels.

In Figure 5.4 we can see that when an image is moved on the monitor, a position of the object's edge within one pixel of the video camera does not change. Furthermore, the coordinate localised using the proposed method has a subpixel shift. The results were compared to the most known methods to confirm the accuracy of the low-frequency filtering method. For this purpose, a mean-square measuring error of the approximated line determined by coordinates was found. More than 100 images of the object were captured and the edge points of several matrix lines were analysed. All the algorithms of the edge point localisation were used in equal conditions and the mean square deviations of the data measured were evaluated by the random error evaluation method for indirect measurements, as given in Table 5.2.

The known ratio of the monitor pixel size to the video camera pixel size enabled to determine an image shift as 0.25 of the pixel size. At that, it was determined that the main source of this error are random errors related to the pixel heterogeneous sensitivity and a distortion of the optical system. Considering that a distribution of an error is normal, a maximum error of the method for edge point localisation was calculated as not exceeding 10% of the interpixel space. Research data confirm the high accuracy of the low-frequency detector in comparison to other known methods, including the zero crossing detector.

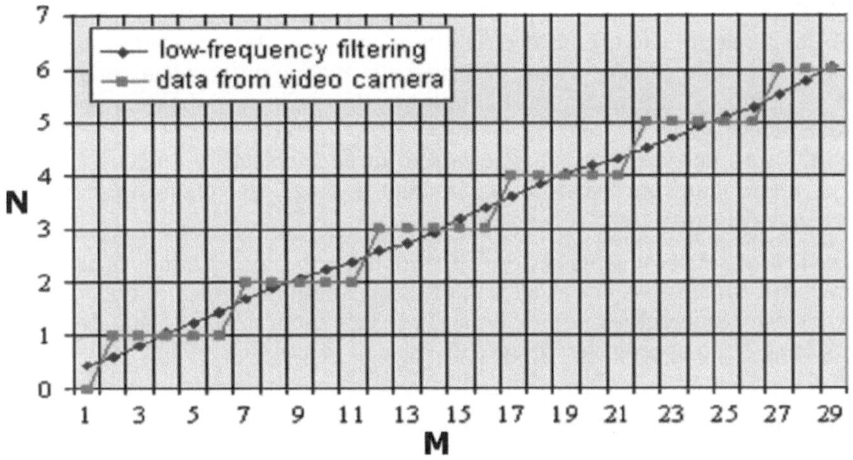

Figure 5.4 Shift of the object's edge position obtained with a video camera and using the proposed method.

Table 5.2 Comparison of the edge localisation results for different methods.

Method	Mean square error
Without subpixel correction	0.2800
Gausse approximation	0.0223
Linear interpolation	0.2100
Parabolic estimation	0.0420
Photometric interpolation	0.1200
Zero crossing	0.0280
Gradient	0.0300
Low-frequency filtering	0.0170

4 METHODS FOR EDGE DETECTION BASED ON LOW-FREQUENCY FILTERING AND ANALYSIS OF PREVIOUS RESEARCH

In a modern theory of digital image processing much attention is paid to the development of edge detection methods, because a detection of contrast differences is one of the main problems of image recognition in many technical vision systems. This is related to the intuitive understanding that the contour lines contain much information. Contour lines are formed in boundary regions of the objects and can be a boundary between not only the objects of a scene and a background, but also between the images of different objects and even the images of adjacent surfaces of the same object. Besides, segmentation algorithms utilising one of two basic characteristics of the intensity, discontinuity and homogeneity, are based on edge detection. The traditional solution of the edge detection problem has four stages: intensification of the intensity differences, selection of the boundary points, skeletonisation and elimination of the gaps. But only intensification of the intensity differences and selection of the boundary points are paid significant attention to. The simplest method for primary edge detection is threshold processing, which runs as follows. If a pixel intensity is higher than a certain threshold, then the pixel is set to binary one. If an intensity is lower than a threshold, then the pixel is set to binary zero. But such an approach can be used only for images on a homogeneous background. The other method for detection of points that differ in intensity consists in finding a two-dimensional 1st derivative (gradient) and setting a certain threshold, above which all the points are considered to be edge points. A connected set of such points, according to the connection criterion, defines the spreading difference in an intensity called the edge. According to the alternative definition, edge points are the points where the 2nd derivative is zero.

Today, a Canny detector is most widely used for edge detection. In general the detector consists of a few algorithms: smoothing, gradient finding, applying a threshold. The main defects of such detectors are as follows:

- possible loss of small elements because of smoothing the corner points in an image;
- incorrect detection of Y-splits as a result of using a limited segmentation;
- minor intensity differences cause multiple fake edges and a small gradient does not allow a quick setting of an appropriate threshold level and identifying the intensity change as the edge.

Modern edge detecting operators cannot be directly used to measure the coordinates of an object on an image because, as a rule, they provide a wide edge. In this case, it is necessary to use special procedures to process a binary image and specify an edge (skeletonisation). Thus, in developing the edge detection method and detectors based on it, ensuring a minimum edge width of 1–2 pixels is still an important problem. The above-considered method for edge point detection based on Gaussian low-frequency filtering with subpixel localisation can also be used for edge detection.

5 DIAGRAM OF THE EDGE DETECTION METHOD

A general defect of the above-mentioned methods is, first of all, a high sensitivity to noise because their principal operation is based on calculating the 1st and 2nd derivatives within the window and their combination. A derivative value is calculated directly in each point, therefore the noise existing in an image is amplified as a transformation result. Both gaps and wide edges can appear on an image. Therefore, there is always a ±1-pixel ambiguity in an edge position. Therefore, a more correct way for edge detection is not the use of a pixel line but a boundary between pixels, as shown in Figure 5.5.

On the other hand, an edge can be defined as a line of a double width between points, where a boundary with subpixel coordinates is located, enabling more accurate detection of the edge pixel. Thus, only edge detectors that more precisely determine an object's coordinates can be used in optoelectronic measuring channels. The proposed edge detection method is based on finding intersection points of object boundary curves in an image, obtained as a result of low-frequency filtering. Such filtering, first of all, suppresses noise in an image and provides characteristic points, some of which belong to an edge. To suppress noise, smoothing Gaussian filters are used. At that, a convolution operation is performed:

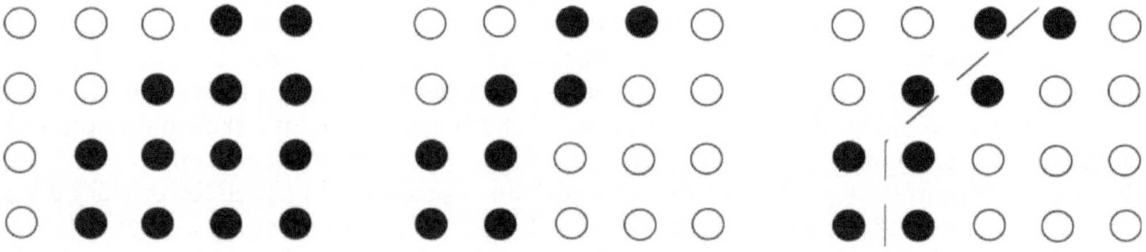

Figure 5.5 Edge detection in a digital image: a) binary image; b) edge fragment; c) fragment of the object's boundary.

$$H^*(n,m) = F(n,m)^{**}G(k_1, k_2). \tag{5.17}$$

Filtering of a discrete image $f(n, m)$ is specified by a weighed mean filter. In the case if a useful signal and a noise are a stationary random sequence with known statistical characteristics, the smoothing level parameter σ can be chosen to obtain a filtered image and ensure minimum errors, i.e. minimise its dispersion. In a general case an edge detection method based on Gaussian low-frequency filtering can be described by the following expression:

$$J(n, m) = p(H^*(n, m)\big|_{\sigma 1} - H^{**}(n, m)\big|_{\sigma 2}, \tag{5.18}$$

where $H^*(n, m)$, $H^{**}(n, m)$ = images obtained as a result of low-frequency filtering for the appropriate blur parameters σ_1 and σ_2; p = scaling coefficient.

Figure 5.6a shows a fragment of one matrix row of a noisy image with a sharp intensity difference and a filtered image. An important feature of the processed image is that a great number of common intersection points appear as a result of filtering and a combination of two images. Part of these points are the object's edge points and a set of such edge points form an image edge. Figure 5.6b shows a fragment of the same matrix row as a result of repeated filtering with a further combination of filtered images. Comparing the images, one can make the conclusion that repeated filtering decreases the number of common points. At that, a gradient value in intersection points of the filtered images, corresponding to the heterogeneity points of a background and an object (and not relating to an edge) is decreased. This means that the additional characteristics of intensity difference can be obtained due to the value of the gradient and the point found in the difference. It means that additional characteristics of an intensity difference can be obtained due to the gradient value, and a point which was found based on this difference can be (or not) classified as an edge point. Edge points, as a rule, are located in the region of interpixel space, i.e. the region between two adjacent pixels, where a sign is changed (plus to minus or vice versa) as a result of an element-wise subtraction of the filtered images. Thus, the problem of finding coordinates of an object's edge consists in identification of these points. A set of common points, which are edge points, can be obtained as a result of an element-wise transformation:

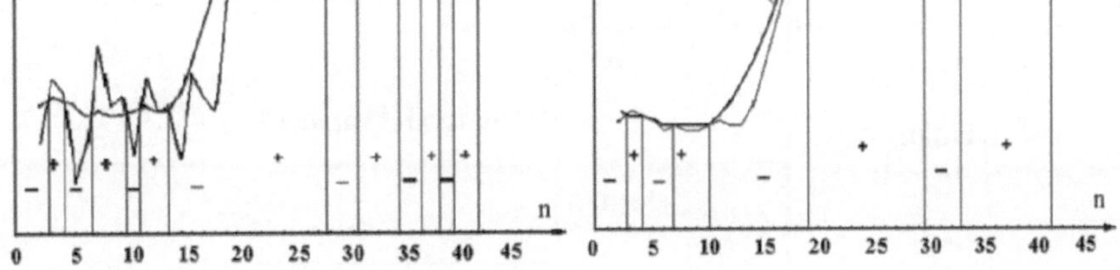

Figure 5.6 Result of low-frequency filtering: a) with further combination of the input and filtered images; b) with further combination of two filtered images.

$$h(n,m)=\begin{cases}1 & npu\;\; J((n-1),m)\cdot J(n,m)<0,\\ 1 & npu\;\; J((n-1),m)\cdot J(n,m)=0|_{J((n-1),m)\neq J(n,m)},\\ 0 & npu\;\; J((n-1),m)\cdot J(n,m)\geq 0.\end{cases} \tag{5.19}$$

The same procedure (5.19) is performed for the m axis. Furthermore, as a result of this transformation, the image edge has a great number of fake edge points caused not only by noise but also by the nonstationarity of the background and the object. In order to decrease the number of non-edge points as much as possible, it is necessary to select a filter with an optimum mask size and perform smoothing and connecting operations repetitively. This means that to detect an edge, the following concepts must be defined:

- the ratio of a difference value in intersection points of the filtered images, i.e. the difference threshold (a gradient remains high in edge pixels and tends to zero in fake edge pixels);
- an optimum low-frequency filter (a number of intensity differences not relating to an edge decreases because of repeated low-frequency filtering).

These properties of the filtered images were used for development of the edge detection method. Its block diagram is given in Figure 5.7. The image $F(n, m)$, corrupted by the noise $\nu(n, m)$, enters a detector input. Afterwards, the sets of image data $H^*(n, m)$ and $H^{**}(n, m)$ are formed as a result of filtering with a known level of smoothing σ_1 and σ_2. The stages of the edge detection using a low-frequency filtering are given in Figure 5.8. One of the main approaches to connect edge points consists in analysis of edge pixel characteristics.

Images in Figure 5.8 show that such a transformation enables getting an outline of a binary image with a great number of pixels with no relation to the edge. Therefore, edge detection algorithms, as a rule, are supplemented with appropriate procedures and additional filtering to form a substantial edge.

A gradient value and a direction of a gradient vector of different implementations are used to determine the similarity of edge pixels. In further research a few edge detectors based on low-frequency filtering have been developed. These detectors use different additional procedures of combining and forming the final contour. For the quantitative evaluation of such filtering the known *PSNR* criterion (peak signal-to-noise ratio) is used:

$$PSNR(n,m)=20Lg\frac{255}{\sqrt{\frac{1}{N}\sum_{i=1,\dots N}d(n_i,m_i)^2}}, \tag{5.20}$$

where N = total number of pixels in each image; n_i, m_i = pixels of two compared images; $d(n_i, m_i)$ = the difference in colour of the corresponding pixels (the difference of pixel values on a greyscale, and the Euclidean distance between pixels in a three-dimensional colour space for

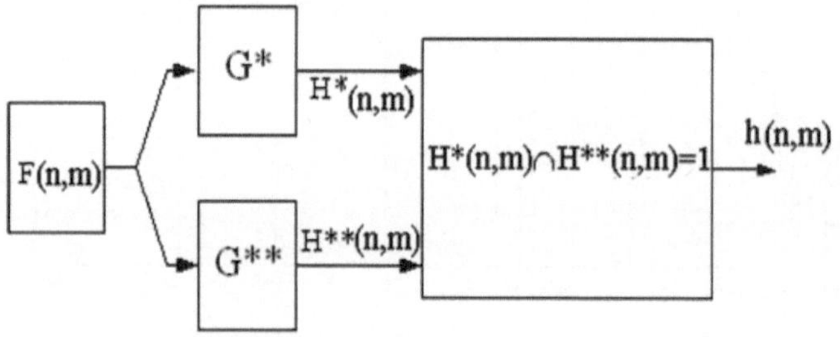

Figure 5.7 Block diagram of the edge detection method.

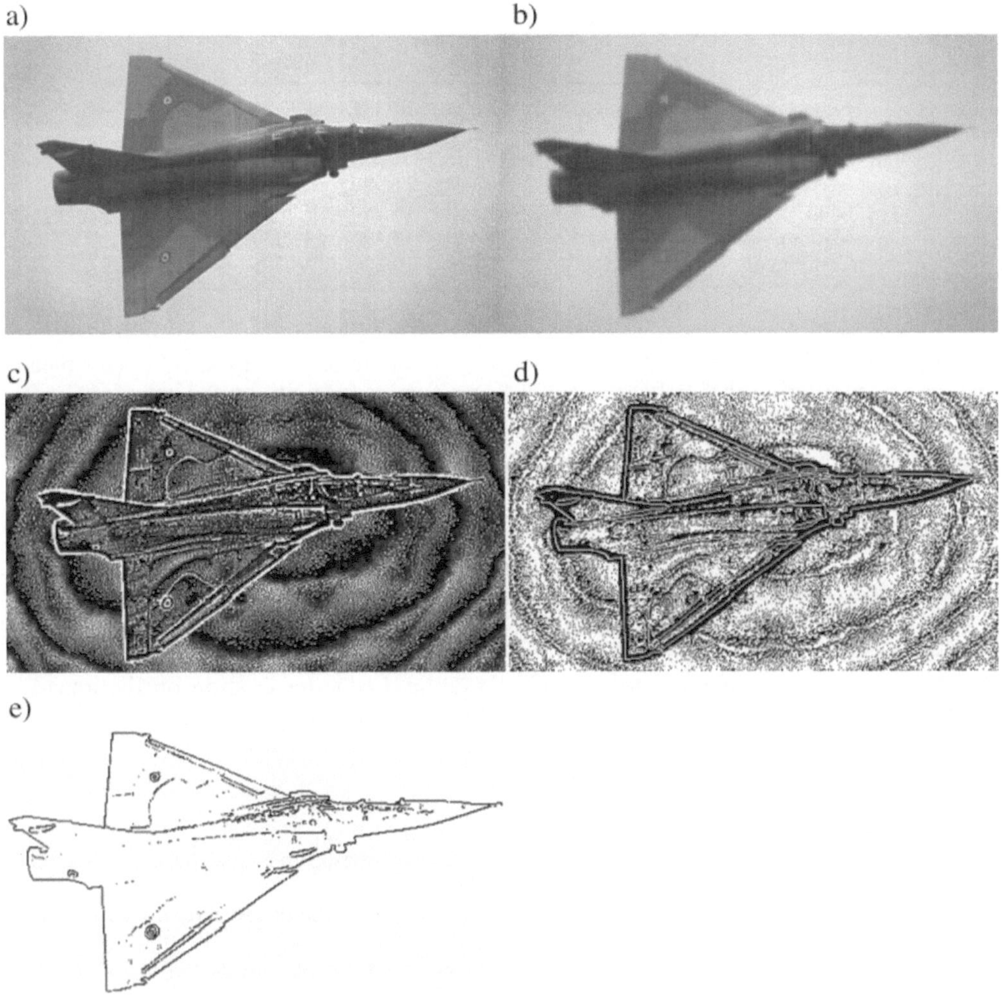

Figure 5.8. Stages of the object's edge detection: a) input image; b) smoothed image; c) subtraction result of the filtered images; d) image of shared points forming the boundary curves; e) outline image.

colour images). According to this criterion, the higher *PSNR* value, the better quality of a filter operation. Besides, a filter operation was evaluated using *RMSE*:

$$RMSE = \sqrt{\frac{\sum_i \sum_j (n(i,j) - m(i,j))^2}{N}}, \tag{5.21}$$

where $n(i, j)$ = initial image; $m(i, j)$ = filtered image; N = number of the processed pixels. According to this criterion, the lower the error value, the better quality of a detector operation. Results of noise suppression by the known and combined filters are given in Table 5.3 below. The results show that the median filter is more efficient in comparison with the linear low-frequency filter at a level of noise above 10%. Furthermore, a combination of the adaptive median filter with a low-frequency filter improves the parameters of the image. The high

Table 5.3 Filtering quality comparison.

	10%		20%		40%	
Filter type	PSNR	RMSE	PSNR	RMSE	PSNR	RMSE
No filtering	29.870	24.550	26.900	34.550	24.960	48.120
Average	38.000	9.560	36.100	11.990	33.290	16.570
Gaussian	35.110	13.420	34.160	14.980	32.000	17.300
Median	36.530	11.400	34.450	14.490	34.830	20.560
Combined	37.639	10.040	37.228	10.520	36.355	11.639

filtering quality of the combined filter remains even at a noise level up to 80%. This means that combined filtering should be used to find an object's edge point on the image.

6 CONCLUSIONS

A new method for edge detection based on low-frequency filtering is proposed. The method uses a polynomial interpolation to reproduce a continuous boundary curve and provides sub-pixel coordinates of the object's edge points on the image. The experimental results clearly showed and confirmed the validity of using the proposed method. An edge detection error in an inerpixel space is less in comparison to the results obtained by the zero crossing method. Based on the proposed method for an object's subpixel edge localisation on the image, a method for edge detection using low-frequency filtering is developed.

REFERENCES

Abdou, I.E. 1979. A quantitative calculation of circuits detectors based on emphasizing the differences of brightness followed thresholds. *TIIER* 67(5): 59–70.

Bertero, M. & Poggio, T. 1988. Incorrect problems in the pre-processing of visual information. *TIIER* 76(8): 17–39.

Bilynskyy, Y.Y. 2007. Mathematical model of localization edge of the image object. *Information Technology and Computer Engineering* 10: 73–79.

Dyakonov, V.P. 2001. *Computer's Mathematica. Theory and Practice*. Moscow: Knowledge.

Furman, Y.A., Krevetskyi, A.V., Peredreev, A.K., et al. 2003. *Introduction to the contour analysis. Application to image processing and signal*. Moscow: FIZMATLIT.

Marr, D. & Hildret, E. 1980. Theory of edge detection. In *Proceedings of the Royal Society of London* B-207(1167): 187–217.

Rusyn, B.P. 1977. *Systems synthesis, processing and recognition of complex structured image*. Lviv: Vertical.

CHAPTER 6

Magnetocardiographic technology for human heart investigation

M.A. Primin & I.V. Nedayvoda
V.M. Glushkov Institute of Cybernetics, Kiev, Ukraine

A. Smolarz & W. Surtel
Lublin University of Technology, Lublin, Poland

B. Suleimenov
Kazakh National Research Technical University after K. I. Satpaev, Almaty, Kazakhstan

1 INTRODUCTION

Upon excitation of the myocardium, there is an electromagnetic field in the human body and in the surrounding area. Magnetocardiography (MCG) realises the registration and analysis of the magnetic component of the field, and the ECG—the electric component. Therefore, the same biophysical model is used in order to explain the nature and characteristics of an MCG signal, as well as the ECG signal. Variation of the magnetic field corresponding to cardiocycles is called an MCG-curve. The MCG-curve has a similar shape and is described by the same set of names of the peaks, segments and intervals as an electrocardiogram. Note that the MCG signal of adults is as low as tens of pT (10^{-12}Tesla), so it is a million times smaller than the external magnetic field of the earth in the measurement point. Thus magnetic signal requires special, more complex and expensive registration systems compared to the ECG. Measurements of the magnetic signal of the heart are provided by using SQUID magnetometer systems. Accordingly, magnetocardiography must possess a high diagnostic efficiency compared to the ECG to ensure "right to use" in a clinical practice. MCG has a diagnostic efficiency, in our opinion, due to fundamental differences between this method and potential methods (ECG, mapping of the body surface potentials—BSPM). Specifically, the MCG measurements are performed not only non-invasive, but non-contact; a magnetometric system itself has no effect on the electrophysiological processes in the heart since under registration of diagnostic information; it does not radiate any energy. It is also known that the conductive volume of the human body is "transparent" to the magnetic field of the heart with a high degree of accuracy and does not affect the signal detected by the magnetometer system. Thus, when measuring using MCG, we obtain a direct information on the currents in the heart, when using ECG—on currents flowing in the human body and intermediary in heart.

In cardiac electrophysiology it was found that almost any reason of pathology is related to the mechanism of ion current density variation across the cell membrane. This density of changing relative to normal—it is the first functional disorders that lead to pathology. Thus, MCG, which is sensitive mainly to the inside and to extracellular ion currents of the heart, provides more earlier diagnostic information than the known potential methods (Electrocardiography—ECG; Body Surface Potentials Mapping—BSPM). Moreover, data of potential measurement (ECG) contain no information about the shape of the current field source elements whose potentials are recorded on the body surface, while magnetometric data contain information about the spatial configuration of the ionic current in the heart.

On the basis of biophysical models adopted in cardiology it is known that the propagation of the wave front of myocardium excitation circulates from epicardium to endocardium and of myocardium depolarisation in the opposite direction, provided in the normal case by the prevalence rate of radial action currents on the tangential. Registration of the potential signals (ECG, BSPM) allows to record and analyse potential changes, associated with predominantly the radial components of the current. By measuring the component of the magnetic field of the heart (MCG), normally to the chest, we actually register the magnetic signal associated with the current of the heart, which is located in a plane parallel to the plane of the measurement (tangential components with respect to the surface of the patient's chest). In other words, the anomalous zones of the tangential components of the current density could be a markers of occurrence of functional and/or pathological changes even with the constant radial component of the vector's current density.

These reasons reasonably allow to assume that the recorded a magnetocardiographic signal more completely and accurately reflects the electrical processes in the heart. Also, magnetocardiography is more sensitive than electrocardiography, primarily to changes in the distribution (including spatial) of the current density vector in the myocardium. In other words, the structure of the magnetic signal is changed in those cases where the electrocardiographic signal is normal.

Thus, by non-contact measurement of the magnetic field parameters of the heart in the air above the human chest and proper restoration of the spatial distribution of its sources in the heart, one can notice the first changes in the spatial structure of ion currents which are precursors of later pathology.

Developing a super-sensitive equipment is only a part of the problem of contactless diagnostics. Another essential component of the high technology which determines the possibility and success of such systems' application is the developing of information technology for the interpretation of the magnetometric measurements data. This requires theoretical studies and the development of new mathematical models and methods to restore the space-time image of the distribution of the field sources in the human heart.

Thus, magnetocardiographic technology is a new medical technology and provides technical and software tools, combined in the developed diagnostic complexes of the "MAGSCAN" series (Primin et al. 2010, Cryoton 2016). Such complexes do not require special equipment and a magnetic shielding room, which opens up the possibility of their wide use in conventional urban clinics. Manufactured diagnostic systems have passed technical and clinical trials.

Additional advantages of magnetocardiography application in the medicine in comparison with, for example, ECG and BSPM include: (a) a quick examination of a large mass of people (screening); (b) MCG registration for patients in a cast or bandages, and patients with burns, where it is impossible or undesirable to use electrodes mounted on the body of the patient.

2 TECHNOLOGY OF MAGNETOCARDIOGRAPHIC STUDY

The procedure of patient examination using magnetocardiography consists of several stages: preparatory; MCG data registration; record of MCG data to database; computer processing of magnetocardiosignal (MCS); space-and-time analysis of MCG and its sources; obtaining the automatic report.

The preparatory stage. Before making the measurements the patient is relieved of part of the outer wear. Special attention should be paid to the lack of metal objects that can interfere with the magnetic field of the heart during the investigation as well as to the availability of places to place the ECG electrodes (usually recorded standard lead II). To perform the examination, the patient is placed on a couch, which provides its positioning in a predetermined position relative to the fixed suspension system with the magnetometric unit of the complex. A magnetocardiograph is shown in Figure 6.1.

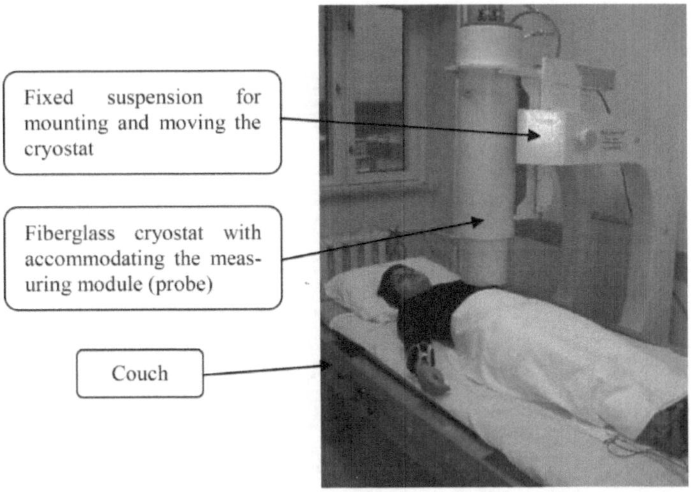

Figure 6.1 Magnetocardiographic complex "MAGSCAN".

The magnetocardiographic complex "MAGSCAN" (Cryoton 2016) provides 9 channels for magnetocardiosignal (MCS) recording and 3 reference channels, which are used in the system of electronic noise suppression. Each channel for MCS registration comprises a magnetic flux transformer in the form of the second order axial gradiometer ($\partial^2 B_z/\partial z^2$), made from NbTi superconducting wires on a cylindrical graphite base 20 mm in diameter. The transformer is connected to the DC-SQUID (direct current SQUID) and placed in a superconducting shield. The reference channels are in the form of a vector SQUID magnetometer, which consists of three separate DC-SQUIDs arranged on the respective sides of the cube to the size of the edge, equal to 12 mm. In the process of the MCG examination, the couch with the patient is moved relative to the fixed cryostat with a measuring module sequentially in 4 spatial positions. The movement is performed in such a way that after the location of centres of the flux transformer of MCG, the recording channels are forming a system of 36 points in the plane (6 × 6 along mutually perpendicular directions with a step of 4 cm). Figure 6.2 shows a diagram of the points of magnetocardiosignal (MCS) registration in relation to the patient's chest and its "binding" to the anatomical landmarks (at *jugular foci*).

Magnetocardiosignal registration takes about one minute in each of the spatial positions for the accumulation of 30–60 cardiocycles. The shape and amplitude of the magnetic field of the heart is different at the points of measurement used, and have a local maximum in the positions closest to the heart. Minimising the distance between the heart and the measuring unit is performed by a preliminary check by moving of the patient in all positions. At the same time there should be no contact between the chest and the cryostat during the patient's breath intake. After performing this procedure, a couch is set and fixed in the first position and ECG electrodes are placed and connected (standard lead II). The patient is ready to conduct the MCG investigation.

MCG registration records magnetocardiosignal (MCS) in all 36 points of the measurement grid (Fig. 6.2). Magnetocardiosignals—values of the parameters of the magnetic field of the heart—are recorded synchronously on all channels sequentially in each of the positions. In the standard mode, the duration of the MCS registration in each of the positions takes 30 seconds. The final step in this phase of the investigation involves recording of MCG registration data to database and executing signals pre-processing in an automatic mode. Such express analysis allows the operator to control the quality of the recorded MCG. If

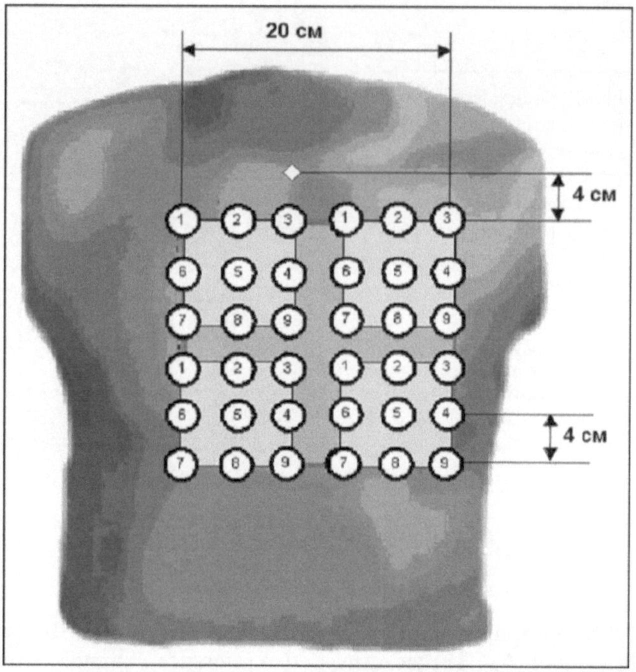

Figure 6.2 Arrangement of MCG recording channels and positions of the measuring module of the 9 recording channels in relation to the patient's chest.

there are significant impulses or low-frequency harmonic noise in averaged MCG results, the operator must return to the registration of the MCS and repeat the recording.

3 PRINCIPLES AND STAGES OF MAGNETOCARDIOSIGNAL ANALYSIS

At the first steps of the MCG development, the MCG Analysis methods are reproducing the ECG analysis methods: all the names of ECG peaks, segments and intervals were used without changes. The morphological features of the MCG at different points of measurements plane were studied and a few amplitude-temporal criteria for the diagnosis of some disease symptoms were found and described. It is necessary to understand that the MCG processing peculiarity is that the object of the study is one averaged cardio complex at given points of measurements plane (in our case the number of points is 36: a 6×6 grid with a distance of 4 cm between the points placed along the mutually perpendicular axis). During the ECG analysis the subject of the study is the temporal sequence of complexes of the determined number of ECG leads. Therefore "the direct transfer" of ECG analysis methods into MCG analysis prevents from using in this case the main advantage of MCG—the high sensitivity of this method to the changes of spatial-temporal distribution of currents density vector or to the changes of distributions of the measured values of the heart magnetic field in the borders of the measurements area.

As a result, the next step in the development of MCG analysis and interpretation methods was the development of new computer analysis methods directed to the study of spatial (in the borders of the measurements area) and temporal (in one or a sequence of discontinuous temporal points of the cardiocycle) characteristics of the MCG signal.

Computer processing of MCG starts from digital filtration and averaging of MCG data (Voytovych et al. 2002). Averaging (accumulation) of MCG cardio-cycles supposes the synchronisation of them with respect to some temporal moment of support at any recurring QRS complex. Moreover, binding to the support point inside already averaged cardio-cycles is necessary for the synchronisation of MCG measurements at different space points made at different time intervals. Since ECG and MCG are caused by the activity of the same electrophysiological sources, the support time moments and cardio-cycle borders are chosen from the second standard of the ECG lead. All the process is made automatically, but in the case of need the manual correction of all the filtration and averaging parameters is possible. As a result of the initial processing, the file with temporal sampling of averaged cardio-cycles is created for every type of the QRS complex and for every 36 points of space where MCG recording was performed (Fig. 6.3).

The cardio-cycle after the averaging includes the complete P-QRS-T complex with the segments of base (zero) line before and after the complex. The averaged cardio-cycles are synchronised in all the measurement points. The sample consisting of all the sampling recordings with the same numbers (equidistant from the start of the cardio-complex) characterises the spatial distribution of the measured field characteristic at a specific moment of the cardio-cycle. The program block Projbma.exe is used for the study of the magnetic field spatial structure and its changing dynamics during the different cardio-cycle intervals. The main functions of this program block are: the visual analysis of the spatial structure of measured magnetic field parameters at any moment of the cardio-cycle; the representation of the map dynamics and correlative estimation of the similarity of the heart magnetic field distribution for any interval of the cardio-cycle; the allocation of the analysis interval and formation of the data files which are the input information for the solution of the inverse problem; numerical estimation of the spatial-temporal MCG signal variations at specific intervals of the cardio-cycle; the record of numerical estimations of average cardio-cycles in the diagnostic parameter files.

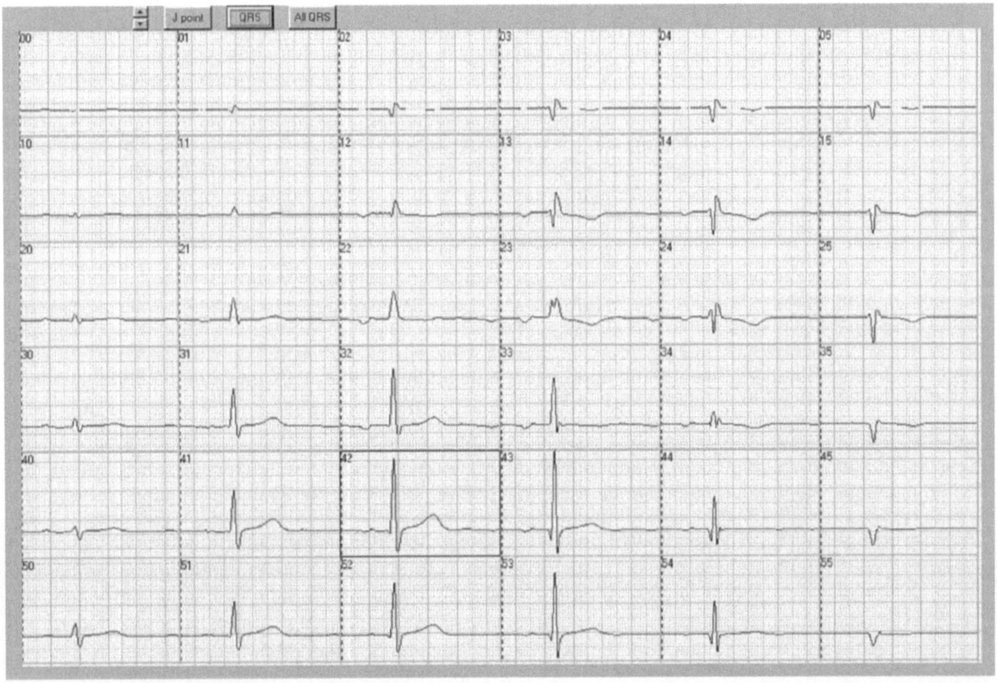

Figure 6.3 Averaged MCG cardio-cycles in 36 points of rectangular measurements grid—an example of the representation on the computer screen.

Figure 6.4, the so called butterfly graph, shows all 36 synchronous MCG cardio complexes. Also shown here are the cursor positions used to fix the (or to correct the automatically obtained) borders of the investigation interval, the location of the base line and the corresponding numerical parameters, the calculation of which is performed by the program Projbma.exe.

The program also calculates the average weighted temporal variations over the measurement subarea of such specific points of the cardio-cycle as the peak locations of "P", "Q"; "R" and "T". The set of calculated parameters and the average weighted variations for several subareas of the measuring grid presented in a numerical view reflects the features of the spatial-temporal structure of the patient's heart's magnetic field is used during the solution of the problem of classification.

Construction and analysis of the dynamic sequence of the spatial-temporal distribution of the parameter value of the patient's heart's magnetic field in the borders of measurement grid (magnetic field map) for the chosen time moments of averaged cardio-cycle is one of the main and obvious stages of the MCG analysis. Figure 6.5 shows as an example of the sequence of the magnetic maps during the ST-T interval for a healthy patient and for a patient with the ischemia heart disease.

Each map presents the measured magnetic field distribution not only in the given 36 points of measurement plane but also in the points of a finer grid. The signal values in these lattice points (not corresponding to the initial 36 points) are calculated using interpolation methods. The magnetic field maps can be generated (calculated and represented) with the time interval of 1 ms. Such MCG signal presentation has the following peculiarities:

- It is possible to study the multi-pole heart generator and get the more precise evaluation of the local electrical activity of the heart muscle;
- The information is presented as the time sequence of magnetic field distribution maps (dynamic sequence), so it is possible to study the de—and repolarisation processes dynamic of, for example, heart ventricular system;
- It is possible to use for MCG study the up-to-date image analysis and pattern recognition methods (solution methods of classification problems).

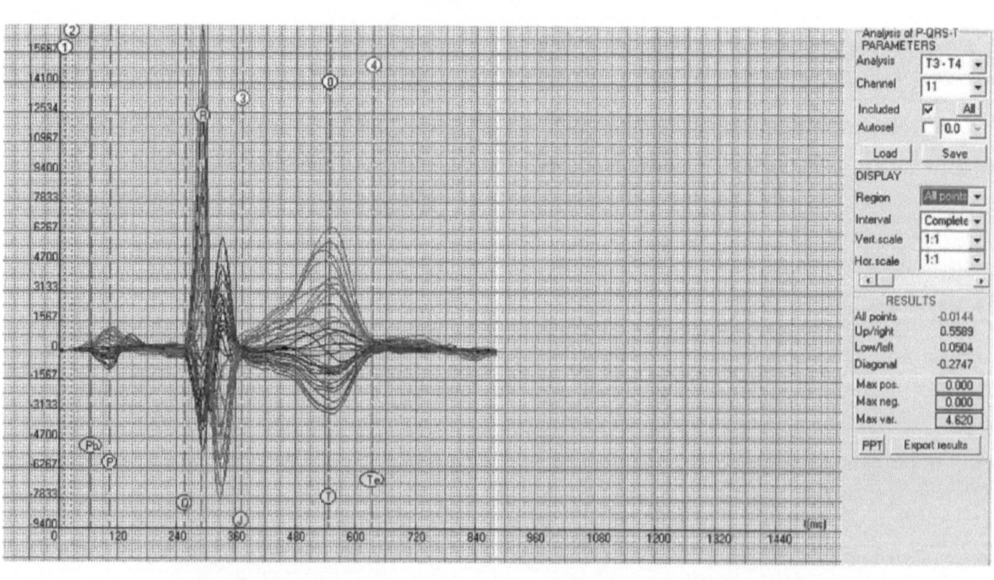

Figure 6.4 "Matched P-QRS-T" cardio-complex with a marked period of repolarisation (an example of the representation on the computer screen).

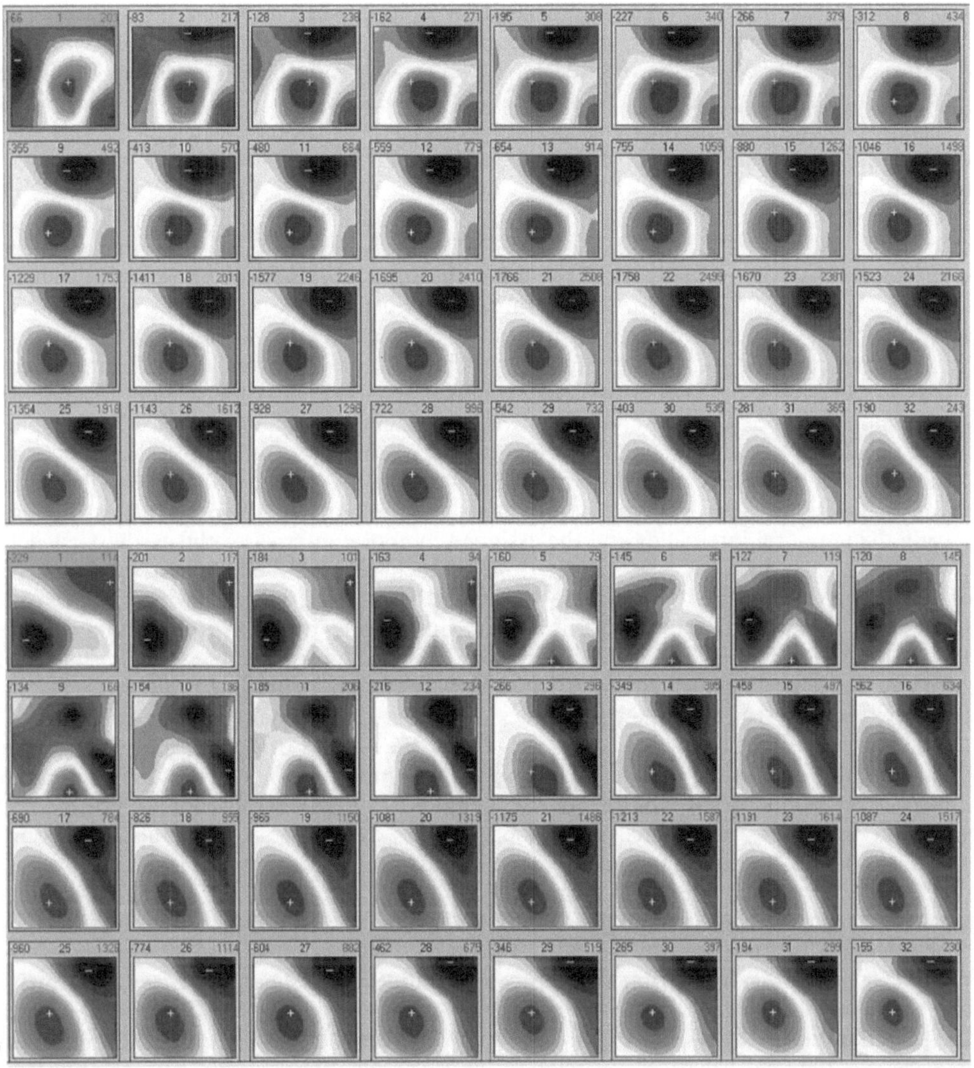

a)

b)

Figure 6.5 Heart magnetic field distribution (ST-T interval) in the norm (a) and in the case of the left coronary artery occlusion (b).

During the study of the ventricular repolarisation process the known electrophysiological model is used as the hypothesis. This model supposes that the beginning of the ST-T interval clashes with the start of the slow repolarisation phase (action potential plateau). If all areas of the myocardium simultaneously enter into this phase, we get the magnetic field map with "normal" structure from the start of ST interval (two extremes—positive and negative, the map is symmetrical with respect to the diagonal, the maximum positive value exceeds the absolute value of the negative in the range 1.3–2.3 on the entire range of ST-T). However, even in the norm we may observe some heterogeneity (dispersion) of the repolarisation on the first part of ST. It becomes apparent in the fact that the first few magnetic field distribution maps (and currents maps as well) have modified (another) structure compared with all other maps from the ST-T interval. At the increase of the heterogeneity level as a result of the change of the action potential shape (for example because of ischemia or other pathological processes), the number of myocardium areas with unfinished depolarisation can increase. It leads to the increase of maps with abnormal field distribution. If after some moments all the myocardium areas are in the same action potential phase then the recovery of the field distribution map structure happens.

It is possible to estimate the heterogeneity durability and the nature of the magnetic maps during the visual analysis of the MCG of the investigated patient and/or using the special magnetocardiograph software.

For the study and analysis of the homogeneity of the heart ventricular repolarisation processes using the magneto-cardiograph MAG-Scan, the program block Spcwin.exe is developed and used (Voytovych et al. 2002). After the start of this program the MCG analysis in the ST-T interval is performed according to a special algorithm. As this is taking place, consistently for each time moment (for every magnetic map) of the investigated section of the averaged cardio-cycle, the intensity value of the human heart magnetic field gradient g {(0,0); (*dx*,0); (2*dx*,0); …; (*Idx*,0)} is determined at given points of the straight line connecting the points of positive (M^+) and negative (M^-) magnetic field extremums. The graphical image of g (*idx*,0) values is named as spectrums lines, and the sequence of these lines is constructed for the analysed cardio-cycle interval using a special algorithm—the spatial spectrum of magneto-cardio-signal. To get the quantitative estimation of the magneto-cardio-signal during the temporal interval dt and the assigned temporal interval of the cardio-cycle let us consider the spectrums for the "current" time moment and for the following (next) moment of time. As a rule, during the considered interval (the ascending segment of ST-T), the magnetic signal amplitude in the "norm" increases from the previous to the following moment of time. After the normalisation of the measurements results it is possible to claim that in the "norm", the ascending segment of ST-T, any following spectrum line must be bigger than the previous one. However, the coordinates (location) of the change of the field source in the heart with respect to the measurements plane, the change of the orientation of current density vectors and/or the change of their spatial distribution can lead to the appearance of the spectrum points where this rule is not realised. In other words, there are points of the spectrum, where at some moment t_k the "spectral line" is equal to zero, but at some moment t_{k+1} it is different from zero and vice versa. The total amount of "inversions" in all points of the spectrum, where at least one of the lines is not equal to zero, can be determined using known algorithms. Thus, we will get a set of spectrums $g(x_i,t_0),...,g(x_i,t_N)$ during the chosen time interval ST-T. On the other hand, for each spectrum point x_i the value of the studied parameter g for every given time moment was found. Presenting all these values in one picture (or on the monitor) gives the spatial-temporal spectrum of the MCG signal. Along with the presentation of the quality picture of the MCG signal changes during the chosen time interval, the founded values of inversion criteria also give the quantity evaluation of these changes.

The present approach of MCG evaluation is realised in the "MAGSCAN" software for the whole ST-T interval and the inversions calculation algorithm, which consists of the following:

- the lengths of the spectrum lines are compared in every point;
- if the length of the spectrum line at some time moment (t_{i+1}) exceeds the length of the spectrum line at moment (t_i), then the inversion number increases by 1 (Rule 1, applied to the growing part of *ST-T segment*);
- if the length of the spectrum line at some time moment (t_{i+1}) falls short of the length of the spectrum line at moment (t_i), then the inversion number increases by 1 (Rule 2, applied to the decreasing part of *ST-T segment*).

Then the algorithm realisation follows the steps below:

1. The angle θ between the perpendicular to line AB connecting the points M^+ and M^-, and the referent line are the coordinate axes OX for every chosen time moment from the analysed interval

2. Taking into account that value of the angle θ can change from 0° to ± 180° during the next step, the program creates the graphical picture of a circle diagram, divided into sectors by line segments, whose direction coincides with the obtained values of the θ angle. The circle is divided into 10 adjacent sectors. Sectors 1–9 have the same area and sector 0 is three times bigger. Each sector has its own weight coefficient, the weight coefficient of sector 0 is zero. The weight coefficient values of sectors 0–6 are positive and those of the other sectors—negative. The coefficient values, which define the spatial position of the magnetic field extremums on the measurements plane during the whole ST-T interval, are determined taking into account the accepted weights of the circle sector.
3. The building and estimation of the spatial spectrum of the magnetic field distribution between the M^+ and M^- points of measurement plane.
4. The building and estimation of the spatial spectrum on the map interval which corresponds to the projection of the M^+ M^- segment on the coordinates axes OX.
5. The building and estimation of the spatial spectrum in the lattice points of the measurements grid.
6. The absolute values of the relations of the maximum value of the magnetic field to the minimum (by absolute) value are calculated for every moment of time of the analysed time interval (in the standard regime 64 or 32 moments of time). The temporal dependence of this value is built in a graphical view for the whole analysed time interval.
7. Calculation of the correlation dependence between the magnetic field map corresponding to the time moment T_{max} and all the other time moments from the interval ST-T (under assumption that the field source is a dipole). The temporal dependence of this value is built for the whole time interval studied.

All the parameters listed (and others (Voytovych et al. 2002, Nedayvoda et al. 2010, Nedayvoda et al. 2009)) are available during the analysis of the MCG signal of each patient in "step-by-step" mode (in this case it is important to analyse visually the graphical presentation of the values characterising the temporal changes of the patient's heart's magnetic field) and during the analysis of groups of patients (numerical parameters are in this case written in special data files).

Figure 6.6 shows an example of one variant of information presentation during the work of the Spcwin.exe program block:

The reconstruction and analysis of the magnetic field sources distributed in the heart volume is performed on the next stage of the MCG study. Maploc.exe is the program block to solve the magnetostatics inverse problem for the dipole model of the MCG signal source. After the start, this program performs the solution and analysis of the magnetostatics inverse problem for the "focal" pathologies for given time moments from a chosen cardio-cycle interval. By mathematical nature the transformation methods of MCG information (for this stage of the study) correspond to the solution of the so called magnetostatics inverse problem for the dipole model of the magnetic signal source. The authors of the "MAGSCAN" information technology have proposed to use as a biomagnetic signal source the so called magnetic dipole and have formulated the solution to the problem in the form of simple algebraic equations (ratios). The developed method (Primin et al. 2009) is realised in the form of *Maploc.exe* program blocks of the magneto-cardiograph and is used successfully in cardio-hospitals to find the location of arrhythmia (fibrillation) sources in the heart. Metal rings 10 mm in diameter were used for connecting the results of of the localisation of the magnetic field source with the anatomical reference points in the heart. These coils were fixed on the patient's thorax over the problem place. The coordinates of this place were calculated during the processing of the measurement data of the MCG signal (after the ***Maploc.exe*** program had been applied). The metal coils are well distinguishable in the X-ray light during the surgery operation (Fig. 6.7).

The accuracy of calculating the coordinates of the magnetic field's focal source of is better than 5 mm.

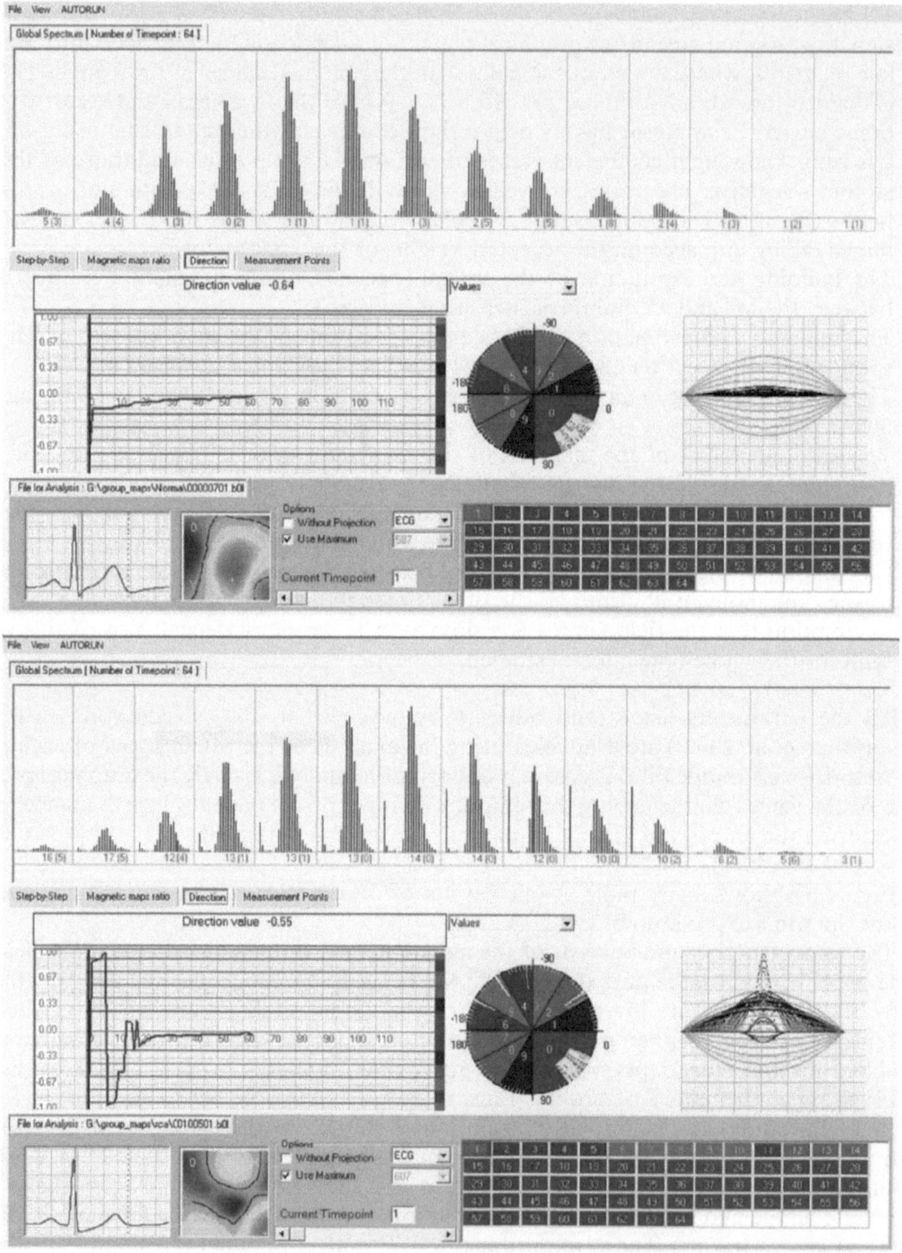

a)

b)

Figure 6.6 Example of presenting information on the computer screen in a "step-by-step" mode of MCG analysis: the homogeneity study of the repolarisation process of the heart's ventricular system – (a) – the norm; (b) – ischemia heart disease.

At the next stage it is possible to find a solution to the magnetostatics inverse problem for several independent magnetic field sources distributed in the heart. In other words, the "MAGSCAN" program makes it possible to find and localise non-invasively the position of several simultaneously existing pathology zones by no-contact method.

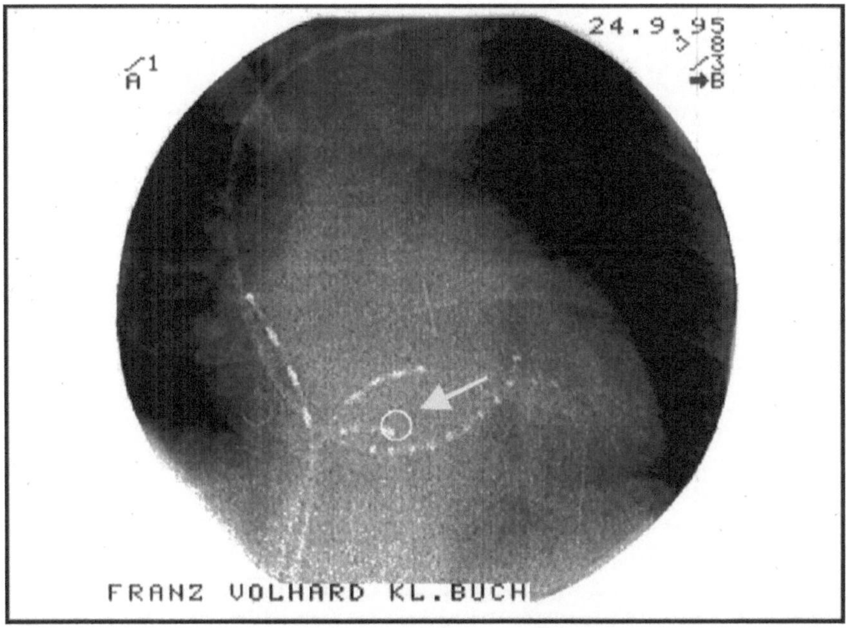

Figure 6.7 View of the X-ray scanner screen during the high frequency ablation of an additional conduction way under WPW syndrome. The arrow shows the position of a 10 mm wide metal coil against the background of the heart. The coordinates of this coil are defined during the MCG signal analysis and the point inside the coil is the catheter position during ablation.

Figure 6.8 demonstrates the view of a few versions of the presentation results of the "MAGSCAN" program complex (block Maploc.exe) in "step-by-step" mode of MCG data processing.

The program block used for MCG signal analysis is called Curwin.exe. This program is intended for the solution of the magnetostatics inverse problem for the bio-magnetic signal source presented as the system of currents distributed on a plane which is cutting the heart and is parallel to the measurements plane (Nedayvoda et al. 2008, Primin et al. 2007). When this program starts the solution and the analysis of magnetostatics inverse problem is performed for the pathologies connected with the changes of electro-physiological properties in the big volume of the myocardium: the revealing of patients with the ischemia disease of the heart (CAD), monitoring of heart-patients after (or during) different courses of treatment, localisation of the part of coronary artery responsible for ischemia, etc.

Figure 6.9 shows as an example a few versions of data representation during the work of the "MAGSCAN" program complex (block Curwin.exe) in the "step-by-step" mode of MCG data processing.

It is clear that to analyse the MCG signal it is possible to use magnetic field distribution maps and the proper current density maps received after the inverse problem solution. Current distribution maps give more complete and correct information in comparison with the maps of magnetic field distribution in the measurement area. On the one hand, the inverse problem solution as found in the spatial distribution of the current density vector over the plane parallel to the measurements plane corresponds uniquely to the measured heart magnetic field for the given moment of the cardio-cycle and decreases the influence of anthropometric variations of different patients on the analysis results. On the other hand, the current distribution map obtained after the inverse problem solution allows to interpret the local

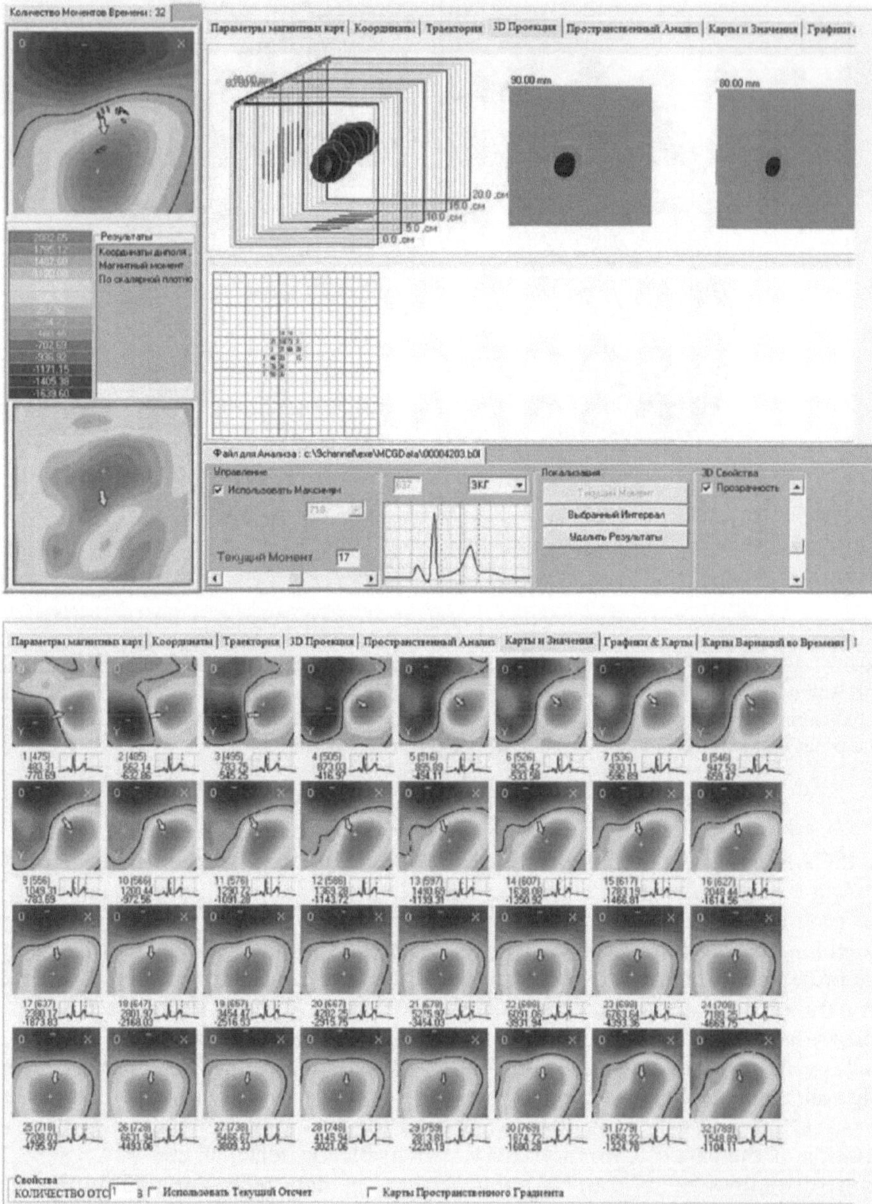

a)

b)

Figure 6.8 Example of MCG data processing presentation on the computer screen during the work of the *Maploc.exe* program in "step-by-step" mode during one of the patient's MCG study.

electrical processes in the myocardium in correspondence with their real distribution. Let us note that the study of the current density vector distribution maps in MCG is not similar to ECG diagnostics. That analysis is most commonly used to generate diagnostic conclusions.

The limits of the map with the distribution of the current density vector correspond to the limits of the measurements area. The distance from the plane where this distribution was found to the measurements plane is determined by the distance to the most "active" zone

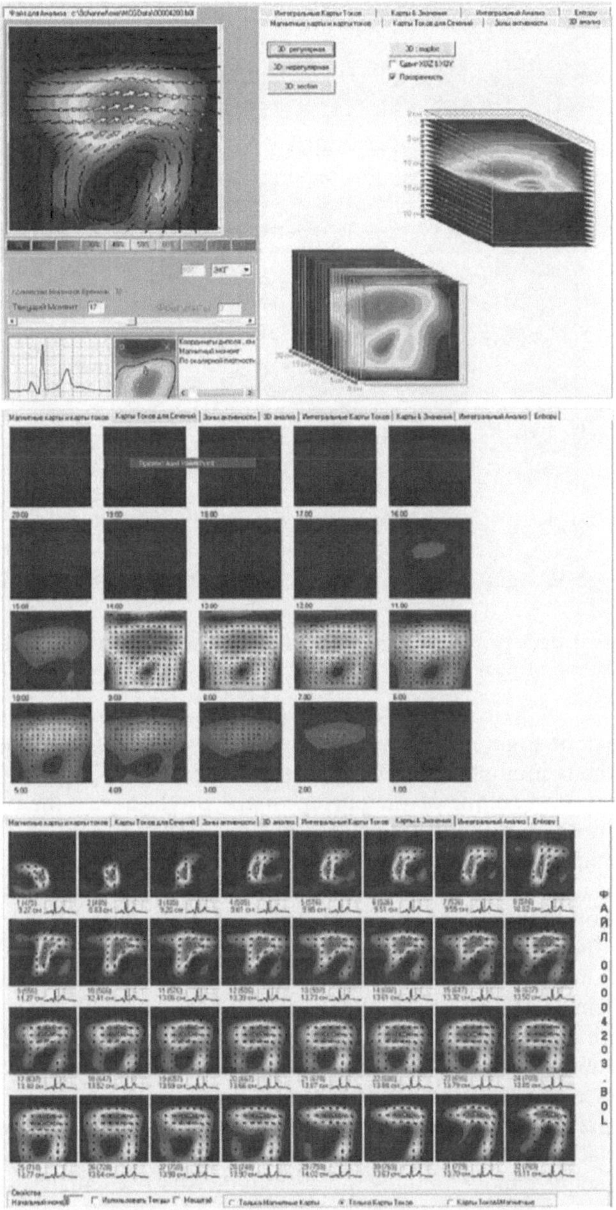

a)

b)

c)

Figure 6.9 Examples of data imaging of MCG processing during the inverse problem solution in "step-by-step" mode of the program Curwin.exe: (a) and (b) – layer-to-layer inverse problem solution for a given cardio-cycle time moment and representation of this solution over the corresponding layers of the tree-dimensional heart volume; (c) –sequence of distribution maps of the current density vectors over the analysed cardio-cycle time interval.

in the heart for the given time moment of the cardio-cycle (determined by the Maploc.exe program). Figure 6.10 demonstrates an example of one map of the current density vector distribution for the time point coincident with the top of the "T" peak of the cardio-cycle.

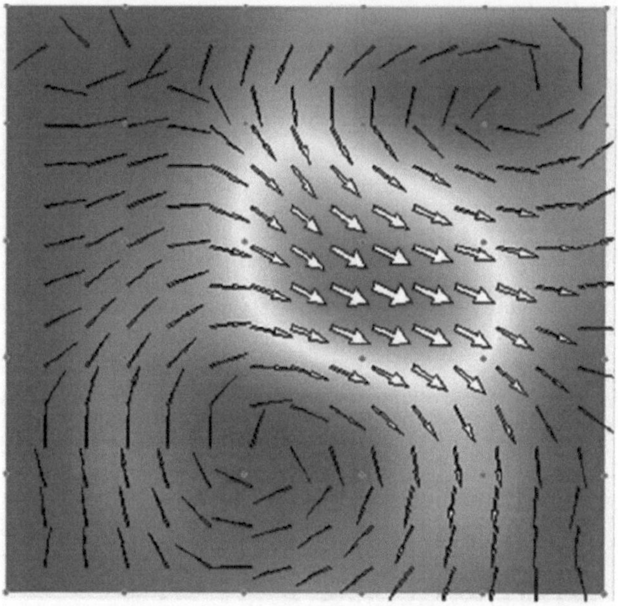

Figure 6.10 Current density vector distribution found after the inverse problem solution: "norm"; time moment of the top of peak "T".

To a certain extent Figure 6.10 presents the picture of currents proportional to real currents in one of the frontal planes transversal to the heart. The arrows' size, their density as well as the background colour of the current map correlate with the projection, value and density of real currents in the heart volume on this plane. The more things the arrows are presenting, the smaller are the values of current density. The increase of the distance between the arrows means a smaller density of values over the distribution plane. The analysis of the current distribution map includes the map structure analysis and the analysis of the values and direction of these vectors. Under the map structure we understand the quantity, relative intensity and mutual arrangement of zones with increased electrical activity (in the limits of the inverse problem solution area). If the current distribution map has a view of Figure 6.10 (has one area with an increased electrical activity in the central part of the map), this map is called homogeneous. Figure 6.11 shows an example of the map for the same time moment (as in Fig. 6.10) for the patient with abnormalities of heart functioning.

On the map presented in Figure 6.11, the areas of maximum vectors are situated not symmetrically relative to the centre of the map and have another direction of vectors. The homogeneity principle can be used for the current density map analysis for any cardio-cycle interval—as the map is more homogeneous as it is closer to the "norm" (as a rule).

Analysis and estimation of the location (coordinates) and direction of the current density vector of the electrical activity area must have an "association" to the considered cardio-cycle interval, which concludes the investigated map. The numerical parameters (coordinates of the vectors with the maximum density, the vector angle in the accepted coordinates system) are determined automatically or after the user inquiry (command) and are written in special table-files. Figure 6.12 shows an example of presenting the location of the myocardium electrical activity areas for the above MCG at the same time moment (top of the "T" peak).

Analysis of the current density distribution vector maps gives the opportunity to estimate simultaneously the structure, direction and relative values of the current vectors for the studied cardio-cycle intervals.

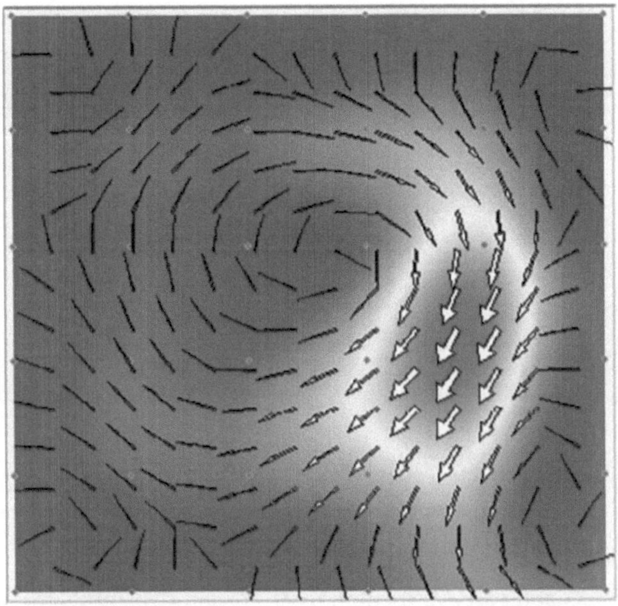

Figure 6.11 Current density vector distribution found after the inverse problem solution: ischemia heart disease (IHT); time moment corresponds to the top of peak "T".

a)

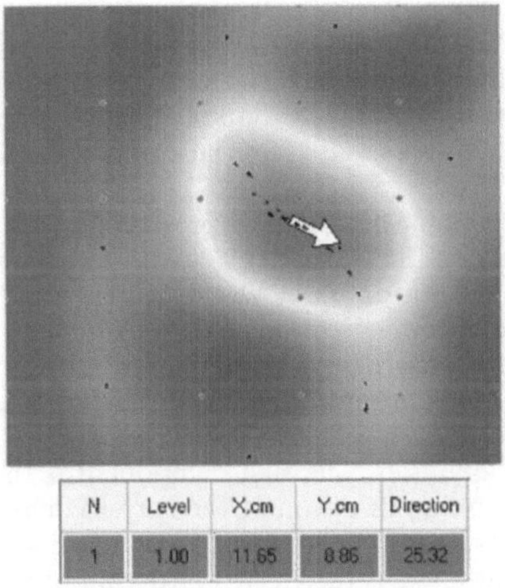

b)

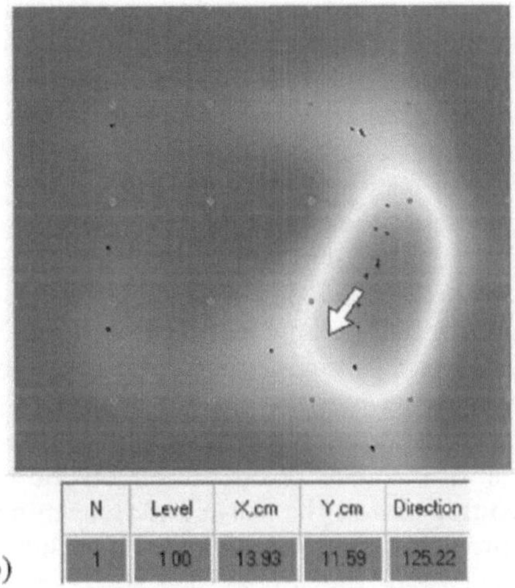

Figure 6.12 Example of the presentation of the zones with the maximum electrical activity during MCG processing: (a) "norm", time moment corresponding to the top of the "T" peak; (b) ischemia heart disease, time moment corresponding to the top of the "T" peak.

The experience of study and analysis of big groups of patients with different diagnosis shows that the parameters (location, relative current density value, current direction in the accepted coordinates system) of the electrical activity zones identified in the heart are important for diagnostics, their visualisation and method of presentation give additional information about the processes in the human heart. This is why one more algorithm of presentation

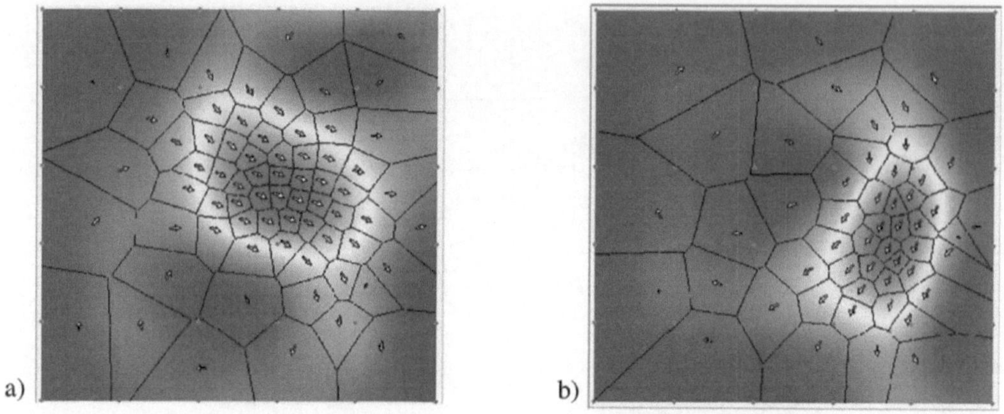

Figure 6.13 Example of the presentation of maximumelectrical activity zones obtained during MCG processing on an irregular grid: (a) "norm", time moment corresponds to the top of the "T" peak; (b) ischemia heart disease, time moment corresponds to the top of the "T" peak.

is realised in the MCG software—presentation of current density vector distribution on an irregular grid (Fig. 6.13).

The quantity and mutual location of irregular lattice points in Figure 6.13 corresponds to the spatial distribution of current density vectors in regular lattice points. The number of irregular grid segments depends of the distribution structure of the current vectors and an average current density vector is shown in the centre of each segment. The variations in the structure and location of the biomagnetic signal source during the cardio-cycle will be mapped under the correct solution of the inverse problem in the change of direction of current density vectors. Therefore such variants of the visualisation of the inverse problem solution can be used for the quality of MCG analysis as well as for the automatic classification of groups of patients. Let us note that, according to the adopted biophysical models of processes, the biomagnetic signal source passing in the heart can be presented as the spatial distribution of the currents in the heart volume on the boundary between the excited and not excited myocardium parts during its depolarisation or between the regenerated and not regenerated myocardium parts in the phase of repolarisation of the ventricular system. The emergent currents can be described as consisting of two components—the "primary current", which are created by the difference of ion concentration on cells membranes, and the second component, which is caused by the gradient of trans-membrane action potential in the volume conductor on the media boundaries. The first component is the main component in the norm and determines the resulting direction of the current density vector. This direction is connected with the appropriating time moment of the cardio-cycle. In the case of the appearance of different type pathologies the electro-physical properties of the myocardium parts change and this can cause the disturbance of the ratio between the first and the second current components. Some homogeneity disturbances of the structure of vectors and their directions and/or additional areas of electrical activity can in this case appear on the map of the current density vector distribution. The direction of the maximum current density vector, in fact, corresponds to the direction of the myocardial tissues in which the summary electrical activity is determined at the appropriate time moment of the cardio-cycle. Change in the direction of the current density vectors is caused by the work or adaptation mechanisms as a consequence of disease. It is possible to suppose that the zone of maximum electrical activity in the myocardial is shifted from one fiber layer to another (with respect to normal, for example). In other words the analysis of the structure of the current distribution maps, the analysis of the currents' values and directions give a real idea about the electrical events in the heart. It is clear that the myocardium is a complicated three-dimensional structure, so it is necessary to take into account the distribution of current density over depth for the analysis of the current map. This analysis can be done by the "layer-to-layer" solution of the inverse problem realised by the SoftMAG program. One version of the presentation of such a solution for one time moment is shown in Figures 6.14a and 6.14b.

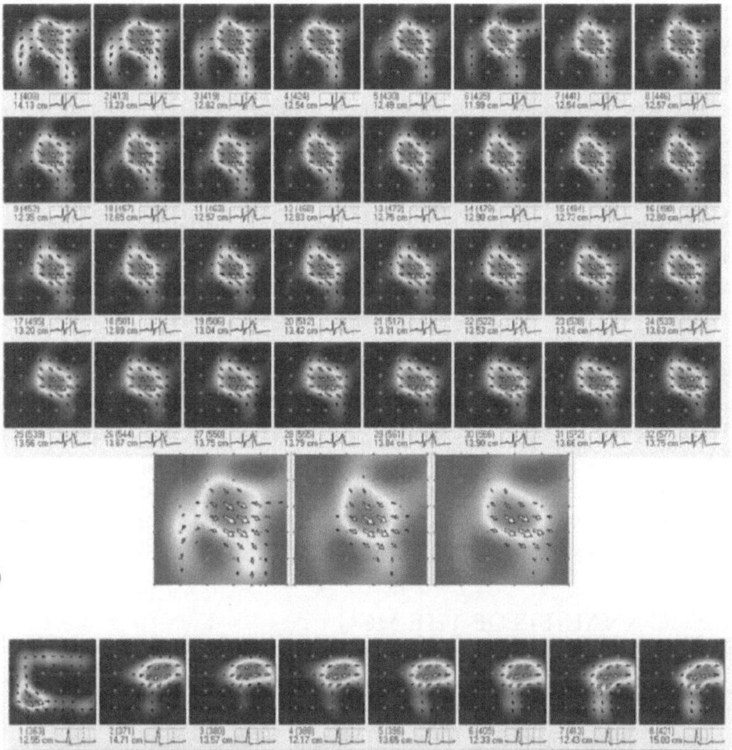

a)

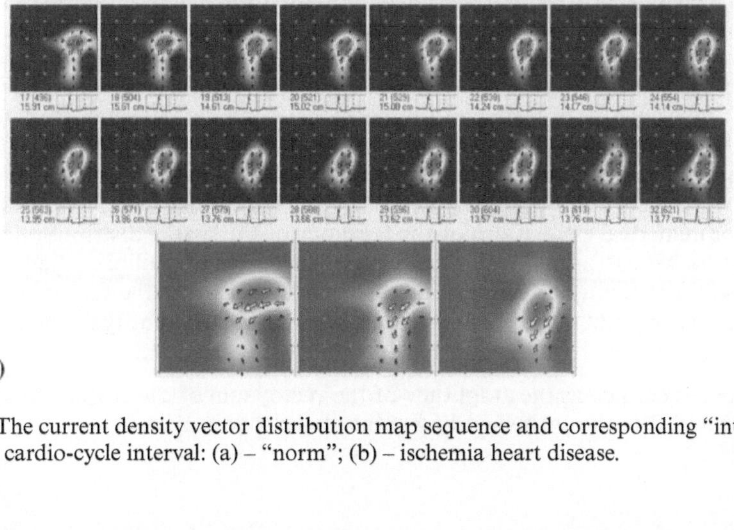

b)

Figure 6.14 The current density vector distribution map sequence and corresponding "integral" maps for the chosen cardio-cycle interval: (a) – "norm"; (b) – ischemia heart disease.

So far, we have considered the analysis of single maps of the current density vectors distribution for a given time moment of the cardio-cycle. It is clear that this is not enough to make a decision about the heart's pathology. To make an MCG conclusion, it is necessary to analyse the whole process of for example de—and/or repolarisation of the heart's ventricular system. The analysis of the sequence of current distribution maps with a given time step form the start until the end of the physiological process gives such an opportunity. In the case of the QRS analysis the first map corresponds the moment of the start of the interval and the last—the moment of point "J". The map's quantity for this time interval can be 32 (the 16-th clashes with the "R"-peak), 104 (the 43-th clashes with the "R"-peak) or any other with a minimum time step of 1 ms (dependent on the analysis algorithm used). Taking into account that MCG is highly sensitive to tangential currents, it must give more significant diagnostic information during the analysis of ventricular repolarisation. This is connected with the fact that, during exactly this interval, current spreads mainly parallel to the chest (tangential to the MCG measurement plane). During the ST-T interval analysis, the first current map corresponds to point "J", and the last map—to the end of peak "T". The time step between the elements of the map sequence is determined by the length of the interval and, depending on the chosen algorithm, can be 32, 64 or any other number (with the time step not smaller than 1 ms in the selected interval). Figure 6.14 demonstrates an example of the current density vector distribution map sequence on the part of the ST-T interval (32 maps). In the lower drawing part it is possible to see the "integral" maps, which are achieved by averaging every 10 following in the map series in the limits of a chosen interval. Such version of data visualisation allows to see the tendency and to appreciate the changes of the current map structure in the "big" intervals of the cardio-cycle (usually QRS and/or ST-T).

The analysis of the sequence of current density vector distribution (in the chosen time interval) is performed for each map (as it was described) for the whole time interval connected with the analysed process (for example, de—or repolarisation of the ventricular system).

4 AUTOMATIC ANALYSIS OF THE MCG

Now it is time to admit that aim, if MCG analysis is the solution of problem classification (or recognition) (Chaikovsky et al. 2006). This problem consists in the attribution of some patient w to one of the groups W_1, W_2,... W_k on the base of measurements of $\boldsymbol{p}$ parameters X_1, X_2, ...X_p. In our case, the measured parameters X_1, X_2, ...X_p are the results of the inverse problem solution in the form of the distribution of the current density vectors found at a discontinuous set of points (the points number is 961: 31 × 31) on a plane which is parallel to the measurements plane. Thus, for one current distribution map we have 961 (in fact 2 × 961, since the current distribution vector is presented in the form of two components) parameter values. Since the analysed cardio-cycle interval can contain tens and hundreds of such maps (signal sampling rate is 1000 Hz), and the patients' number in the group can also be tens and hundreds, for the analysis of such multi-dimensional input data it is necessary to use the special methods of receiving high informative variables.

Compare the spatial configuration of the distribution of the current vector density to "pair" the MCG records for a single point in time of the cardiac cycle. Let us denote them as α and Ω. For numerical estimations of the topology of the spatial distribution of the current density vectors we use an algorithm of entropy calculation (Kullback-Leibler algorithm). Suppose that the structure of the current density distribution of the vector systems α and Ω is described at each point of the plane by the value of a scalar quantity ε_α and ε_Ω, correspondingly, and is determined by the following algorithm:

- parameter ε is defined as the amplitude of the vector sum of the current density vector for systems α and Ω in the corresponding point of the source plane:

$$\xi = \sqrt{(j_{x\alpha}(i,j) + j_{x\Omega}(i,j))^2 + (j_{y\alpha}(i,j) + j_{y\Omega}(i,j))^2};$$

- the integral (on the plane of the source) value of the scalar parameter ε is calculated for each of the current systems α and Ω;
- for each system both α and Ω compute "normalised" distribution of scalar parameter so that the total amplitude is equal to 1;
- calculate the following parameter by obtained values:

$$\Delta = \sum_{i=1,31} \sum_{j=1,31} \varepsilon_\alpha(i,j) \ln\left[\frac{\varepsilon_\alpha(i,j)}{\varepsilon_\Omega(i,j)}\right].$$

The Δ parameter ("entropy") has only values positive or equal to zero, if the distribution of the vector current density is identical for the studied map pair.

Thus, the proposed algorithm (described here as an example) of topology evaluation for the distribution maps of current density vectors is implemented in the magnetocardiograph software (Primin et al. 2010). The algorithm allows describing the spatial distribution of the magnetic field and the corresponding two-dimensional source by one numerical parameter.

The number of points in the plane where components of the vector current density were found is discrete and fixed. Considering this, the following algorithm is used for a quantitative description of the "map" of the current distribution:

1. Sub-regions with a characteristic distribution of the current density vector (patterns) are allocated in the source plane;
2. Set the reference angle θ (zero angle is determined by the OX axis of the laboratory coordinate system).

The algorithm of numerical estimation involves the following:

- A plane S (current distribution map), in which the solution of the inverse problem is found, is divided into three subdomains—S0, S1, S2. And S0 corresponds to the main pattern of the currents distribution of the "norm";
- The sum of the scalar products of the unit vectors of the main directions of the basic pattern for the current "norm" and the found current density vector is determined in each of the constituent subdomains S0, S1, S2. This takes into account the square of the elementary rectangle, centre of the rectangle is the application point of this vector. As a result, each of the maps of the current distribution of the investigated interval will be described by three numbers.
- The time-dependent integral characteristics, which represent the coefficients of correlation between parameters S0 = f (j,S0), S1 = f (j,S1), S2 = f (j,S2) for "normal", and the patient under examination are determined. Thus, we obtain a set of parameters for assessing the degree of closeness to the current rate of current distributions to "norm" for different sectors of the map and for different time intervals.

Other algorithms for estimating the two-dimensional distribution of the current density vector include: evaluation of the vector density of solutions; assessment of "integral" maps of the distribution of the current density vector; analysis of the distribution of the current density vector with the help of the Voronoi diagrams; estimates of the solution of the inverse problem in the nodes of a non-uniform grid. Obtained numerical parameters after MCG analyses are recorded to special filetables and used to obtain the rules of classification of groups of patients.

In one of our studies we have performed the analysis of MCG data for two groups of patients. The first group was composed of 53 MCG recordings of healthy volunteers which had "no history" of heart decease. It was performed for them by complex medical studies and established the absence of malfunctions in their heart activity. The second group was composed of 69 MCG records of patients who had heart decease. Moreover, none of these patients had a diagnosis of "myocardial infarction".

After the MCG measurements of the patients and data analysis by the "MAGSCAN" magnetocardiograph software in automatic regime, the parameter files were received. This set of parameters were studied with the help of the statistical processing program "STATISTICA". The classification rule for the verified patient groups was obtained by the method of step-by-step discriminant analysis. The stability of the classification algorithm was proved by the test samples and with the help of standard cross-estimation algorithms.

The use of the newly found rule in the software of the "MAG-SCAN" diagnostic system gives the opportunity to get an automatic conclusion. The first page of the report includes the general information about the patient and the results of the study of the patient's ECG over the second standard lead. The second page includes the results of the classification ("group 1" – "norm"; "group 2" – some deviations from the "norm", additional investigations are required; "group 3" – boundary state) of the patient and the graphical parameters presentation in the case of "norm". For the current study (the decision about the affiliation of the patient with the appropriate group was made on the base of such a comparison). Figure 6.15 demonstrates an example of automatic report after a patient's MCG data processing.

Note that the visual analysis ("step-by-step" mode of data processing) allows to evaluate the structure of the field maps and distribution of the current density vectors, analyse the zones of high and low electrical activity in the myocardium in a more complete and detailed way than in the automatic mode, when only numerical criteria and estimations are implemented. Moreover, by using a visual analysis a physician-expert, with time (and experience), forms for himself 'images' of maps of the norm and maps of various pathologies by "his

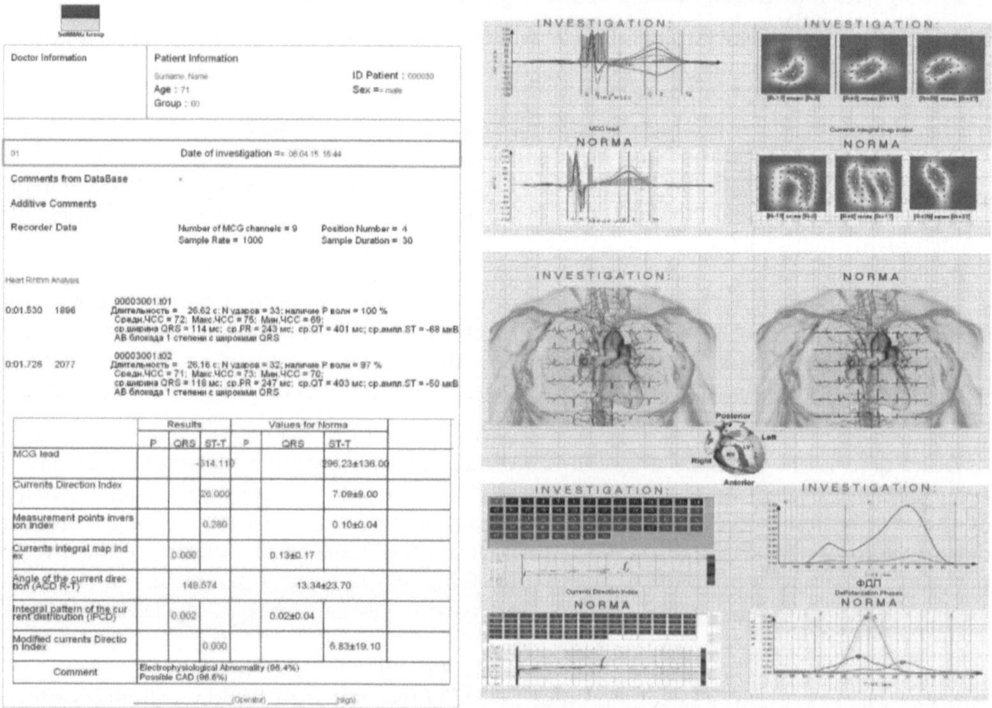

Figure 6.15 Example of automatic report after performing the classification procedure.

Table 6.1 The averaged values of analysed MCG parameters (in relative units) and their deviation.

Parameters	Groups		Statistical significance (p-value)
	Norm group	Heart disease group	
CDI	6.615 ± 6.261	38.276 ± 21.458	2.0×10^{-11}
IPCD	0.176 ± 0.112	0.068 ± 0.093	2.7×10^{-5}
E_{RT}	3.821 ± 1.525	6.529 ± 3.351	3.0×10^{-4}

Table 6.2 The results of automatic classification of investigated groups of patients.

Result	Indicator	Formula	Value
TP = 67	Sensitivity	Se = TP\(TP + FN)	89.33%
FN = 8	Positive Predictivity	+P = TP\(TP + FP)	100.00%
TN = 27	Specificity	Sp = TN\(TN + FP)	100.00%
FP = 0	False Positive Rate	FPR = FP\(TN + FP)	0.00%
	Negative Predictivity	–P = TN\(TN + FN)	76.47%

Table 6.3 The diagnosis value indexes in the heart disease group.

Parameters	Sensitivity	Specificity
	Se = TP/(TP + FN)	Sp = TN/(TN + FP)
CDI (<22.34)	73%	100
IPCD (>0.12)	81%	65
E_{RT} (<5.17)	60%	73
All three parameters	89%	100

own" signs and rules that are difficult to formalise. However, this approach requires considerable training of the physician and may have a lower frequency of occurrence in the evaluation of the same pathologies. Automatic analysis has advantages in the analysis of groups of patients; however, the numerical classification parameters used do not always reflect the characteristics of the processes for a particular individual. Therefore, these types of analysis of the MCG, if possible, should be used simultaneously.

5 CONCLUSIONS

The MCG study is not only non-invasive, it is also non-contact. The MCG system applies no influence on the patient or on the physiological processes in his heart, or other organs, since during the registration of diagnostic information the system radiates no energy (MCG is essentially a "passive system for object location"). Thus the magnetocardiographic technology of heart investigation excludes any possibility of complications for the patient caused by the MCG study.

This is a new, rapidly developing area of medicine. Therefore, the "MAGSCAN" diagnostic complex software allows to study verified representative groups of patients with various cardiac diagnoses in automatic regime, get tables of numerical data, find the decision rule, enter this rule (as a text file) into the SoftMag complex and also use it in patient investigation. Note that the current version of the software allows operation in conjunction with the classification of the two rules.

In one of our studies we have performed the analysis of MCG data for two groups of patients. The first group was composed of 27 MCG recordings of healthy volunteers. The second group was composed of 75 MCG records of patients who had heart decease. The developed classification rule included three parameters: a) Current Direction Index (CDI) – it characterises the homogeneity of ventricular repolarisation process; b) Integral Pattern of Current Distribution (IPCD) – spatial distribution of currents density vector in the central part of the map with respect to a given direction (single vector of 50° direction with respect to axes OX); (c) – the energy ratio index E_{RT}—it characterises the ratio of the energy of the magnetic field of the heart within the boundaries of the field measurements for the time corresponding to the maximum wave "R" and the end of wave "T" of the cardiac cycle. The results of analysis of patient groups are shown in Tables 6.1, 6.2 and 6.3.

To test the stability of the classification rules (apart from the standard cross-validation-checks), the test group was formed, which included 41 MCG records. Automatic analysis showed that 40 MCG records (from 41) were classified correctly.

The results of the practical application of information technology developed on the basis of the "MAGSCAN" complex were tested after a public approval by discussions of biophysics and cardiology experts and received a positive assessment of experts in many countries.

REFERENCES

Chaikovsky, I., Hugenholtz, P., Primin, M. et al. 2006. Methodical approaches for the clinical interpretation of the magnetocardiogram. *USiM* 2: 33–43.

Cryoton UK Ltd. 2016. *Cryoton UK Ltd. – Squid Systems.* http://www.cryoton.com/squid.php.

Primin, M. A., Nedaivoda, I. V., Maslennikov, Yu. V., and Gulyaev, Yu. V. 2010. Software for the magnetocardiographic complex for the early diagnostics and monitoring of heart diseases. *Journal of Communications Technology and Electronics* 55 (10):1169–1186.

Nedayvoda, I. V., Primin, M. A., and Vassylyev, V. E. 2008. An Algorithm of Estimating the Topology of Spatial Maps of Current Density Vector in Magnetocardiography. *USiM* 2: 11–19.

Nedayvoda, I.V., Primin M.A. and Vassylyev V.E. 2009. An Algorithm of Topology Estimation of Spatial Maps of Current Density Vector in Magnetocardiography. *USiM* 3: 7–14.

Nedayvoda, I.V. and Primin, M.A. 2010. The Algorithm of the Estimation and Analysis of Space-and-Time Characteristics of the Magnetic Field in Magnetocardiography. *USiM* 4: 15–20.

Primin, M.A., Nedayvoda, I.V. and Vassylyev V.E. 2007. A Method and the Algorithm of Reconstruction of a Spatial Structure of Current Density Vectors in Magnetocardiography. *USiM* 5: 5–16.

Primin M. and Nedayvoda I. 2009. Inverse problem solution algorithms in magnetocardiography: new analytical approaches and some results. International Journal of Applied Electromagnetics and Mechanics 29 (2): 65–81.

Voytovych, I.D., Chaikovsky, I.A., Primin, M.A., Kozlovsky, V.I., Sosnitsky, V.M. and Stadnyuk, L.A. 2002. *Diagnostic Criteria for Chronic Ishemic Heart Disease Based on the Registry and Analyses of Magnetocardiograms*. Kiev: V.M. Glushkov Institute of Cybernetics.

CHAPTER 7

Processing laser beam images using parallel-hierarchical FPGA-based transformations

L.I. Timchenko, N.S. Petrovskiy, N.I. Kokryatskaya & A.A. Yarovyi
State University of Transport Economy and Technologies, Kyiv, Ukraine

R. Romaniuk
Warsaw University of Technology, Warsaw, Poland

P. Kisała
Lublin University of Technology, Lublin, Poland

S. Smailova
D.Serikbayev East Kazakhstan State Technical University, Ust-Kamenogorsk, Kazakhstan

1 INTRODUCTION

One of the fastest spreading methods of modern communication is satellite laser optical links (Buck & Washington 2013, Borovoy et al. 1988). There are two reasons why we turn our attention to these systems:

1. Energy efficiency—Laser communications links use significantly less power than classical radio systems for transmissions over the same distance through small beam divergence.
2. Speed—At the same power levels, laser systems allow for the transmission of significantly more information, which is needed for future studies of the solar system.

However, the small beam divergence is also one of the major technical hurdles in constructing such systems, since the beams need to get to the receiver over a distance of millions of kilometres, while the transmitter is constantly moving. This in turns means that the receiver needs to constantly track the transmitter's position. For these types of systems, there must be a high degree of accuracy in determining the coordinates of the transmitter satellite. However, passing the laser beam through the atmosphere presents significant obstacles. If the energy attenuation of the laser beam propagating through the atmosphere leads to range restrictions of the laser communications and navigation devices, its impact on the structure of the beam path and its distribution determines to some extent the accuracy parameters of such devices. Light waves propagating in the atmosphere not only experience energy loss, but are also subject to amplitude and phase fluctuations. These fluctuations occur due to the random temporal distribution of the refractive index, which in turn is caused by turbulent motions in the atmosphere, entailing random temperature changes. Atmospheric turbulence causes a curvature in the wave front of the light wave, which leads to the expansion of the laser beam, the redistribution of energy within the beam and changes to its "centre of energy", as well as fluctuations of the total intensity (Weichel 1990, Medina et al. 2011a).

Of course, measuring the coordinates of objects takes place with the help of geometric moments (Medina et al. 2011b, Fernandez et al. 2008], the use of which in the problem of measuring the centre of energy of laser images which are deformed in the atmosphere, results in a significant measurement error. The measurement error in the coordinates of the energy centre of the laser image can be up to 10 pixels. Therefore, the actual problem becomes the classification of extended laser trail images, in the cases where the images are subject to a number of deforming factors, while maintaining parity between the energy efficiency and computational speed. Also it has not always been a simple task to create specialised hardware that can implement certain methods. Even well-known methods or algorithms which already have parallelism on the level of mathematical operations still require additional analysis or a complete change in the order of operations.

A more precise classification requires the use of more sophisticated algorithms which apply techniques capable of adapting to channel noise. To implement this step parallel-hierarchical networks may be used (Timchenko 2000), which have the property of adaptability while maintaining a simple mathematical apparatus, which is advantageous for implementation on a FPGA. This is described in works on the usage of FPGA, for example Apopei & Dodd 2012, or Palagin 2013.

2 THEORETICAL FOUNDATIONS OF ORGANISING PARALLEL-HIERARCHICAL NETWORKS ON THE BASIS OF FUNCTIONAL SETS

It is necessary, when implementing parallel-hierarchical networks, to determine the character of interacting elements in the network, shown in Figure 7.1. The concept central to the multistage processing is parallel-consequential interaction of data streams. As shown in Figure 7.1, at the first processing level the multiprocessor network decomposes the input data into temporal intermediate sequences $\{a^1_{st}\}$. At the second level the processor elements (PEs) form the second series of intermediate signals. Such intermediate series are generated at all subsequent levels if different PEs are activated simultaneously, similarly to the associative coincidence in the cerebral cortex. An output result a^j_{11} is produced at each level on condition that no simultaneous activations of different PEs occur. This mechanism is analogous to the formation of cortical coalitions which are isolated from the others in space and time (Livingstone & Hubel 1984).

In general, the interactive characteristics of the multiprocessor network (Fig. 7.1), which implements the multistage structure, can be described by six types of functional series. These series represent interactions between the parallel channels at different levels of the hierarchical network. The first series is defined as:

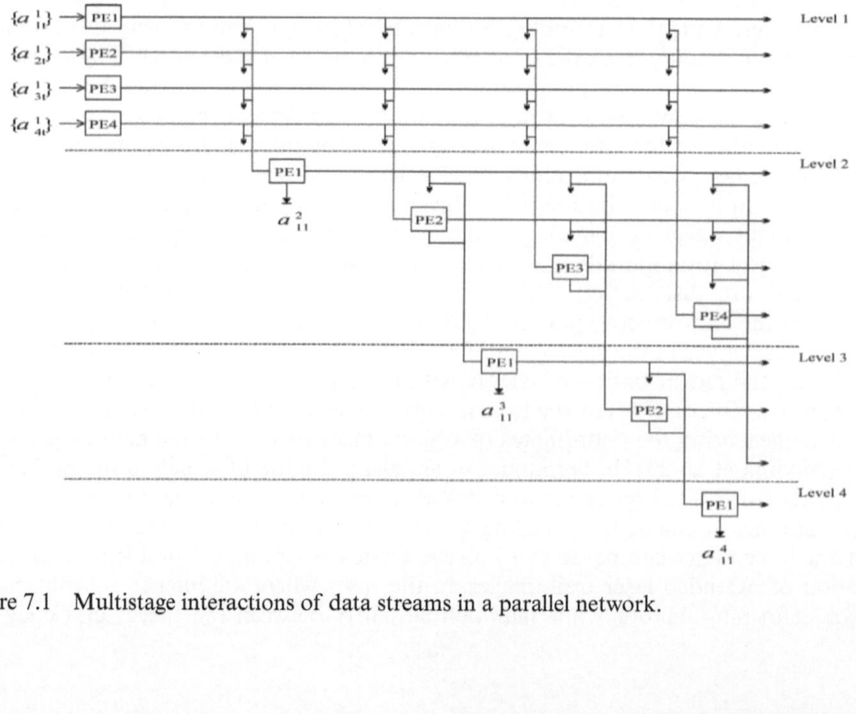

Figure 7.1 Multistage interactions of data streams in a parallel network.

$$N_1(i',j') = \bigcup_{i'=1}^{n} \bigcup_{j'=1}^{n} \left(A \left] \frac{n-(i'-1)}{j'} \right[\right), \tag{7.1}$$

where n denotes the number of stages at the first processing level, notion i' represents the stage of the process, j' represents the level of the hierarchy, and][denotes the equal or least bigger integer function.

The easiest way to describe all the subsequent series is by arranging them in pairs.

$$\begin{aligned} N_2(i',j') &= \bigcup_{i'=n+1}^{2n-1} A(2n-i') \quad j'=1 \\ N_3(i',j') &= \bigcup_{i'=n+1}^{2n-1} \bigcup_{j'=2}^{i'} \left(A \left] \frac{i'}{j'} \right[\right) \end{aligned}, \tag{7.2}$$

The second series is defined by the first part of expression (7.2) for $j'=1$ and by the second part of (7.2) for $j'=2,3,\cdots,2n-1$. It partially describes the first level of the network by $N_2(i',j')$ at each i'-th stage. At the higher levels of the hierarchy, the second series is represented by $N_3(i',j')$. This pair wise description is also applied to the other series, given in expressions (7.3) to (7.6).

The third series is:

$$\begin{aligned} N_4(i',j') &= \bigcup_{i'=2n}^{3(n-1)} A(3n-2-i') \quad j'=3 \\ N_5(i',j') &= \bigcup_{i'=2n}^{3(n-1)} \bigcup_{i'=4}^{i'} A \left] \frac{i'}{j'} \right[\end{aligned}, \tag{7.3}$$

The fourth series is:

$$\begin{aligned} N_6(i',j') &= A(1), i'=3n-2, j'=3,4 \\ N_7(i',j') &= \bigcup_{i'=5}^{i'} \left(A \left] \frac{i'}{j'} \right[\right), i'=3n-2' \end{aligned} \tag{7.4}$$

The fifth series is:

$$\begin{aligned} & N_8(i',j') = A(1) \\ & (3n-1) \le i' \le (3n-2)+(n-3)^2 \\ & 5 \le j' \le 4+(n-3)^2 \\ & N_9(i',j') = \bigcup_{i'=3n-1}^{(3n-2)+(n-3)^2} \bigcup_{j'=i'+(7-3n)}^{i'} \left(A \left] \frac{i'}{j'} \right[\right) \end{aligned}, \tag{7.5}$$

The sixth series is:

$$\begin{aligned} & N_{10}(i',j') = A(1), (3n-1)+(n-3)^2 \le i' \le n^2 \\ & (n-3)^2+6 \le j' \le (n-3)^2+2(3n-5) \\ & 5 \le j' \le 4+(n-3)^2 \\ & N_{11}(i',j') = \bigcup_{i'=(3n-1)+(n-3)^2}^{n^2} \bigcup_{j'=2i'-(n-3)^2+9-6n}^{i'} \left(A \left] \frac{i'}{j'} \right[\right) \end{aligned}, \tag{7.6}$$

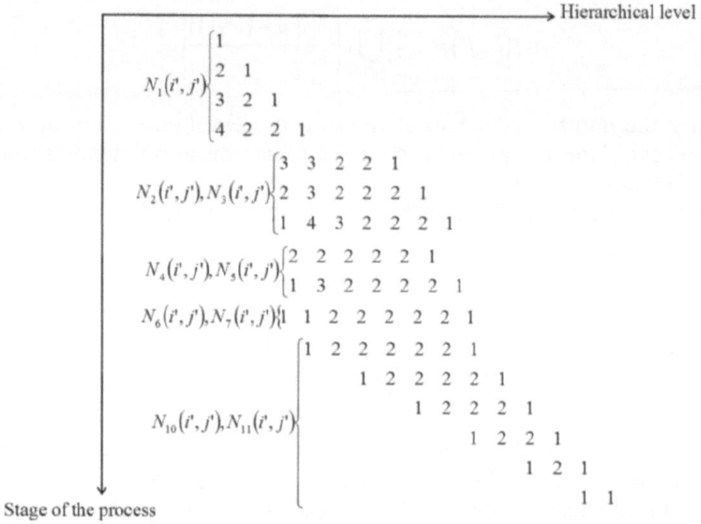

Figure 7.2 Interactions between the four parallel channels of the network at different hierarchical levels. Processing at the first level involves four stages.

These six series organise a functional parallel-hierarchical structure and describe the spatial-temporal interaction in the multiprocessor network.

Expressions (7.1) to (7.6) are validated on a simple example of calculating the processor interactions in the multiprocessor network with network dimensions $S \times n = 4 \times 4$, where S denotes the number of initial image segments and n denotes the number of processing stages at the first level (Fig. 7.2).

Expressions (7.1–7.6) describe the spatial-temporal interaction of certain parameters of the image elements. The numerical series $N_1(i',j') \div N_{11}(i',j')$ illustrate the dynamic correlation at different levels of the multistage hierarchy. This mechanism is very similar to various neurophysiologic processes, such as associative learning (Kandel & Hawkins 1992), spatial summation of postsynaptic potentials (Sherrington 1961), and various interconnection pathways between the specialised visual cortical areas (Livingstone & Hubel 1984). Implementation of the spatial-temporal image processing and multistage integration of the results may be very promising when realising real-time artificial neural structures.

3 DIRECT PARALLEL-HIERARCHICAL TRANSFORMATION

Usually, to correct the "centre of energy" a number of well-developed methods are used, such as filtration and image classification, which does not require complex calculations. However, large distances need adaptive filtering, which can be used for a class of classification methods like neural networks. Parallel-hierarchical networks can be used for laser beam spot images processing, which due to the atmospheric influence experience significant deformation (Fig. 7.3).

The G algorithm conversion implements the pyramidal process of parallel data summation in the branches of the parallel-hierarchical network. A pyramidal decomposition of the mathematical model of the set $\mu=\{a_i\},\ i=\overline{1,n}$ has the form:

$$\sum_{i=1}^{n} a_i = \sum_{j=1}^{R}\left(n - \sum_{k=0}^{j-1} n_k\right)\left(a^j - a^{j-1}\right), \tag{7.7}$$

where $a_i \neq 0, R$ is a dimensionality of a given set. Let us form subsets from the same elements, the elements of one set we denote by $a^k,\ k=\overline{1,R}$, n^k is a number of elements in the kth

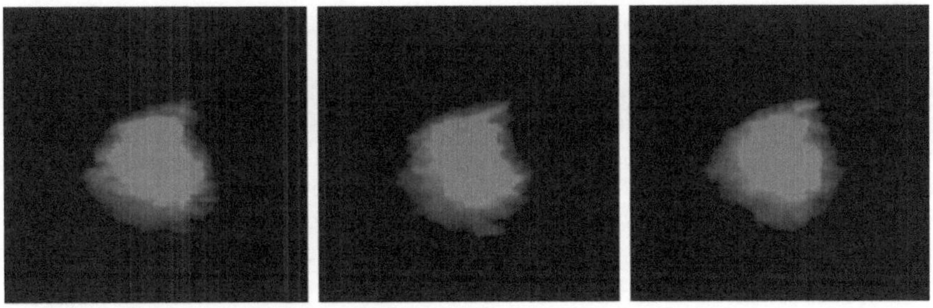

Figure 7.3 Laser beam trace image, 128 × 128 pixels.

subset (i.e. multiplicity of a_k), a^j is a random element of the set $\{a^k\}$ selected at the jth step, $j=\overline{1,R}, a^0=0, n_0=0$. Having analysed the pyramidal processing of numeric information in (7), we can conclude that in this process a number of elements decreases with each step. The PH transformation algorithm is:

Let us consider the transformation $G(M)=\{a_j \mid j=1,2,...,m_1\}$, applied at each processing channel. Let us represent the original image M with n segments, over which runs transformation G in each processing channel i, $i=1,...,n$ simultaneously (Timchenko et al. 2011). Then, consider the i-segment of the image $M_i^1=\{a_{ij}^1 \mid j=1,2,...,m_i^1\}$, where m_i^1 is the number of components in the i-th channel of the first level, and all the segments under consideration can be represented in matrix A_1:

$$A_1=\begin{bmatrix} M_1^1 \\ M_2^1 \\ \cdots \\ M_i^1 \\ \cdots \\ M_n^1 \end{bmatrix}=\begin{bmatrix} a_{11}^1 & a_{12}^1 & \cdots & a_{1m_1^1}^1 & x & x & \cdots & x \\ a_{21}^1 & a_{22}^1 & \cdots & \cdots & a_{2m_2^1}^1 & x & \cdots & x \\ \cdots & \cdots & \cdots & \cdots & \cdots & \cdots & \cdots & x \\ a_{i1}^1 & a_{i2}^1 & \cdots & \cdots & \cdots & \cdots & \cdots & a_{im_i^1}^1 \\ \cdots & \cdots & \cdots & \cdots & \cdots & \cdots & \cdots & x \\ a_{n1}^1 & a_{n2}^1 & \cdots & a_{nm_n^1}^1 & x & x & \cdots & x \end{bmatrix}, \tag{7.8}$$

where x means the absence of the component. The index of the column indicates the step of component extraction and the line index indicates the channel from which this component is extracted. Let us reflect on the data analysis, given the matrix A_1 in operator form at the second level by the operation of transposition T. That is, the initial matrix of the second level will be introduced as $A_1^m=T(A_1)$. After performing the transposition, the row index indicates the number of steps for the component extraction.

At the second processing level, conversion G is organised so that it is possible to study the correlation between the components, which have been simultaneously extracted from various channels of the first level. This procedure is applied to the rows of matrix A_1^T.

$$A_2=G(A_1^T)=G(T(G(M)))=\begin{bmatrix} a_{11}^2 & a_{12}^2 & \cdots & \cdots & a_{1m_1^2}^2 & x & \cdots & x \\ a_{21}^2 & a_{22}^2 & \cdots & a_{2m_2^2}^2 & x & x & \cdots & x \\ \cdots & \cdots & \cdots & \cdots & \cdots & \cdots & \cdots & x \\ a_{i1}^2 & a_{i2}^2 & \cdots & \cdots & \cdots & \cdots & \cdots & a_{im^2}^2 \\ \cdots & \cdots & \cdots & \cdots & \cdots & \cdots & \cdots & x \\ a_{n^21}^2 & a_{n^22}^2 & \cdots & a_{n^2m_{n^2}^2}^2 & x & x & \cdots & x \end{bmatrix}, \tag{7.9}$$

where $n^2 = m^1, m^2$ respectively denotes the number of parallel channels and the number of processing steps at the second level.

Matrix A_2 is formed at the second processing level after the temporal decomposition in which each component a_{ij}^2 is extracted at the stage $t = i + j - 1$. If matrix A_2 is formed so that the column index indicates the component extraction step, then the same processing procedure can be applied at each subsequent level of the hierarchy. This procedure is implemented as a horizontal alignment of the rows of the matrix A_2 and puts the first non-empty cell in each row on the main diagonal. The resulting matrix is designated as $A_2^\bullet$, and $A_2^\bullet = \mathrm{P}(A_2)$, where P denotes the operator of row shift.

$$A_2^\bullet = \begin{bmatrix} a_{11}^2 & a_{12}^2 & \dots & \dots & \dots & a_{1m_1^2}^2 & x & \dots & \dots & \dots & \dots & x \\ x & a_{21}^2 & a_{22}^2 & \dots & a_{2m_2^2}^2 & x & x & \dots & \dots & \dots & \dots & x \\ \dots & \dots & \dots & \dots & \dots & \dots & \dots & \dots & \dots & \dots & \dots & x \\ x & x & x & a_{i1}^2 & a_{i2}^2 & \dots & \dots & \dots & \dots & \dots & \dots & a_{im^2}^2 \\ \dots & \dots & \dots & \dots & \dots & \dots & \dots & \dots & \dots & \dots & \dots & x \\ x & x & x & x & x & a_{n^21}^2 & a_{n^22}^2 & \dots & a_{n^2m_{n^1}^2}^2 & x & \dots & x \end{bmatrix}, \quad (7.10)$$

The component a_{11}^2 is the only one and that's why it can be extracted at the first stage of second level processing. This component is not associated in time with any of the other components of the second level and is therefore the source. It is also the intermediate result of network processing and the only component which was extracted as a result of multistage pro-cessing at the second level. This component is formed from the matrix by removing its first column, and the remaining components are saved in matrix $A_2^{\bullet\bullet}$. This procedure is performed by applying the operator L, i.e. $\mathrm{L}(A_2^\bullet) = a_{11}^2 + A_2^{\bullet\bullet}$. The third level matrix A_2^T is formed after T matrix transposition: $A_2^T = \mathrm{T}(\mathrm{L}(\mathrm{P}(A_2)))$.

The described procedure is performed at each next hierarchical level to the last level—k_{max}, in which matrix $A_{k_{max}}$ contains a single element. Then $\mathrm{T}(\mathrm{L}(\mathrm{P}(A_{k_{max}}))) = \varnothing$. Consistent use of operators G, P, L, and T can be represented as the execution of operator F:

$$F(A_k^T) = T\Big(L\Big(P\Big(G\big(A_k^T\big)\Big)\Big)\Big) = A_{k+1}^T. \quad (7.11)$$

Consistent use of operator F can be represented as $F^k(A_1^T) = F^{k-1}\left[F(A_1^T)\right]$. Then all the multistage process can be represented in next operator form:

$$F^{k_{max}-1} = \left[T\left(G\left(\bigcup_{i=1}^{n} M_i\right)\right)\right] = \{a_{11}^k \mid k = 2,3,\dots,k_{max}\}. \quad (7.12)$$

Thus, the result of processing in PH network is presented as image vector.

4 IMPLEMENTATION OF PARALLEL-HIERARCHICAL NETWORKS FOR PROCESSING LASER BEAM SPOT IMAGES

To solve the problem of laser beam processing, we can use a two-stage algorithm of classification of laser beam spots. The first stage gives us coordinates and performs segmentation of laser beam spot images, and at the second stage we will use a parallel-hierarchical network. Laser beam spot images have a drop in brightness which is clearly seen in the histogram of Figure 7.4.

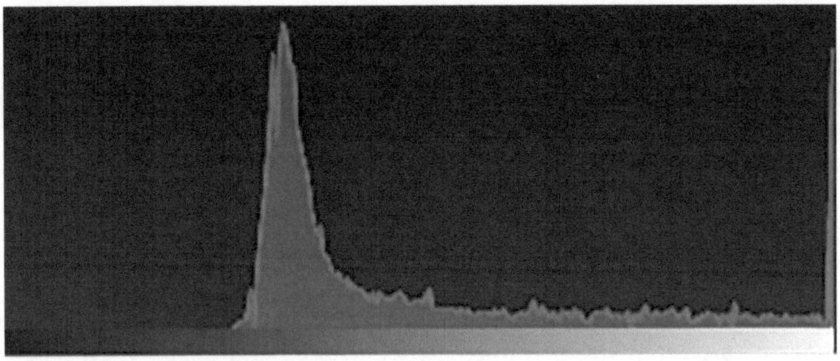

Figure 7.4 Histogram of brightness.

The left histogram has noise, which does not carry any relevant information for PH transformation. This means segmentation can use a threshold filter with a double border, according to the following formula:

$$\begin{cases} w(f(x,y)) = 0, w(f(x,y)) \le W_{0.5} \\ w(f(x,y)) = w(f(x,y)) - W_{0.5}, W_{0.5} < w(f(x,y)) \le W_{0.75} \\ w(f(x,y)) = 0, w(f(x,y)) \le W_{0.75} \\ W_{0.75} = W_{\max} \cdot 0.75, W_{0.5} = W_{\max} \cdot 0.5 \end{cases} \quad (7.13)$$

where $w(f(x,y))$ is the luminance value point and $W_{\max}$ is the max luminance of the image.

For the second stage, we find correlating scores for tail-end elements of the image using PH transformation.

Thus, the overall highest-accuracy classification algorithm for laser beam spots is as follows:

1. Find the image coordinates, and perform segmentation.
2. Find the tail-end elements to save for direct PH transformation.
3. Form a reference image—the average tail-end elements of the first twenty images.
4. Compute the correlation coefficient between the tail elements of the reference image and the next image.
5. If the correlation coefficient is above 0.9, then the picture is "good".
6. Repeat steps 4–6 for each successive image.

In order to identify the important characteristics of the images, and to create an image processing schema, we performed a computer simulation of the algorithm on real images of laser beams. As a consequence, the simulation of direct PH transformation showed the maximum number of rows of the original matrix of the transformation should not exceed 120, and the maximum number should be less than 210. Thus, we can use these initial parameters for creating the PH transformation schema. We will use 16-bit terms. Since the original image has the size of 128 * 128, then the maximum number of rows for the G transformation is also 128.

However, making hardware for processing the parallel-hierarchical networks at the second stage is not a simple task and is described in the authors' article (Timchenko et al. 2014). But it has not solved the problem of working with memory, which is the "bottleneck" for many systems. Parallel-hierarchical networks that require recurrent access to the data matrix are not an exception either.

4.1 *The concept of P and T operators processing*

However, the basic operations for working with memory are the operators of P and T transformations which are inherently read operations, and hence it is possible to carry out some optimisations considering the structure of RAM devices. The only operation that requires a full cycle, i.e. read-modify-write is the G operator (or G conversion).

It should be noted that each level of direct parallel-hierarchical transformation requires the allocation of new memory capacity, whereby the memory capacity required for the PH transformation is 100 to 1000 times more than the size of the original matrix (meaning that the previous PH levels are not removed until the transformation is done).

However, the size of the required memory will be substantially reduced if the necessary matrix memory of a certain size is immediately allocated and overwritten on every level of the PH transformation.

Table 7.1 shows the estimation of the maximum matrix size for the algorithm of the G transformation. It was carried out on a computer in Visual Studio 2010 (Hejlsberg et al. 2010) in the programming language C#. The artificially-generated images via RNG (Random 2016) were used as test images. The colour of the images has a depth of 8 bit grey.

The following also reduces the number of operations for P and T operators:

1. T-operator, or the matrix transposition operation, requires the rewriting of each member of the matrix in accordance with the (7.2) into a new matrix M^T.

Since data storage in most RAM devices is also in the form of a matrix (Karbo 2002), it is quite clear that transposition can be replaced by a simple rearrangement of the column and row address pointers. As a result, the rewriting operation is simply not needed.

At the same time the control unit of such memory also stores data about the matrix size, in order to handle only the specified memory region.

2. P-operator, or shift operator. Requires (according to (7.10) rewriting of each next row that is one position to the right from the previous. This operator can be accelerated, as, in fact, it also requires read only. And since there are operators L and T (7.11) going after it, then it is possible to perform these operators in a single pass with simple rearrangement of the address pointers.

An important consequence of this operation is the required memory reduction. The maximum number of diagonal sets does not exceed the number of columns, and therefore in the transposition of such a matrix the number of rows does not exceed $2 \times N^k_d$.

Then, the maximum size of the memory is defined as:

$$M = (r_{\max})^2, \tag{7.14}$$

where M – memory capacity, $r_{\max}$ – the maximum number of rows in the PH matrix decomposition of a certain size (Table 7.1).

Table 7.1 Characteristics of the PH transformation using the minimal element in operator G.

Parameter	Matrix 4 × 4	16 × 16	64 × 64	128 × 128	256 × 256
Number of levels	15	144	578	1150	2140
Maximum number of rows	6	56	253	512	964
Maximum number of columns	10	110	504	1022	1926
Maximum value	447	1680	4032	16000	64512
Execution time (ms)	41	189	4710	36000	251000

Thus, the algorithm of working with memory in the PH transformation can be written in a C-like language (we assume that the data are written into memory and the ranges of the matrix are known):

1. Reading operation in the first transposition:

```
for (x=0;x<Endx;x++)
{
  for (y=0; y<Endy;y++)
    {
    G[x,y] =read (x,y);
    }
}
```

where x, y are addresses of the memory cells' elements in columns and rows respectively, *Endx*, *Endy* are matrix ranges, *Read* denotes reading from memory operation and G[x, y] is the vector, which performs the G transformation on the matrix row (in fact, it is the interface to the calculator).

If we assume that the operation of each cell reading is performed for 1 beat, then the total reading time of the matrix (in beats) is equal to the product of matrix ranges.

2. Combined reading operation at S and T.

```
// Reading the first half of the matrix (up to the main diagonal and including it)
for (x=1;x<=Endx;x++)
{
  for (y=0; y<=Endy;y++)
  {
    if (y>x)
    break;
    G[x,y]=read (x-y,y);
  }
}
// Reading the second half of the matrix (after the main diagonal)
for (y=1;y=<Endy;y++)
{
  for (x=Endx; x>=0;x--)
  {
    if (x<y)
    break;
    G[x,y]=read (x,Endx-x+y);
  }
}
```

Figure 7.5 shows the matrix of the first transpose (a) and the combined reading (b).

If we assume that the operation of each cell reading is performed for 1 beat [18], then the total reading time of such a matrix is:

$$T = E_{ndx} \cdot E_{ndy} - 1. \tag{7.15}$$

Thus, the operation of a combined reading allows to reduce the amount of RAM accesses approximatelytwice.

4.2 *Development of parallel structures of P and T transformation*

The main task while parallelising the memory access processes is increasing the memory speed as well as ithe size of the access bus. Under this approach, there are two kinds of work with memory:

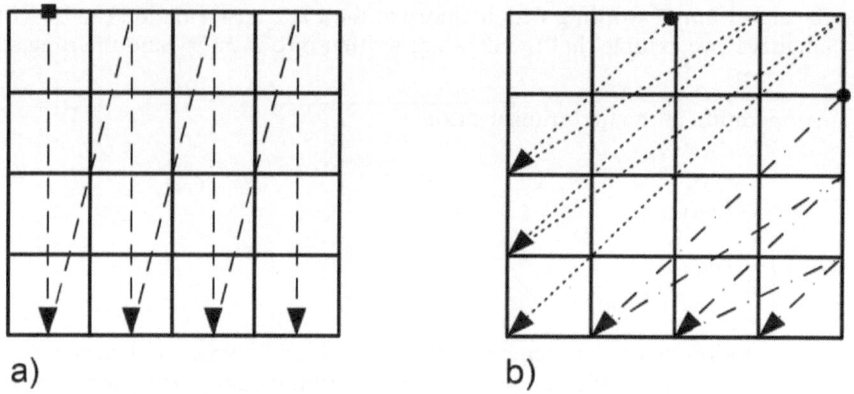

Figure 7.5 Diagram of data reading.

- using serial EC of RAM;
- creation of a dedicated RAM device on PLD.

1. Modern PLD micro schemes are equipped with a specialised interfaces for work with external memory chips (SRAM, SSRAM, QDR, DDR, etc.). Moreover, depending on the PLD type, it may have several such interfaces. Thus, it is possible to create an external memory with quite a large bus width. For example, the chip Stratix V (Altera 2016) supports up to 4 DDR3 SDRAM x72 DIMM, which gives the resultant data bus of 288 bits. Or, if we set the size of the cell for the PH transformation to 16-bit (a word), then we will get immediate access to up to 18 words. However, as can be seen from Table 7.1, even for a 16 × 16 matrix, that is not enough to display one row. Thus, between the devices that perform the G operation there must be an inserted storage buffer that will form the input and output data.

Another problem of serial IP is that their original state is not defined, and to get a "0" in the cell it is necessary to clean it beforehand. This problem occurs not only at the beginning of the work, but also after each level of the PH network. If at the time a new entry reading of the matrix has not finished, there may be a collision when the new data erase the data that have not been read yet. So before recording a new row into memory, the matrix must be completely read, and the previous row should be erased.

Since the G transformation is inherently an asynchronous process, then according to this approach the G transformation device must have enough memory to store the entire matrix.

However, large amounts of memory in modern chips make this task easier. Just select 2 memory areas of the same size, one of which is used for reading and one for writing. At the next level of the PH network, they change places with each other. In addition, the presence of two (or more) physically separated memory IP allows us to make the processes of reading and writing simultaneous. This approach is necessary as reading the data also erases it. Thus, parallel access to the external memory is determined by the ratio of the data bus width to a bit of the words used in the system.

2. When using the external memory, the major problems are: the width of the data transmission bus and the need to erase the cell after reading.

However, the PLD allows creating logic circuits that are the most relevant to the problem. So to solve the problem of access speed to the RAM it is possible to create a dedicated register cell of the RAM device. The circuit of such a cell is shown in Figure 7.6.

The cell consists of two registers: RG1 – entry register, RG2 – read register, and the output buffer with three states—TBF. The read bus and write bus are separated, as well as their

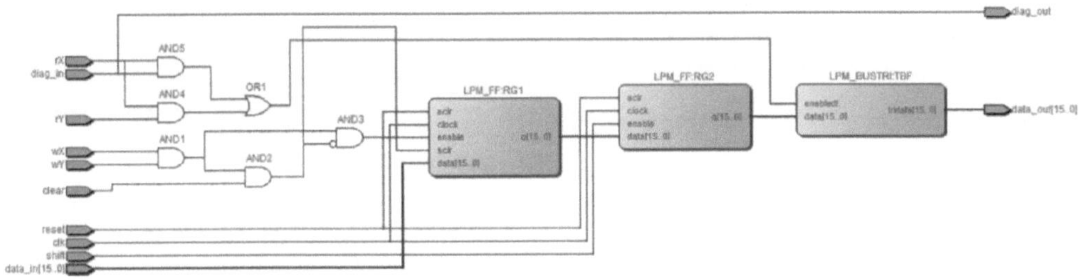

Figure 7.6 The circuit of the register memory cell.

Table 7.2 Description of the register memory cell outputs.

Output name	Direction	Description
Reset	Input	Reset
Clear	Input	Simultaneous cleaning of the entry register
Shift	Input	Command of data transferring from register 1 to register 2
wX, wY	Input	Address inputs of column and row respectively, for write operation
rX, rY	Input	Address inputs of column and row respectively, for read operation
Clk	Input	The clock frequency
data_in	Input	The input data bus
data_out	Output	The output data bus
diag_in	Input	The input of read command when transposing
diag_out	Output	The output of read command when transposing

address inputs, so the read and write operations can be done simultaneously (description of the cell inputs is shown in Table 7.2).

The cell operates as follows. After setting «1» to the input of Reset the scheme is put to its original state. If set «1» to the input of wX, wY, then data from the input bus may be written down. Further, if set «1» during the one beat to the input of Shift, then data from the first register are transferred into the second register.

Further, if set «1» to the input of rX, rY, then data from the second register on the output bus can be read. When there is «0» at the inputs of rX, rY, the output is in high-impedance state because of the tri-state buffer. The diagram of the cell work is shown in Figure 7.7.

Simulation in an Altera Quartus 14.0 environment for the 16-bit bus showed that for one such cell 35 logical elements are needed, 32 of them are triggers. The maximum operating frequency is 250 MHz.

It is further proposed to build out of these cells memory arrays of any dimension (limit is the PLD size and the specificity of its organisation). And the reading buses combine together horizontally, forming a reading vector. And the recording buses combine together vertically, forming a recording vector. Thus, the circuit forms a static vector RAM device (Goodman 1984). There are also row and column control devices (address decoders) attached to the circuit separately for reading and writing address inputs (Fig. 7.8).

Inputs Shift of all the cells are combined into one signal, and so are inputs Reset, Clear and Clk. The outputs diag_out are connected to the inputs diag_in diagonally by the formulas:

$$X_{in} = X + 1, \quad Y_{in} = Y - 1 \tag{7.16}$$

where X_{in} and Y_{in} – the “coordinates” of *diag_in* input, X and Y – the “coordinates” of *diag_out* output.

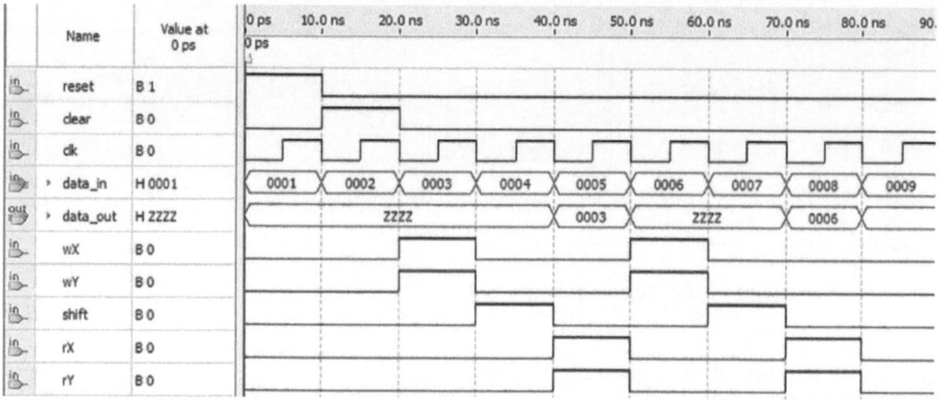

Figure 7.7 The diagram of the register cell work.

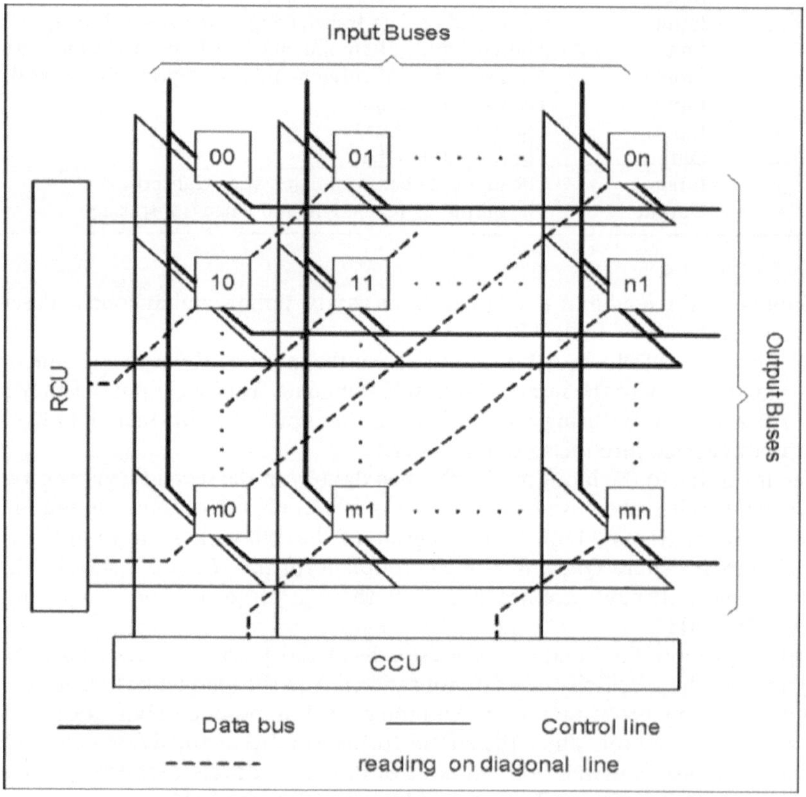

Figure 7.8 The scheme of register memory module (RCU – row control unit, CCU – column control unit).

The advantages of such a memory device are:

- simultaneous and independent operation of reading and writing.
- the ability to conduct both scalar and vector operations.
- transfer of data from the recording register to the reading register for 1 beat.

- the possibility of both scalar and vector erase of the recording registers.
- common data buses may also be combined in order to reduce the dimensionality of the input and output vectors. This reduces performance, but operations with other units of smaller dimension become possible.
- due to the diag input the vector reading of matrix diagonals is possible.

4.3 *The development of a specialised computer system for coordinates calculation and classification of laser beam spot images using a direct parallel-hierarchical transformation*

The above developments allow creation of image classification scheme based on a parallel-hierarchical network. A generalised scheme of the developed device is shown in Figure 7.9.

The algorithm for computing the coordinates and classification of laser beam spots using the method of direct parallel-hierarchical transformation for one frame is presented in Figure 7.10.

The simulation was performed on the basis of DE1-SoC PCB, the layout of which is shown in Figure 7.11.

The simulation data:

- total logic elements (ALM) 9.632
- total registers: 13822
- total memory bits: 163619
- DSP Blocks: 21

Performance of a complete circuit when processing real laser beam spot images is (at the main operating frequency of 100 MHz):

- using IC of serial memory—up to 25 ms/frame;
- using register memory—up to 7 ms/frame (an incomplete matrix of memory was used due to the limited resources of the used PLD).

5 RESULTS

The boundaries for the classification were chosen by the minimum average error relative to the centre of the real image (for the image sequences presented the real centre belongs to the

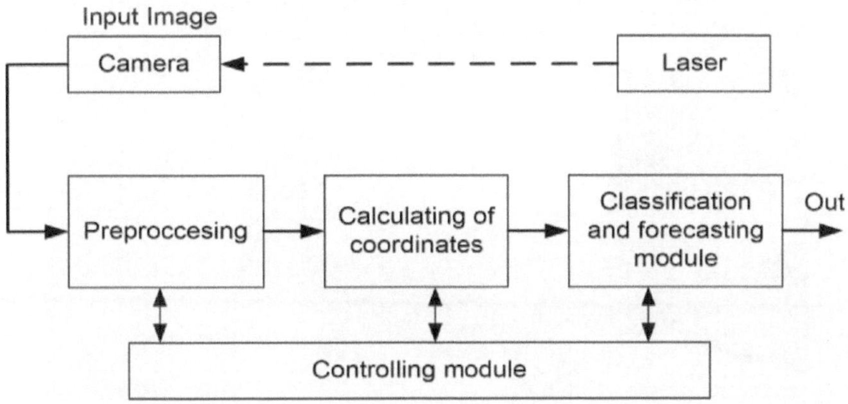

Figure 7.9 Generalised scheme of the laser beams spot image processing.

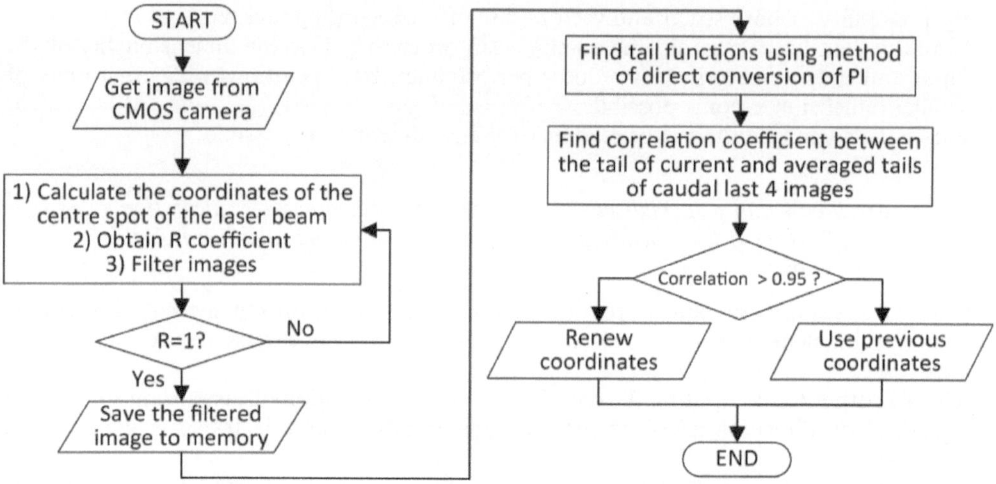

Figure 7.10 The algorithm of the combined method for the coordinates computing and classification of laser beam spots using the method of direct parallel-hierarchical transformation.

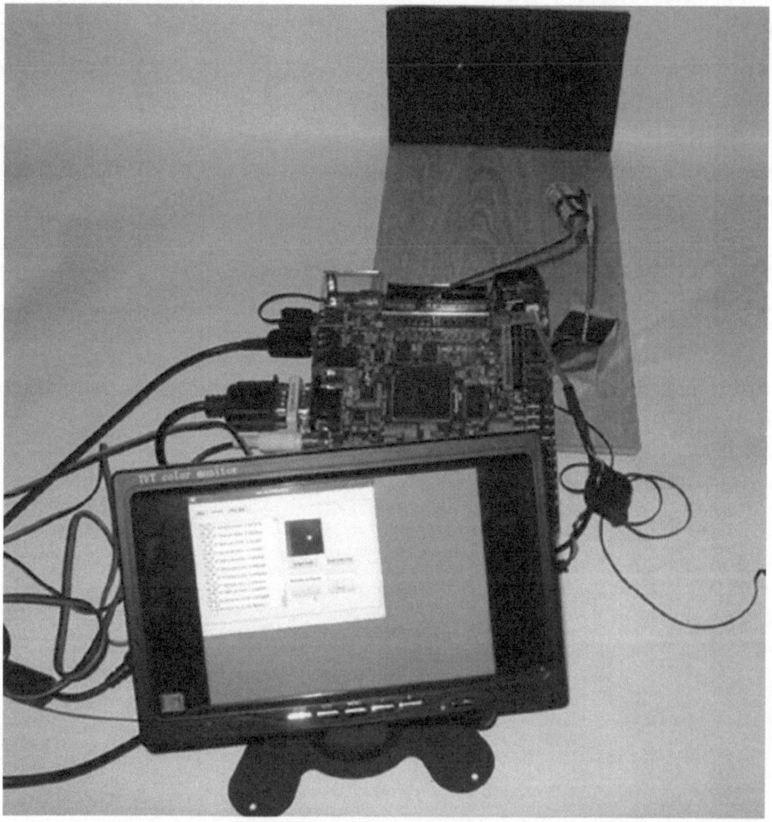

Figure 7.11 The layout form on the basis of DE1-SoC PCB.

point at X = 64, Y = 64). Thus in order to identify the optimal limits, an average error evaluation was made for various boundary distances depending on the correlation coefficient of the combined method. An average error graph, depending on the threshold selection for one of the tracks is shown in Figure 7.12.

The graph clearly shows that the method has the smallest error value at some minimum point, after which the threshold expansion error value increases again.

The quality of classification was also tested by ROC (Swets 1996); the graph is shown in Figure 7.13. The operating points for the developed method are TPR = 71%, FPR = 23%. Thus, the average error of the developed method is 0.47%, the maximum error is 1.6%, standard deviation – 0.36. The graph of errors compared to the method of contour tape [Statix 2016] for the track segment on the example of the X coordinate is shown in Figure 7.14.

The graph shows that the combined method has a more stable low average error than the method of contour tape and it can more accurately calculate the trajectory. For data transmission systems using a laser beam, it is important to not only know the specific current location of the transmitter at a given moment of time, but also to be able to predict its position at the next moment of time. In order to verify the quality of the developed algorithm classification a simulation was made about the received coordinate's treatment with some prediction methods to the actual track images provided by JSC "KIA Systems" (Moscow, Russia).

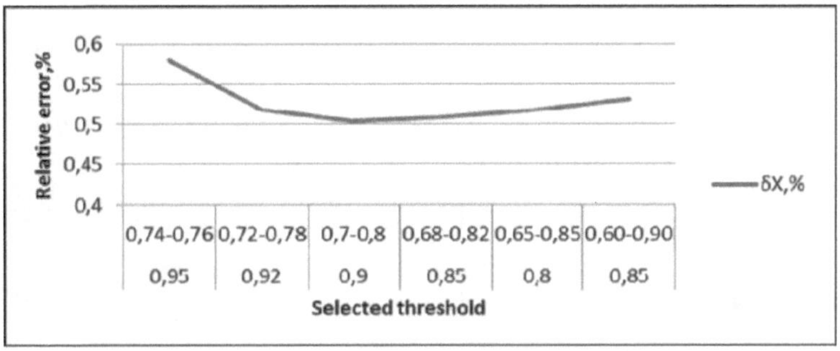

Figure 7.12 The dependence of the average error of coordinate X from the selected threshold of classification.

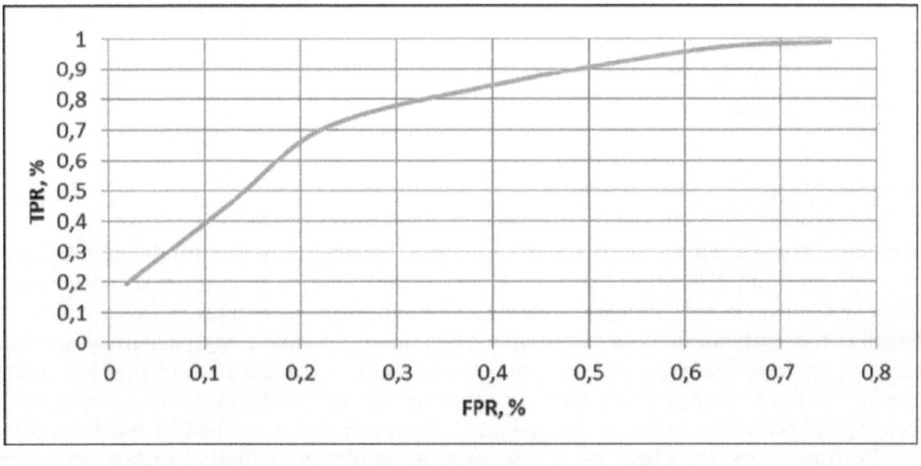

Figure 7.13 The ROC graph for the developed method.

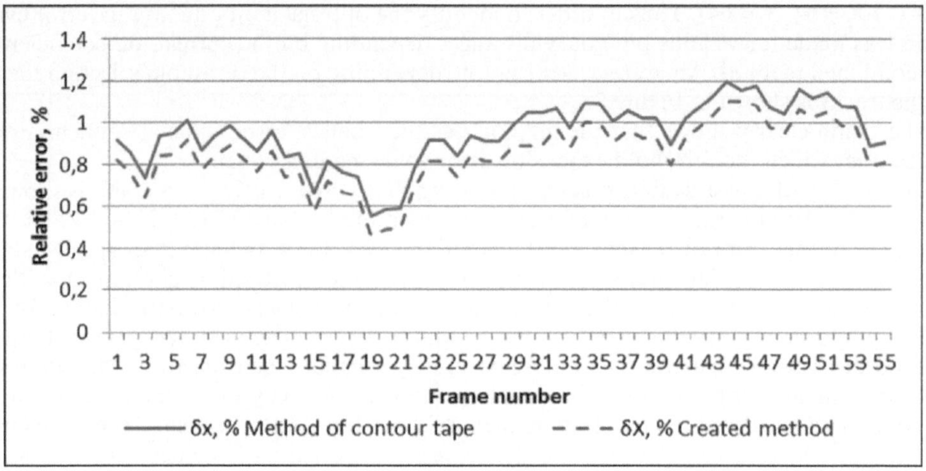

Figure 7.14 The comparative graph of the relative errors.

Table 7.3 The comparative analysis of some prediction methods for various kinds of data preprocessing.

Name of the method	"contour tape" method δxav,%	proposed method δxav,%
	Numerical methods (Box & Jenkins 1994)	
Exponential smoothing, additive model	0,87	0,85
Exponential smoothing with damping	0.69	0.66
AR model	1,43	0,97
	Neural networks (Haykin 1999)	
Radial basis function RBF S5	0,51	0,43
Linear network S5	0,46	0,37
Multi-layer perceptron MP5–2-1	0,47	0,38

Table 7.3 shows data for the average prediction error of some forecasting methods for pre-treatment for both the developed method and contour tape method (Timchenko et al. 2011) (δxav is the average relative error of the method, calculated between the actual and the predicted value). As can be seen from the table, the proposed method is 15–20% better than the contour tape one.

6 CONCLUSIONS

This chapter considered the problem of sending a laser beam in the atmosphere for atmospheric optical communication. It is established that for positioning transmitter-receiver devices, they must classify images in order to highlight non-noisy ones.

To solve the problem of laser beam image classification with a high accuracy, we recommend the proposed method of direct parallel-hierarchical transformation that has adaptive properties similar to neural networks. In order to accelerate the operations of laser beam spots processing, a specialised memory device and its implementation on FPGA has been offered. Also, the framework for checking the theoretical results is created. Further development resulted in the method of direct parallel-hierarchical transformation, which combines the shift and transposition operators for parallel-hierarchical network in order to reduce the amount of memory accesses by half. The improved reading operation of 2-port memory allows for rapid-forming parallel-hierarchical transformation displacement vector in one clock cycle.

REFERENCES

Altera. 2016. AN 461: *Design Guidelines for Implementing QDRII+ and QDRII SRAM Interfaces in Stratix III and Stratix IV Devices*: http://www.altera.com/literature/an/an461.pdf.

Apopei, B. Dodd, T.J. 2012. Automatic parallelisation for LTI MIMO state space systems using FPGAs. An optimisation for cost & performance. *Journal of Parallel and Distributed Computing* 72(8): 990–1007.

Borovoy, A.G. Patrushev, G.Y. & Petrov, A.I. 1988. Laser beam propagation through the turbulent atmosphere with precipitation. *Applied Optics* 27(17): 3704–3714.

Box, G. Jenkins, G. 1994. Time series analysis: forecasting and control: 592. Canada: John Willey & Sons.

Buck, J. & Washington, D. 2013. *NASA Laser Communication System Sets Record with Data Transmissions to and from Moon*, https://www.nasa.gov/press/2013/october/nasa-laser-communication-system-sets-record-with-data-transmissions-to-and-from/#.WJ9 s2vnhCM8

Fernández-García, N.L. Carmona-Poyato, A. Medina-Carnicer, R. & Madrid-Cuevas, F.J. 2008. Automatic generation of consensus ground truth for the comparison of edge detection techniques. *Image and Vision Computing* 26(4): 496–511.

Goodman, J. 1984. The use of static column ram as a memory hierarchy. In R.G James, Ch. Menchow (eds) *ISCA '84 Proceedings of the 11th annual international symposium on Computer architecture*: 167–173. New York.

Haykin S. 1999. Neural Networks: 1104. New Jersey: Prentice Hall.

Hejlsberg, A. Torgersen, M. at all. 2010. The C# Programming Language. *Addison-Wesley Professional* 4: 864.

Kandel, R. & Hawkins, R. 1992. The Biological Basis of Learning and Individuality. *Journal Scientific* American 267(3): 53–60.

Karbo, M. 2002. PC Architecture. *Know Ware—Competence Micro*: 386.

Livingstone, M.S. & Hubel, D.H. 1984. Anatomy in the Primate Visual Cortex. *Journal of Neuroscience* 4: 309–356.

Medina-Carnicer, R. Muñoz-Salinas, R. Carmona-Poyato, A. & Madrid-Cuevas, F.J. 2011. A novel histogram transformation to improve the performance of thresholding methods in edge detection. *Pattern Recognition Letters* 32(5): 676–693.

Medina-Carnicer, R. Muñoz-Salinas, R. Yeguas-Bolivar, E. & Diaz-Mas, L. 2011. A novel method to look for the hysteresis thresholds for the Canny edge detector. *Pattern Recognition* 44(6): 1201–1211.

Palagin, A. 2013. The structure of FPGA-based cyclic-code converters. In A. Palagin, V. Opanasenko, & S. Krivoi (eds), *Optical Memory & Neural Networks (Information Optics)* 22(4): 207–216. Springer.

Random Integer Generator / Randomness and Integrity Services Ltd.: http://www.random.org/integers/

Sherrington, G.E. 1961. The Integrative Action of the Nervous System. New Haven: Yale University Press.

Stratix V Feature Overview: www.altera.com/products/fpga/stratix-series/stratix-v/features.html

Swets, J.A. 1996. Signal detection theory and ROC analysis in psychology and diagnostics. *Lawrence Erlbaum Associates*: 332.

Timchenko L. Poplavskyy, A. Petrovskyi, N. Kokriatskaia, N. & Kutaev, Y. 2011. Method of reference tunnel formation for improving forecast results of the laser beams spot images behaviour. *Optical Engineering* 50(11): 117007.

Timchenko, L.I. 2000. A multistage parallel-hierarchic network as a model of a neurolike computation scheme. *Cybernetics and Systems Analysis* 36(2): 251–267.

Timchenko, L.I. Melnikov, V.V. & Kokryatskaya, N.I. 2011. Parallel-hierarchical network learning methods and their application to pattern recognition. *Cybernetics and Systems Analysis* 47(6): 986–994.

Timchenko, L.I. Petrovskyi, N.S. & Kokriatskaia, N.I. 2014. Laser beam image classification methods with the use of parallel-hierarchical networks running on a programmable logic device, *Optical Engineering* 53(10): 103–106.

Weichel, H. 1990. Laser Beam Propagation in the Atmosphere, *Proceedings of SPIE* TT03: 108.

CHAPTER 8

The conjugated null space method of blind deconvolution

R.N. Kvyetnyy, O.Yu. Sofina & Y.A. Bunyak
Vinnitsia National Technical University, Vinnytsia, Ukraine

W. Wójcik & P. Komada
Lublin University of Technology, Lublin, Poland

A. Kalizhanova
Al-Farabi Kazakh National University, Almaty, Kazakhstan

N.A. Orshubekov
Kazakh University of Railways and Communications, Almaty, Kazakhstan

1 INTRODUCTION

Many modern applications need real time reconstruction of high resolution images of some millions pixels in size, which are corrupted by defocusing, medium penetration, camera jitter and other factors. Usually, the model of corruption is presented as convolution of the original image signal and the point spread function (PSF) (Biemond et al. 1990, Jiang & Wang 2003b, Kundur & Hatzinakos 1996). The exact PSF shape is in most cases unknown. Thus, the image reconstruction problem includes the blind identification of the PSF and deconvolution. Both problems are ill-posed and their solution is approximate in accordance with the chosen optimisation criterion.

The principal possibility of a solution to the PSF estimation problem was proven analytically by Lane and Bates (1987). They have shown that convolved components of any multidimensional signal can be separated on condition the signal dimension is greater than one. Their conclusions are based on the analytic properties of the Z-Transform (ZT) in multiple dimensions. The zeros of the ZT of multi dimensional components lie on a hypersurface which can be separated, and the zeros of the individual components can be recognised up to complex scale factors. The general approach to zero-sheet separation is based on finding combinations of some mutually dependent zeros belonging to each of the separate ZT coordinates. The required combination creates the singularity of a Vandermonde like matrix (Aogaki et al. 2006, Lane & Bates 1987). This condition points to the presence of a polynomial substructure in a polynomial structure of higher order. Such a solution is equivalent to finding a null space (NS) of the mentioned matrix. The zero-sheet separation approach is very complicated for implementation because zeros accuracy evaluation depends on the resolution of spectral image presentation, which is limited by the available combinations of the number of spectral components and must not be enormously large. The model of image signal can be used instead of the image itself to reduce the problem complexity. As shown in Biemond et al. (1988), and Lagendijk et al. (1990), the autoregressive and moving average (MA) model enables to separate the original image and the PSF as parts which correspond to the AR and MA models accordingly. The AR model characteristic polynomial contains zeros, exact or fuzzy, that are equal to ZT zeros. But this zeros set includes original image zeros as well PSF zeros because the AR model parameters can be estimated only by means of a measured degraded image. An elimination of the PSF zeros influence can be reached by using some number of images obtained as different degradations of the same original image. As was shown in Pai & Bovik (1997), if there are at least three differently degraded images, then the original image can be reconstructed exactly as the right side NS of the operator which acts as convolution of the AR parameters and the image data vector. The AR model of a higher order was used, whose size is compatible with image size. It was defined correctly using some blurred images. Therefore the image in the manner of a set of different planes with sharp edges was exactly reconstructed as NS in Pai & Bovik (1997). The NS may be presented by a single eigenvector or by optimised sum of some eigenvectors (Pai et al. 1997, Pai & Bovik 2001) which correspond to least eigenvalues of the AR model operator. This approach is useful in cases of strongly noised and blurred images. The eigenvector or the sum of eigenvectors are the lexicographical presentation of the original image signal matrix and so the NS approach is appropriate to the reconstruction of relatively small images for a time far from the usual period of image frames stored by a camera.

When the PSF is known, the problem of deblurring can be considered as an inverse filtration of the observed image. Methods of inverse filter implementation are direct, mainly in spectral domain, and indirect, by using maximum likelihood, Bayesian and variational approaches. The Wiener spectral method (Biemond et al. 1990, Kundur & Hatzinakos 1996) lies at the base of most methods of inverse filtration (Carasso et al. 2006, Michailovich & Tannenbaum 2007, Ng et al. 2000). The designed methods are intended for regularisation of spectrum inversion and optimisation of the PSF spectrum shape with the aim of eliminating the noise influence.

There are some approaches to simultaneous iterative deconvolution and PSF estimation. The Lucy-Richardson (LR) maximum likelihood (ML) method (Lucy 1974, Richardson 1972) of deconvolution was supplemented in (Holmes 1992) by an iterative schema of PSF estimation and was developed in Biggs & Andrews (1997), Fish et al. (1995), Jiang & Wang (2003a), and Singh et al. (2008) in an extended manner. The LR method has some limitations, such as slow convergence, sensitivity to noise, image artefacts presence. The methods of variational optimisation (Chan & Wong 1998, Chan et al. 2005, Hao & Qinzhang 2007, Molina et al. 2006, You & Kaveh 1996, Zhu & Chan 2012), statistical Bayesian and maximum posterior models of blur (Babacan et al. 2009, Bronstein et al. 2005, Liao & Ng 2011, Levin et al. 2011, Likas & Galatsanos 2004, Michailovich & Tannenbaum 2007, Money & Kang 2008, Tzikas et al. 2009) are used to obtain the iterative schemas of the image sought and the PSF estimates. Limitations and advantages of the variational method depend on the estimated prior model of the PSF and the regularisation operator. In the case of a large image, its implementation is difficult because it uses operators in the manner of a matrix with row size equal to the size of the lexicographical presentation of the processed image. The parametrisation of least square, Bayesian or Euler-Lagrange (EL) optimisation problems in accordance with gradient methods give appropriate schemas for iterative optimisation of the original image estimate (Bar et al. 2007b, Donatelli et al. 2006, Han et al. 2009, Katsaggelos et al. 2009, Landweber 1951, Liang & Xu 2003, Rudin et al. 1992, Yang et al. 1999). These schemas are not always stable and convergent, and usually require hundreds of iterations for attaining the convergence limit condition.

We consider the problem of arbitrary size image series reconstruction from the point of view of their real time processing. This aim means that the original image estimate can be found by one step deconvolution using the inverse point spread function (IPSF) characteristic and it is allowable to use some optimisation iterations. It is assumed that the blur characteristic changes slowly and the IPSF can be estimated without real time restriction. Therefore, the problem solution includes PSF estimation, definition of the optimal IPSF and evaluation of primary image estimate and optimisation of a given estimate by some number of iterations.

2 THE CONJUGATED NS METHOD OF PSF ESTIMATION

2.1 *The problem formulation*

The linear model of a degraded measured image $X = X(x,y) \subset \Omega$, where Ω is an image space, x,y – image pixel coordinates; in noise-free case it has the form of a convolution

$$X = H * S \tag{8.1}$$

of blur characteristic PSF $H \subset \Xi \subset \Omega$: $Power(\Xi) << Power(\Omega)$, and original image $S \subset \Omega$ (Biemond et al. 1990, Kundur & Hatzinakos 1996). It is required to obtain the inverse expression

$$S = G * X \tag{8.2}$$

for image reconstruction on condition that the blur function H is unknown. The IPSF is defined in Ξ or it can be defined in Ω too.

One of the ways of solving the problem is based on the assumption that original and degraded images possess algebraic structure which is invariant to blur operator (8.1) action. Such common algebraic structure may be defined as operator A, whose NS is constituted by the image matrices X and S:

$$\int_{\Omega} A(x,y;\varsigma,\xi)S(\varsigma,\xi)d\varsigma d\xi \cong 0 \tag{8.3}$$

$$\int_{\Omega} A(x,y;\varsigma,\xi)X(\varsigma,\xi)d\varsigma d\xi \cong 0 \tag{8.4}$$

The transforms (8.3) and (8.4) are linear and so degradation transform (8.1) and inverse transform (8.2) do not influence their result. The operator A can be complemented by conjugated null space (CNS) $F \subset \Xi$:

$$\int_{\Xi} F'(\varsigma,\xi)A(\varsigma,\xi;x,y)d\varsigma d\xi \cong 0 \tag{8.5}$$

where •′ – the conjugation. In general, the exact NS does not exist and so we used approximate equality in (8.3)–(8.5).

We shall show that matrix convolution transforms, which correspond to expressions (8.1), (8.3) and (8.5), on the condition of model operator shift invariance: $A(x, y; \varsigma, \xi) = A(x-\varsigma, y-\xi)$, are commutative and can be joined in matrix transform corresponding to (8.4). Therefore the CNS in (8.5) can be considered an estimate of the PSF in (8.1): $F \cong H$.

2.2 *The null space method of image deblurring*

The NS method (Pai & Bovik 1997) includes four steps of original image reconstruction.

At the first step the extended matrix is created

$$\mathbf{X} = \left[\mathbf{x}_{i+k,l+m}\right]_{i=1...P,\ l=1...q}^{k=0...N_x-P-1,\ m=0...N_y-Q-1} \tag{8.6}$$

where low indices point to image matrix columns and high indices point to rows, $N_x \times N_y$ – image matrix X size, P, Q – algebraic structure parameters, $\mathbf{x}_{i,k}$ – pixels of matrix X, or vectors of pixels of a series of matrices like X, with indices i and k along coordinates x and y.

The second step, the NS vector $\mathbf{a} = \mathbf{vec}(A)$ – the lexicographical presentation of matrix $A = [a_{i,k}]_{i=1...P}^{k=1...Q}$, has to be found:

$$\mathbf{X} \cdot \mathbf{a} \cong \mathbf{0} \tag{8.7}$$

At the third step the matrix is formed

$$\mathbf{A} = \begin{bmatrix} \mathbf{A}_1\mathbf{A}_2...\mathbf{A}_P\mathbf{0}\ ...\mathbf{0} \\ \mathbf{0}\ \mathbf{A}_1\mathbf{A}_2...\mathbf{A}_P...\mathbf{0} \\ \vdots \quad \ddots \quad \vdots \\ \mathbf{0}\ ...\mathbf{0}\ \mathbf{A}_1\mathbf{A}_2...\mathbf{A}_P \end{bmatrix}; \mathbf{A}_k = \begin{bmatrix} a_{k,1}a_{k,2}...a_{k,Q}0\ ...0 \\ 0\ a_{k,1}a_{k,2}...a_{k,Q}...0 \\ \vdots \quad \ddots \quad \vdots \\ 0\ ...0\ a_{k,1}a_{k,2}...a_{k,Q} \end{bmatrix}, \tag{8.8}$$

where $\mathbf{0}$ – null matrix. Matrix (8.8) includes $N_x \cdot N_y$ columns, minimal number of rows $P \cdot Q$.

The fourth step, NS vector $\mathbf{s}$ has to be found:

$$\mathbf{A} \cdot \mathbf{s} \cong \mathbf{0}. \tag{8.9}$$

The vector

$$\mathbf{s} = \mathbf{vec}(S). \tag{8.10}$$

is the lexicographical presentation of the required original image S or its estimate.

2.3 *Null space of the PSF*

We can rewrite the expression (8.7) as the 2D AR model

$$\sum_{i=1}^{P} \sum_{k=1}^{Q} \mathbf{x}_{i+n,k+m} a_{i,k} \approx 0, \tag{8.11}$$

where $\mathbf{x}_{i,k}$ – image signal samples or RGB vectors, $n = 0...N_x - P$, $m = 0...N_y - Q$. As was shown in Pai & Bovik (1997), matrix $\mathbf{X}$ (8.6) and the analogous extended original image matrix $\mathbf{S}$ have the same NS or, in other words, the same AR model (8.11). This assumption was used in Biemond et al. (1988), and Lagendijk et al. (1990) too. We will consider matrix $\mathbf{A}$ (8.8) as the discrete presentation of the algebraic structure A in (8.3)–(8.5).

As image (8.1) is the convolution of the original image and the PSF, model (8.11) is common with respect to these components. But there is one sufficient difference, the images $X,S \subset \Omega$, the PSF $H \subset \Xi \subset \Omega$. The PSF space Ξ can be presented with the help of δ-function window,

$$\Xi = W * \Omega, W = W(x,t;y,\tau) = \delta(x-t,\varsigma)\delta(y-\tau,\xi) : x,y,t,\tau \in \Omega; \varsigma,\xi \in \Xi. \tag{8.12}$$

If we suppose that $H \subset \tilde{H}$: $Power(\tilde{H}) = Power(\Omega)$; $H = W * \tilde{H}$; $X \subset \tilde{H} * S$, then

$$A * X = A * \tilde{H} * S = (W * \tilde{H})' * A * S = H' * A * S = 0, \tag{8.13}$$

The formulation of rearranging (8.13) in discrete matrix form has the following manner:

$$\mathbf{A}\left[\mathbf{x}^{(1)}\mathbf{x}^{(2)}...\mathbf{x}^{(K)}\right]^T = \mathbf{A}\left[\tilde{\mathbf{H}}^{(1)}\tilde{\mathbf{H}}^{(2)}...\tilde{\mathbf{H}}^{(K)}\right]^T \mathbf{s} = \left[\mathbf{H}^{(1)}\mathbf{H}^{(2)}...\mathbf{H}^{(K)}\right]\mathbf{A} \cdot \mathbf{s} \cong \mathbf{0}, \tag{8.14}$$

where T – the transposition, $\mathbf{x}^{(i)} = \mathbf{vec}(X^{(i)})$ – data of $i = 1\ ..\ K$ degradation filters, $\mathbf{s}$ – vector (8.10) of the original image, $\tilde{\mathbf{H}}^{(i)}$ and $\mathbf{H}^{(i)}$ – the i-th PSF filter operators with similar structure

$$\mathbf{H} = \begin{bmatrix} \mathbf{H}_1\mathbf{H}_2...\mathbf{H}_L\mathbf{0}\ ...\mathbf{0} \\ \mathbf{0}\ \mathbf{H}_1\mathbf{H}_2...\mathbf{H}_L...\mathbf{0} \\ \vdots \quad \ddots \quad \vdots \\ \mathbf{0}\ ...\mathbf{0}\ \mathbf{H}_1\mathbf{H}_2...\mathbf{H}_L \end{bmatrix}; \mathbf{H}_k = \begin{bmatrix} h_{k,1}h_{k,2}...h_{k,M}0\ ...0 \\ 0\ h_{k,1}h_{k,2}...h_{k,M}...0 \\ \vdots \quad \ddots \quad \vdots \\ 0\ ...0\ h_{k,1}h_{k,2}...h_{k,M} \end{bmatrix} \tag{8.15}$$

and with different size—the size of the first one being $N_xN_y \times N_xN_y$ and the size of the second one – $L{\cdot}M \times P{\cdot}Q$, $L \times M = Power(\Xi)$. As follows from the structure of matrices (8.8) and (8.15), transform (8.14) implicitly includes the convolution with the space window in (8.12). The rearrangement in (8.13) allows to omit the PSF matrices in (8.14) and define the original image as NS vector (8.10). The NS method (Pai & Bovik 1997) demands absence of coherence between K degradation filters. The filters influence is minimal in equation (8.7) and it is equivalent to equation (8.9) in such conditions.

In accordance with (8.9) $\mathbf{A} \cdot \mathbf{s} \cong \mathbf{0}$ in (8.14), vector $\mathbf{h} = \mathbf{vec}(H)$ of the operator (8.15) in (8.13) and (8.14) can be arbitrary, but on the condition that it is on the left side of the NS,

$$\mathbf{h}^T \cdot \mathbf{A} \cong 0, \tag{8.16}$$

vector $\mathbf{h}$ is the PSF because it was defined with the help of splitting the image matrix X and rearranging the convolved components of (8.13), which are at the symmetric positions in the AR model (8.11). Vector $\mathbf{h}$ becomes independent with respect to the image vector $\mathbf{s}$ as an observation characteristic on condition (8.16). Matrix $\mathbf{A}$ in (8.16) is sufficiently smaller than the same matrix in (8.9). It includes $L \cdot M$ rows and $(P + L - 1) \cdot (Q + M - 1)$ columns, $L < P$ and $M < Q$.

In the account of the structure of matrix (8.15), expression (8.16) can be rewritten as

$$\mathbf{H} \cdot \mathbf{a} \cong 0, \tag{8.17}$$

where $\mathbf{a} = \mathbf{vec}(A)$. The PSF and original image can be matched in Z-space as polynomial substructures of the general polynomial $A(Z)$ related to the AR model (8.11). The polynomial has local and fuzzy roots which form the zero hypersurface $Z_A{:}A(Z_A) = 0$. Expressions (8.7) and (8.17) are different equations for estimation of the same vector $\mathbf{a}$. Thus, the ZT of X and H forms hypersurfaces $Z_X \subset Z_A{:}A(Z_X) = 0$ and $Z_H \subset Z_A{:}A(Z_H) = 0$. However, $Z_H \subset Z_X$ and $Z_X = Z_S \cup Z_H$. The hypersurfaces Z_S and Z_H are mutually independent (incoherent) – $Z_S \cap Z_H = 0$, because they are defined by ZT in different spaces—correspondingly Ω and Ξ. Thus hypersurfaces Z_S and Z_H can be separated using a single image fragment. On the other hand, the original image S was coherent with the measured image X and so $K \geq 3$ degraded images with incoherent blur functions were used for reconstruction of S in Pai & Bovik (1997).

In accordance with expressions (8.11) and (8.17), the bound elements of matrix H must vanish because they interact with few elements of matrix $\mathbf{A}$ which, in general, are far from zero. Conversely, the central elements of matrix H must neutralise the most significant part of matrix $\mathbf{A}$. These conditions determine the convex shape with vanishing bounds of matrix H.

3 DECONVOLUTION OPTIMISATION

3.1 *Inverse PSF estimation*

The IPSF estimation is based on Wiener's spectral method (Biemond et al. 1990, Jiang & Wang 2003b), which includes division by the PSF spectrum and hence needs regularisation. However, even a regularised inverse spectrum gives image boundary fluctuations. Also, the regularisation eliminates filtered image resolution. These deficiencies are caused by the discrepancy of the image and PSF spaces Ω and Ξ. The artificial matching of the PSF into Ω in spectral transforms by supplementation of zeros creates a spectrum leakage with fluctuations, whose influence is intensified by division. We shall find the IPSF without exceeding the bounds of Ξ to avoid these defects.

Letus write expressions (8.1) and (8.2) in a discrete manner.

$$\mathbf{x}_{i,k} = \sum_{l=1}^{L} \sum_{m=1}^{M} \mathbf{s}_{i+l,k+m} h_{l,m}, \tag{8.18}$$

$$\mathbf{s}_{i,k} = \sum_{l=1}^{L} \sum_{m=1}^{M} \mathbf{x}_{i+l,k+m} g_{l,m}, \tag{8.19}$$

where $\mathbf{x}_{i,k}$ and $\mathbf{s}_{i,k}$ are the samples or RGB vectors of the observed distorted image X and the original image S sought, $h_{l,m}$, $g_{l,m}$ –elements of the PSF and IPSF, $i = 0 \ldots N_x - L - 1$, $k = 0 \ldots N_y - M - 1$. The substitution of (8.19) into (8.18) gives the equation for evaluation of the IPSF.

$$\mathbf{x}_{i,k} = \sum_{l=1}^{L} \sum_{m=1}^{M} g_{l,m} \left(\sum_{l'=1}^{L} \sum_{m'=1}^{M} x_{i+l-l',k+m-m'} h_{l',m'} \right). \tag{8.20}$$

The expression in brackets yields once more the degradation of the observed image by filtering. The indices of $\mathbf{x}_{\bullet}$ in the right part of equation (8.20) are symmetrised relatively to the left part indices due to symmetry of convolution. Equation (8.20) is ill-posed because $N_x >> L$ and $N_y >> M$. It needs regularisation which applies restrictions on its solution.

We suppose that the PSF and IPSF belong to a class of smooth functions. We choose the surface area of the IPSF as a criterion of smoothness because the minimal surface area corresponds to the maximally smooth flat surface. The smoothness of the sought IPSF means a minimisation of fluctuations caused by image degradation factors. The surface area as regularisation functional was used in solving the image denoising problem (Bar et al. 2007a, Tschumperle & Deriche 2005). However, it was not met in formulations of problems of convolutional type with the same aim as in (8.20).

The surface area of the function $G(x,y)$ is defined as in Dubrovin et al. (1992)

$$\Sigma_G = \int_{\Xi} \sqrt{1 + G_x^2 + G_y^2}(x,y)dxdy, \tag{8.21}$$

where $G_{x(y)} = \partial G(x, y)/\partial x(y)$. The general functional, which includes the least squares solution of (8.20) and the regularisation term (8.21), can be written as

$$I_G = \arg\min_{G} \left[\frac{1}{2} \int_{\Xi} \|G * Y - \mathbf{x}\|^2 (x,y)dxdy + \lambda \cdot \Sigma_G \right], \tag{8.22}$$

where $Y = H^* X$ – the matrix defined by the expression in brackets in (8.20), λ – the regularisation parameter.

Euler-Lagrange variational derivative (Dubrovin et al. 1992) for functional (8.22) minimum finding looks as follows:

$$\frac{\partial \|G * Y - \mathbf{x}\|^2}{2\partial G} - \lambda \cdot \left(\frac{\partial}{\partial x} \frac{\partial \Sigma_G}{\partial G_x} + \frac{\partial}{\partial y} \frac{\partial \Sigma_G}{\partial G_y} \right) = 0. \tag{8.23}$$

We also have in mind the fulfilment of the zero Neumann boundary condition (Dubrovin et al. 1992). In account of (8.21), the expression (8.23) takes the following form.

$$Y' * (G * Y - \mathbf{x}) - \lambda \cdot \mathbf{L}_{\Sigma}(G) = 0, \tag{8.24}$$

where

$$\mathbf{L}_\Sigma(G) = \left(1+G_x^2+G_y^2\right)^{-3/2}\left(\left(1+G_y^2\right)G_{xx}+\left(1+G_x^2\right)G_{yy}-2G_xG_yG_{xy}\right). \tag{8.25}$$

The discrete iterative schema of the solution to equation (8.24) is as follows:

$$\mathbf{g}^{(k+1)} = \left(R_{YY} - \lambda\cdot\delta R\left(\mathbf{g}^{(k)}\right)\right)^{-1}\mathbf{r}_{YX}, \tag{8.26}$$

where $\mathbf{g} = \mathbf{vec}(G)$, $\mathbf{g}; R_{YY}; \mathbf{r}_{YX} \subset \Xi$,

$$\begin{aligned} R_{YY} &= Y' * Y, \mathbf{r}_{YX} = Y' * \mathbf{x}, \\ \delta R\left(\mathbf{g}^{(k)}\right) &= diag\left[\mathbf{I}+\left(D_x\mathbf{g}^{(k)}\right)^2+\left(D_y\mathbf{g}^{(k)}\right)^2\right]^{-3/2} \\ &\times\left(diag\left[\mathbf{I}+\left(D_y\mathbf{g}^{(k)}\right)^2\right]D_{xx}+diag\left[\mathbf{I}+\left(D_x\mathbf{g}^{(k)}\right)^2\right]D_{yy}\right. \\ &\left.-2\cdot diag\left[D_x\mathbf{g}^{(k)}\right]\cdot diag\left[D_y\mathbf{g}^{(k)}\right]D_{xy}\right), \end{aligned} \tag{8.27}$$

$\mathbf{I}$ – the identity matrix, $D_\bullet$ – the differential operator with indices pointed by variables and degree, *diag*[•] – diagonal matrix, created by the vector in brackets. The parameter λ can be chosen as the maximum possible value that provides convergence of schema (8.26) at first q iterations:

$$\left\langle\left\|\mathbf{g}^{(k+1)}-\mathbf{g}^{(k)}\right\|^2\right\rangle \le \theta\left\langle\left\|\mathbf{g}^{(k)}-\mathbf{g}^{(k-1)}\right\|^2\right\rangle, \tag{8.28}$$

where $k = 0 \ldots q-1$, θ – positive value, $\langle\bullet\rangle$ – the averaging. The iteration process can be stopped if

$$\left\langle\left\|\mathbf{g}^{(k+1)}-\mathbf{g}^{(k)}\right\|^2\right\rangle < \varepsilon \tag{8.29}$$

– a small value.

The IPSF (8.26) can be used for primary estimation of the original image sought in accordance with equation (8.19). Of course, the spectral method can be used too, but in this case the division by the IPSF spectrum is not necessary and the influence of spectrum leakage is insignificant.

The principal distinction of problem (8.22) and similar denoising and deconvolution problems consists in the fact that the arguments are defined in different spaces—the argument of problem (8.22) $G \subset \Xi$ and the argument of the second one? belongs to image space Ω. We project $\Omega \to \Xi$ by convolution operations (8.27) and in that way create a unified problem presentation space.

3.2 *Lucy-Richardson deconvolution schema and its development*

The iterative LR algorithm (Lucy 1974, Richardson 1972)

$$S^{(k+1)} = S^{(k)}\left(H'^{(k)} * \frac{X}{S^{(k)} * H^{(k)}}\right) \tag{8.30}$$

gives the solution of the deconvolution problem in accordance with the ML criterion of the observed X and the original images S sought. In the expression (8.30), $S^{(k)}$ and $H^{(k)}$ – k-th image and PSF estimates, and $S^{(0)} = X$. The iterative estimation of the PSF was introduced in (Holmes 1992) as

$$H^{(k+1)} = H^{(k)}\left(S'^{(k+1)} * \frac{X}{S^{(k+1)} * H^{(k)}}\right) \tag{8.31}$$

and was used when the exact PSF is unknown. The iterations number of the LR schema (8.30)–(8.31) can amount to several hundred. This caused the designing of some methods of iteration acceleration (8.30), for example Biggs & Andrews (1997), or Singh et al. (2008).

The LR algorithm is based on the maximisation of conditional probability distribution (PD) of blurred and initial images using Bayes equation. This equation includes division, so schema (8.30) is unstable, since zero neighborhood zones are inherent to images. The efficiency of the LR algorithm depends on image signal PD type too. Therefore, schema (8.30) demands regularisation and statistical generalisation. The last request is achievable by the assumption of maximum entropy (ME) of image PD. This property is provided by Gaussian PD. The regularised and generalised iterative LRME schema was suggested in Dey et al. (2004), and looks as follows:

$$S^{(k+1)} = S^{(k)} + \delta t \cdot \left(H' * X - (H' * H) * S^{(k)} + \lambda \cdot \mathbf{L}(S^{(k)})\right), \tag{8.32}$$

where δt and λ – the parameters of relaxation and regularisation, $\mathbf{L}(S)$ – the regularisation operator obtained as the EL equation of a regularisation functional. The total variation (TV) regularisation functional (Rudin et al. 1992)

$$\mathbf{R}_{TV}(S) = \int_\Omega \sqrt{S_x^2 + S_y^2}\, dxdy \tag{8.33}$$

was used in Dey et al. (2004). Other linear and nonlinear regularisation functionals are also used in deconvolution optimisation as well as in denoising—Tikhonov, Tikhonov-Miller (TM), TV with additional β-factor – $\sqrt{S_x^2 + S_y^2 + \beta}$, $0 < \beta << 1$, in the expression (8.33), surface area and surface energy, mean curvature, image Laplacian, Laplacian in curved space (Beltrami operator) etc. (Bar et al. 2007a, Brito-Loeza & Chen 2010, Chambolle et al. 2004, Chan & Wong 1998, Chan et al. 2005, Keren & Gotlib 1998, Lysaker et al. 2004).

3.3 *The method of deconvolution optimisation by balanced variations and dynamic regularisation (BVDR)*

The ME generalisation of the sought and blurred images conditional PD gives the trivial functional (Dey et al. 2004)

$$I = \frac{1}{2}\int_\Omega \|X - H * S\|^2 (x, y)\, dxdy, \tag{8.34}$$

which can be optimised by using additional constraints defined by the regularisation functional $\mathbf{R}(S)$. Then deconvolution optimisation means the minimisation of the functional:

$$I_S = \arg\min_S \left[\frac{1}{2}\int_\Omega \|X - H * S\|^2 (x, y)\, dxdy + \lambda \cdot \mathbf{R}(S)\right], \tag{8.35}$$

where λ – the regularisation parameter, a positive value or function. The EL equation gives the expression

$$H' * (X - H * S) + \lambda \cdot \mathbf{L}(S) = 0, \tag{8.36}$$

where $\mathbf{L}(S) = \delta\mathbf{R}(S)/\delta S$ – the variational derivative that is analogous to the second term in (8.23). We suppose that IPSF G is found by (8.20) or (8.26) and convolution $G * H'$ gives a trivial operator. Then the convolution of the IPSF with components of (8.36) gives the next equation:

$$X - H * S + \lambda \cdot G * \mathbf{L}(S) = 0. \tag{8.37}$$

We can parameterise equation (8.37) and present it as an evolutional equation in accordance with the gradient descent method (Landweber 1951, Rudin et al. 1992),

$$S_t = X - H * S + \lambda(t) \cdot G * \mathbf{L}(S), \tag{8.38}$$

where t – the evolution parameter. Neumann boundary conditions are assumed. The regularisation parameter $\lambda(t)$ can be defined such that equation (8.38) has to be convergent.

The convergence of iterative problems in image processing was considered in a review paper by Katsaggelos et al. (2009) and some other papers (Bar et al. 2007b, Cai et al. 2009, Han et al. 2009, Jiang & Wang 2003a, Liang & Xu 2003). We can define the convergence process with the help of l_1 norm as $\langle |S_{t+\tau} - S_t| \rangle \leq \langle |S_t - S_{t-\tau}| \rangle$, or as parametric derivative

$$\langle |S_t|_t \rangle = -\chi, \tag{8.39}$$

where χ is a positive small value. We can write expression (8.39) for (8.38) as follows:

$$\langle |-H * S_t + \lambda_t(t) \cdot G * \mathbf{L}(S) + \lambda(t) \cdot G * \mathbf{L}_t(S)| \rangle = \chi. \tag{8.40}$$

Since we have found the regularisation parameter as a positive function, equation (8.40) can be rewritten as the inequality

$$\lambda_t(t) \cdot \langle |G * \mathbf{L}(S)| \rangle + \lambda(t) \cdot \langle |G * \mathbf{L}_t(S)| \rangle + \langle |-H * S_t| \rangle \geq \chi. \tag{8.41}$$

The χ is an arbitrary value and so expression (8.41) can be transformed into the differential equation

$$\lambda_t(t) + \lambda(t) \frac{\langle |G * \mathbf{L}_t(S)| \rangle}{\langle |G * \mathbf{L}(S)| \rangle} = \frac{\langle |H * S_t| \rangle - \chi}{\langle |G * \mathbf{L}(S)| \rangle}, \tag{8.42}$$

whose solution yields the upper bound of $\lambda(t)$:

$$\begin{aligned} \sup(\lambda(t)) = \lim_{\chi \to 0} \int_0^t \exp\left(-\int_\tau^t \frac{\langle |G * \mathbf{L}_\varsigma(S)| \rangle}{\langle |G * \mathbf{L}(S)| \rangle}(\varsigma) d\varsigma \right) \frac{\langle |H * S_\tau| \rangle - \chi}{\langle |G * \mathbf{L}(S)| \rangle}(\tau) d\tau \\ + \lambda(0) \exp\left(-\int_0^t \frac{\langle |G * \mathbf{L}_\tau(S)| \rangle}{\langle |G * \mathbf{L}(S)| \rangle}(\tau) d\tau \right). \end{aligned} \tag{8.43}$$

The convergence condition (8.39) in a discrete manner means that $\langle |S^{(k+1)} - S^{(k)}| \rangle < \langle |S^{(k)} - S^{(k-1)}| \rangle$. This condition provides the fulfilment of the convergence condition with the l_2 norm of residuals like (8.28)

$$\langle \|S^{(k+1)} - S^{(k)}\|^2 \rangle \leq \theta \langle \|S^{(k)} - S^{(k-1)}\|^2 \rangle \tag{8.44}$$

as the image is a positive function. Formula (8.43) in discrete form is the following:

$$\lambda^{(0)} = \frac{\langle |H*(S^{(0)} - X)| \rangle}{\delta t \langle |G*\mathbf{L}(S^{(0)})| \rangle} \left(\exp\left(\frac{\langle |G*(\mathbf{L}(S^{(0)}) - \mathbf{L}(X))| \rangle}{\delta t \langle |G*\mathbf{L}(S^{(0)})| \rangle} \right) - 1 \right)^{-1};$$
$$\lambda^{(k)} = \left(\lambda^{(k-1)} + \frac{\langle |H*(S^{(k)} - S^{(k-1)})| \rangle}{\delta t \langle |G*\mathbf{L}(S^{(k)})| \rangle} \right) \exp\left(-\frac{\langle |G*(\mathbf{L}(S^{(k)}) - \mathbf{L}(S^{(k-1)}))| \rangle}{\delta t \langle |G*\mathbf{L}(S^{(k)})| \rangle} \right), \tag{8.45}$$

where $S^{(-1)} = X$ and $S^{(0)} = G * X$. The discrete form of equation (8.38) looks as follows:

$$S^{(k+1)} = S^{(k)} + \delta t \cdot \left(X - H*S^{(k)} + \lambda^{(k)} \cdot G*\mathbf{L}(S^{(k)}) \right), \tag{8.46}$$

where δt – the relaxation parameter.

The iterative schema (8.46), in contrast to the known ones like (8.32), includes convolutions with the PSF and IPSF. There are competitive processes of the smoothing and peaking of image shape. If we assume that $\lambda_t(t >> 0) \approx 0$ in (8.40), then the approximate estimate of the regularisation parameter will be:

$$\lambda^{(k)} \approx \frac{\langle |H*(S^{(k)} - S^{(k-1)})| \rangle}{\langle |G*(\mathbf{L}(S^{(k)}) - \mathbf{L}(S^{(k-1)}))| \rangle}. \tag{8.47}$$

Expression (8.47) shows that equation (8.37) constitutes a balance of variations which are caused by convolutions of the PSF and IPSF with the sought image estimate and regularisation term. The first one smoothes the variation of the image surface and the second one sharpens its contours since the regularisation operator is a function of image derivatives. The dynamic character of the schema (8.45)–(8.46) consists in that the regularisation parameter depends on current and previous variations of the image estimate.

3.4 *The method of deconvolution optimisation in curved space (CS)*

The target of optimisation of a functional like (8.34) is to define such S_{opt} that (Dubrovin et al. 1992)

$$\frac{\delta I(S_{opt})}{\delta S} \equiv 0. \tag{8.48}$$

In other words, the optimal value of the functional must be an invariant of argument fluctuation. Let us consider the functional (8.34) in discrete form for $S = S_{opt}$

$$\lim_{\Delta S_{opt} \to 0} \frac{1}{2} \sum_{i,j} \left\| X - H*S_{opt} \right\|^2 \mathrm{P}(\Delta S_{opt})(x_i, y_j) = \min, \tag{8.49}$$

where $\mathrm{P}(\Delta S_{opt}) = \Delta x \Delta y$ – the projection of image surface element on the plane XOY. The variation of expression (8.49) in account of (8.48) yields the nonzero term

$$\lim_{\Delta S_{opt} \to 0} \frac{1}{2} \sum_{i,j} \left\| X - H*S_{opt} \right\|^2 \frac{\partial \mathrm{P}(\Delta S_{opt})}{\partial \delta S}(x_i, y_j) \neq 0. \tag{8.50}$$

The condition (8.48) will be met for each surface element in (8.50) if it is included fully, not by its projection. The surface element in CS with a metric induced by the surface is an invariant of variational transforms which cause corresponding tensor transforms of coordinates. It has the following manner (Dubrovin et al. 1992): $\Delta S_{opt} = \sqrt{\sigma(S_{opt})} \Delta x \Delta y$, where $\sigma(S) = 1 + S_x^2 + S_y^2$ – the determinant of metric tensor at a point of ΔS_{opt}.

The problem of functional (8.34) optimisation with the account of space curvature can be written as

$$I_S = \arg\min_S \left[\frac{1}{2} \int_\Omega \|X - H * S\|^2 \sqrt{\sigma(S)}(x, y)\, dxdy \right]. \tag{8.51}$$

The condition (8.48) provides the convexity of the functional (8.51), and so the existence of a local minimum. The EL equation gives (8.51) the next expression:

$$H' * (X - H * S) - \frac{1}{4\sigma(S)}(X - H * S)^2 \left(\frac{\partial}{\partial x} \frac{\partial \sigma(S)}{\partial S_x} + \frac{\partial}{\partial y} \frac{\partial \sigma(S)}{\partial S_y} \right) = 0. \tag{8.52}$$

The convolution of (8.52) with the IPSF and its parameterisation give the iterative schema for the problem (8.51).

$$S^{(k+1)} = S^{(k)} + \delta t \cdot \left(X - H * S^{(k)} + G * \left(\Lambda(H, S^{(k)}) \cdot \mathbf{L}_\Sigma(S^{(k)})\right)\right), \tag{8.53}$$

where

$$\Lambda(H, S^{(k)}) = \frac{1}{2\sigma(S^{(k)})}\left(X - H * S^{(k)}\right)^2, \tag{8.54}$$

the operator $\mathbf{L}_\Sigma(S^{(k)})$ is similar to (8.25). As follows from expressions (8.53) and (8.54), the iterative process in every point of image surface is assigned by its own parameter—the corresponding element of the regularisation surface Λ. Thus, we have obtained the schema of total optimisation—optimisation in each image point, in contrast to schemas of integral values optimisation like (8.32) and (8.46).

We can rewrite the expression (8.53) relative to $\Delta X^{(k)} = X - H * S^{(k)}$ as

$$(\Delta X^{(k)})^2 + \frac{2\sigma(S^{(k)})}{\mathbf{L}_\Sigma(S^{(k)})} \left(\Delta X_H^{(k)} - \frac{\Delta S_H^{(k)}}{\delta t} \right) = 0, \tag{8.55}$$

where $\Delta X_H^{(k)} = H' * \Delta X^{(k)}$, $\Delta S_H^{(k)} = H' * \Delta S^{(k)}$, $\Delta S^{(k)} = S^{(k+1)} - S^{(k)}$. Let $\Delta X_H^{(k)} \approx \Delta X^{(k)}$ and $\Delta S_H^{(k)} \approx \Delta S^{(k)}$, then expression (8.55) is a quadratic equation and the local minimum of the functional (8.51) will be met in a neighbourhood of its roots or, approximately, in the vicinity of

$$S^{(opt)} \approx G * \left(X - \sqrt{\frac{2\sigma(S^{(opt)})}{\mathbf{L}_\Sigma(S^{(opt)})} \frac{\Delta S^{(opt)}}{\delta t}} \right), \tag{8.56}$$

As follows from (8.56), the precision of evaluation of the optimal estimate S_{opt} in (8.48) is conditioned by the relaxation parameter in (8.56), as well as in (8.53). The choosing of δt has to be made in view that the values of function $\mathbf{L}_\Sigma(S^{(k)})$ can belong to the zero neighbourhood. Thus, the point of $S^{(opt)}$ will be stable on condition that the corresponding values of $\Delta S^{(k)}/\delta t$ belong to the zero neighbourhood too. This condition gives the lower bound of the relaxation parameter a region of allowable values:

$$\delta t \geq \frac{\left\langle \left| S^{(k+1)} - S^{(k)} \right| \right\rangle}{\left\langle \left| \mathbf{L}_\Sigma(S^{(k)}) \right| \right\rangle}. \tag{8.57}$$

Remark. The functional (8.51) cannot be used for optimisation of the IPSF instead of (8.22), because in this case the condition of the unified problem presentation space is violated, the regularisation surface (8.54) meets $\Lambda(G,S) \subset \Omega$ and operator (8.25) $\mathbf{L}_\Sigma(G) \subset \Xi$ concurrently.

4 METHOD IMPLEMENTATION AND TEST EXAMPLES

4.1 *PSF estimation*

The PSF estimation includes the following steps:

1. Evaluation of matrix A using equation (8.10) with vector in the right part, which corresponds to matrix A's central element that is assumed as equal to one. The least squares solution of equation (8.10) can be optimised similarly to procedure (8.22)–(8.27) if the image is noised. The presentable part of the image of a size not less than $2 \cdot P \cdot Q \times 2 \cdot P \cdot Q$ may be used for evaluation of the matrix A elements if the blur is uniform.
2. Creation of the extended matrix $\mathbf{A}$ (8.8) and singular value decomposition (SVD) of the product $\mathbf{A} \cdot \mathbf{A}^T$.
3. The PSF matrix H of the size of the $L \times M$ compilation by means of its lexicographical presentation by the vector of a least singular value.
4. Normalisations of the PSF: $\sum_{l=1}^{L} \sum_{m=1}^{M} h_{l,m} = 1$.

Figure 8.1 shows the three types of estimated PSF. The first one from the left has symmetrical Gaussian shape and displays degradation by defocusing, haze and medium penetration. The next PSF is Gaussian too, but not symmetrical, because it displays degradation by moving along one of the coordinates, in this case—the horizontal one. The third one corresponds to fast moving on the angle, or vibration.

4.2 *IPSF estimation*

We shall consider examples of some image deblurring with different types of blur functions presented in Figure 8.1. The results of deblurring were obtained by convolution with the IPSF. The results of iterative LR deconvolution schema (8.30)–(8.31) and of the APEX method (Carasso et al. 2006) are presented too for comparative analysis.

The image in Figure 8.2 (top left) is an example of aerial photography blurred by haze and vibration. Its PSF is like unsymmetrical Gaussian. The AR model of size $P \times Q = 25 \times 25$ was used to evaluate the PSF of size $L \times M = 9 \times 9$. The haze can be considered as noise and so the AR model optimisation was used accordingly to schema (8.22)–(8.27) with parameters: $\lambda = 0.001$; $q = 3$; $\varepsilon = 1.e - 8$. The convergence of schema (8.26) was fast, the parameter θ in (8.28) amounted to 10. The next two top images in Figure 8.2 show two IPSFs that are found by equations (8.20) and (8.26) correspondingly. The optimised IFPS was reached by seven iterations (8.26). The parameters in expressions (8.26)–(8.29) are: $\lambda = 0.01$; $q = 3$; $\theta \leq 2$; $\varepsilon = 1.e - 8$. The two obtained IPSFs essentially differ and so the results of filtering differ too; they are presented in lower images. It is evident that the convolution with the optimised IPSF gives deblurred image (lower right), small details are recognised but the contours are excessively sharp and the colours are faded.

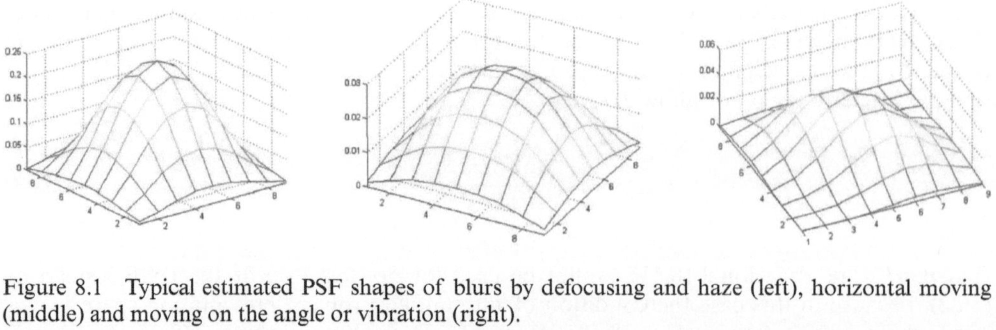

Figure 8.1 Typical estimated PSF shapes of blurs by defocusing and haze (left), horizontal moving (middle) and moving on the angle or vibration (right).

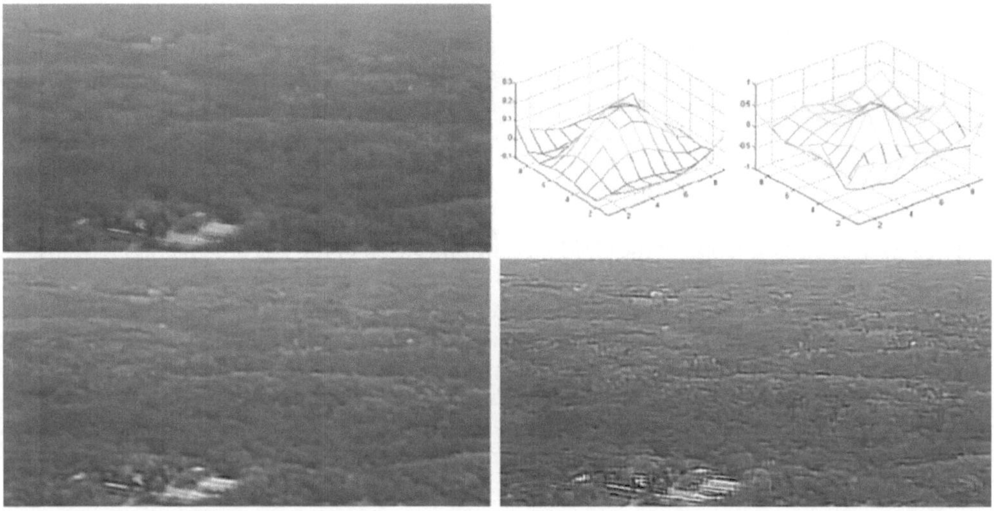

Figure 8.2 Blurred aerial photo (top left), IPSF and optimised IPSF (top center and right), filtered images using IPSF and optimised IPSF (lower left and right correspondingly).

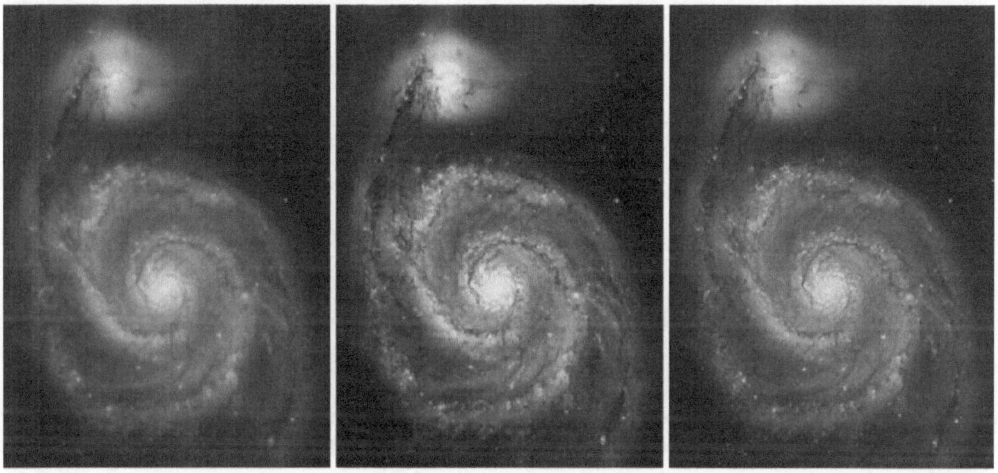

Figure 8.3 The results of one-step deconvolution of an astronomical photo (left) by the method of Carasso et al. (2006) (centre) and by using the optimised IPSF (right).

The first two images in Figure 8.3 were presented in Carasso et al. (2006) – the first one is a camera image, the second is the result of one-step filtering by the APEX method.

The third image was defined by convolution of the first one with the optimised IPSF of size $L \times M = 7 \times 7$, $P \times Q = 17 \times 17$. Obviously, we have obtained the contrast image like before, but without light speckles in the centres of the astronomical objects.

Figure 8.4 presents results of deblurring of images corrupted by defocusing and camera moving, camera and object moving, and fast moving of a gas medium. The original images are unknown but the naturalness and small details of the reconstructed images can be appreciated. The LR schema (8.30)–(8.31) and convolution (8.19) with the IPSF (8.26) in the spectral domain were used. In the case of images in Figure 8.4 in the lower row, the search of the regularisation parameter which provides the convergence condition (8.28) at first $q = 3$

steps in the region $0.01 \geq \lambda \geq 0.0001$ was unsuccessful. Thus, the result of the least square solution of equation (8.20) with the help of the SVD was used. The order of the AR model (8.11) $P \times Q = 17 \times 17$ and the size of the PSF $L \times M = 7 \times 7$ for images in middle and lower rows, $P \times Q = 25 \times 25$, and $L \times M = 9 \times 9$ for top image. The parameters of the AR model and the IPSF optimisation are the same as presented above. The PSF of the first type in Figure 8.1 corresponds to the blurred images in Figure 8.3, the PSF of the second type corresponds to the top and middle images in Figure 8.4 and the PSF of the third type corresponds to the lower image in Figure 8.4.

The PSF (8.16), estimated by the CNS method, was used in the LR schema (8.30)–(8.31) as initial one. The convergence process of the LR schema (8.30) was stopped at the achievement of 100 iteration steps in the case of two top images in Figure 8.4. It was stopped at violation of the convergence condition (8.44) after 41 iteration steps in the case of the lower image in Figure 8.4. The relative change of the PSF shape by 100 consecutive transforms (8.31) was less than 0.1%. On the other hand, the image shape change by transforms (8.30) was up to 5%. This fact confirms that equation (8.16) gives the estimate of the PSF. The images obtained by the LR method have clear contours, but contain artefacts which are inherent for this method—mosaic colours and corrupted bounds.

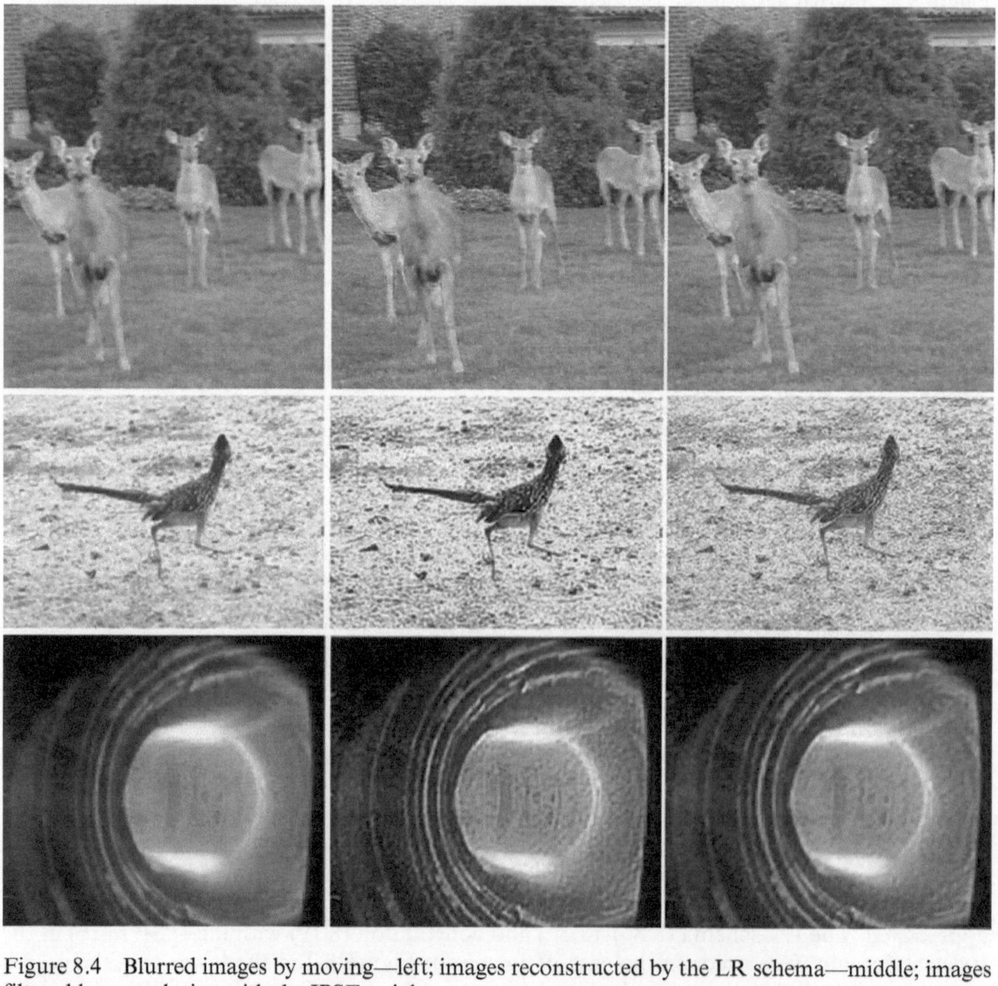

Figure 8.4 Blurred images by moving—left; images reconstructed by the LR schema—middle; images filtered by convolution with the IPSF—right.

We can see that a single convolution transform is enough with the optimised IPSF for blur removing. The result of convolution with the optimised IPSF is reachable by the LR method using not less than 10 iterations (8.30). Thus, we have a single convolution transform opposite to more than twenty ones.

Numerical experiments have shown that if the least square solution of equation (8.20) yields an estimate of the IPSF near to the optimal one, then its further optimisation is not possible, because the search of a regularisation parameter in accordance with convergence condition (8.28) is unsuccessful ($\theta = 1$), an appropriate $\lambda \approx 0$.

The images in Figures 8.2 and 8.4 need colour reconstruction. Thus they can serve as primary estimates for further optimisation with the aim of contour clearing and colour reconstruction.

4.3 *Examples of deconvolution optimisation*

The primary estimates of images in Figures 8.2 and 8.4 were optimised by the schemas LR ME (8.32), BVDR (8.45)–(8.46) and CS (8.53)–(8.54). We used the dynamic regularisation approach (8.39)–(8.42) to estimate the regularisation parameter in (8.32) with the aim to investigate the role of variation balancing in (8.46).

The surface area regularisation functional (SARF) like (8.21)

$$\Sigma_S = \int_\Omega \sqrt{1 + S_x^2 + S_y^2}(x,y)dxdy. \tag{8.58}$$

can be used as regularisation term in (8.35) because its minimisation means maximum possible flatness of image contour neighbourhood and, consequently, sharpness of contours. Thus, we can define the term of regularisation functional in (8.35) as

$$\mathbf{R}_S(S) = \Sigma_S. \tag{8.59}$$

If the problem consists in elimination of image surface fluctuation, the action of regularisation functional (8.59) can be reinforced by using area (8.58) of image surface divergence or Laplacian. The corresponding functionals can be presented as follows:

$$\mathbf{R}_J(S) = \Sigma_J : J = div(S) = S_x + S_y; \tag{8.60}$$

$$\mathbf{R}_G(S) = \Sigma_G : G = \nabla S = S_{xx} + S_{yy}. \tag{8.61}$$

The minimisation of functionals (8.60) and (8.61) means the minimisation of the change and fluctuation of image surface.

The numerical experiments have shown that in all examples schema (8.32) reaches the condition of convergence termination

$$\left\langle \left\| S^{(k+1)} - S^{(k)} \right\|^2 \right\rangle < \varepsilon \tag{8.62}$$

in 2–3 iteration steps at $\varepsilon = 10^{-8}$ without sufficient influence on the primary estimate $S^{(0)} = G * X$. This happens because the schema contains only smoothing convolution transforms. The results of optimisation are presented in Figure 8.5 (left column).

The results of image estimate optimisation by the BVDR and CS schemas are shown in Figures 8.5. In both cases the iterative process was restricted to 10 first iteration steps, violation of the condition (8.44) and the condition (8.58). The SARF (8.59) was used in the BVDR schema. The optimisation procedures (8.46) and (8.53) change colours drawing near them to natural and clearing contours. Different textures and small details of faces show quality of colour tints and contour reconstruction. The BVDR schema is characterised by sharper

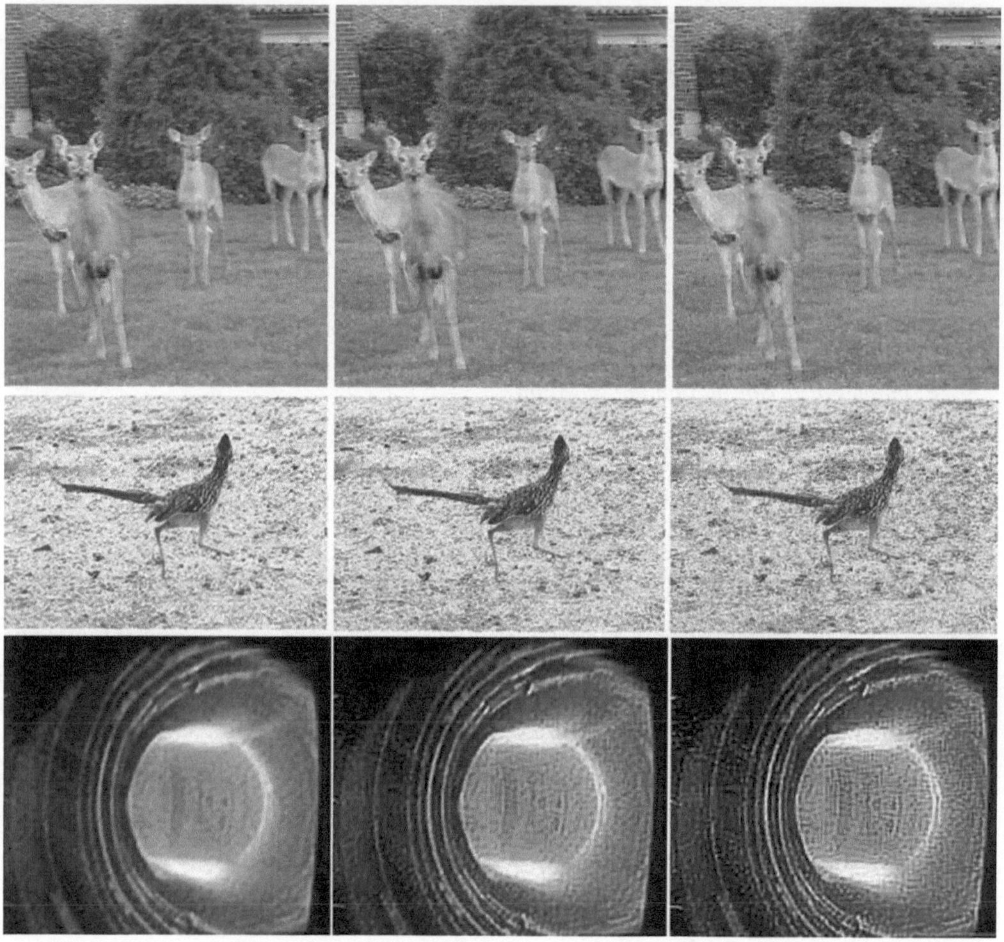

Figure 8.5 Images that are given by optimisation of primary estimate (Figure 8.4, on the right) by using LR ME (8.32), the BVDR (8.46) and the CS (8.53) iterative schemas (from left to right correspondingly).

contours in comparison with the CS schema at the same value of relaxation parameter δt. The CS schema gives tints closest to the blurred image. This is important in video-based measurements, for example in an aggressive medium such as plasma in Figures 8.4 and 8.5 (lower rows). Fast movement of the gas medium hides texture, discontinuities and corrupts colours, which relate to turbulence, density and temperature. These features are important for control processes (Wagner 2007).

The process of convergence of schemas (8.46) and (8.53) is different.

Schema (8.46) has some transition period at the first iteration steps. Initially λ (8.45) grows up to the some maximum value and then monotonically reduces. The residual in (8.58) repeats λ dynamic with one step lag. The transition period duration amounts to 10 iteration steps depending on image structure and relaxation parameter. If an image has many sharp contours, then the period is long, if an image is mainly smooth, then the period amounts to 2–4 iteration steps. The transition period amounts to 20 steps and more when relaxation parameter $\delta t > 0.1$. Thus, we used $\delta t = 0.1$ in estimation of images in Figures 8.6 and 8.7. The transition period did not exceed 5 iteration steps and the convergence process was terminated by restriction in the number of iteration steps. The convergence of schema (8.46) is conditioned

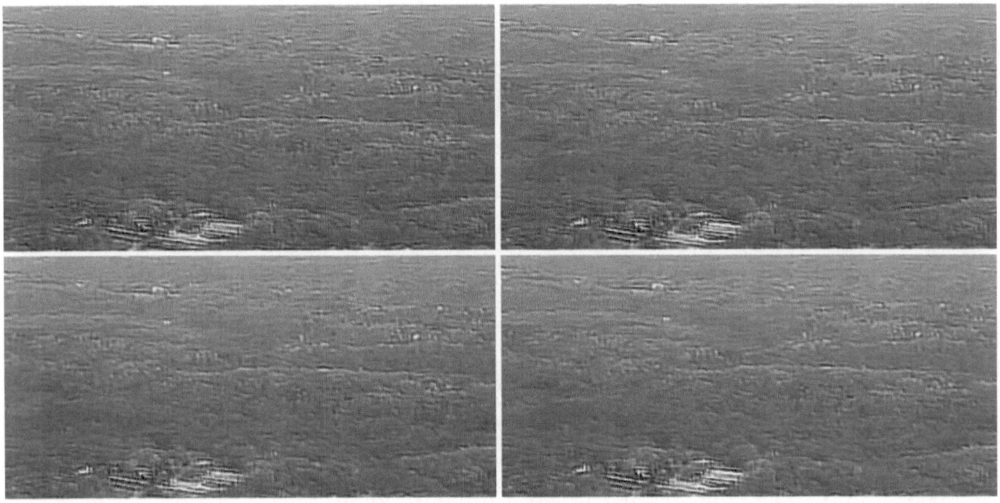

Figure 8.6 The aerial photo in Figure 8.2 optimised by the BVDR schema with SARF (8.59), (8.60), (8.61) and CS schema (from top to low and from left to right correspondingly).

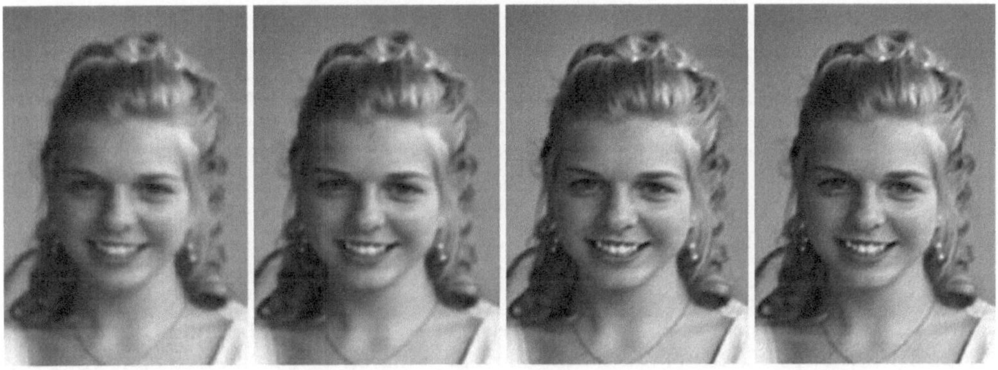

Figure 8.7 Image blurred and corrupted by impulsive noise (first from left), denoised image by the prior IPSF, primary image estimate by the optimised IPSF, optimised estimate by 20 iteration steps of the BVDR schema.

by $\lambda^{(k+1)} \leq \lambda^{(k)}$ (k>>1) in (8.45), since the l_1 norm of smoothed variation in the numerator of expression (8.45) terms? is less than the same norm of the excited variation of the derivative function in the denominator. The reduction of the regularisation parameter causes a decrease of the residual in (8.62). The presence of a transition period is caused by the initial difference between X and $S^{(0)}$ and by the dynamic nature of the regularisation parameter (8.45).

The convergence of schema (8.53) is monotonous, but not unlimited. It reaches some lowest point of the residual in (8.62) and then the convergence condition (8.44) is violated. The point of convergence termination in accordance with (8.56) relates to image structure, filter order and relaxation parameter. For example, in the case of the image in the lower row in Figure 8.6 the condition (8.44) is violated after the 27-th iteration step at $\delta t = 0.1$, after the 9-th step at $\delta t = 0.5$ and after the 6-th step at $\delta t = 1.0$. The result of the last case is shown in Figure 8.6. The number of iteration steps did not exceed 6 for the otherexamples in Figures 8.6 and 8.7 at $\delta t = 1.0$. The relaxation parameter restriction (8.57) was not violated in all examples. As it constitutes the lower bound, the ratio

$$\delta t \cdot \max\left|S^{(k+1)} - S^{(k)}\right| \leq \gamma. \tag{8.63}$$

was used as the higher bound of the relaxation parameter for avoidance of image degradation, the parameter $\gamma = 0.01$.

The parameter of convergence velocity θ did not exceed 1.0001 in (8.44) for both schemas (8.46) and (8.53).

The SARF (8.59) provides a better convergence of the iterative schema (8.46) in comparison with TM, TV and TV with β-factor functionals. Schema (8.46) with the regularisation functionals mentioned is stable and convergent at $\delta t << 0.1$. Therefore, these functionals essentially do not allow to change the primary image estimate by iteration steps.

Figure 8.6 shows optimised estimates of the aerial photo in Figure 8.2 which are obtained by the optimisation procedure (8.46) with SARF (8.59), (8.60), (8.61) and by procedure (8.53). The parameters of schemas (8.46) and (8.53) are as follows: $\delta t = 0.1$; $\gamma = 0.01$ in (8.63); $\varepsilon = 10^{-6}$ in (8.62). The chosen relaxation parameter satisfied both conditions (8.57) and (8.63). There were not more than ten iteration steps of schemas for the achievement of condition (8.62) fulfilment. The parameter of convergence velocity θ in (8.12) was in the range of 1.0005…1.001. The estimates given slightly differ by colour tints. The estimates of the CS and BVDR with SARF (8.61) schemas are closest to the initial image. In comparison with images in Figure 8.2 the optimised images have clearer contours and smoother shape. The image obtained by the schema with SARF (8.61), evolving higher derivatives, has less jitter.

4.4 *Deblurring of noisy images*

Iterative schemas (8.46) and (8.53) are not appropriate for estimation of blurred and noised images because they sharpen all image surface curves and so reinforce noise influence, especially when noise is impulsive. It is necessary to use a prior image denoised estimate X_{pr} instead of X in (8.46) and (8.53). A denoised estimate can be obtained by filtering with regularisation in spectral region (Biemond et al. 1990, Carasso et al. 2006, Kundur & Hatzinakos 1996, Michailovich & Tannenbaum 2007, Ng et al. 2000) or by the iterative schemas as a special procedure (Brito-Loeza & Chen 2010, Chan et al. 2005, Katsaggelos et al. 2009, Keren & Gotlib 1998, Lysaker et al. 2004, Rudin et al. 1992) or as a procedure joined with deconvolution (Bar et al. 2007a, Bar et al. 2007b, Katsaggelos et al. 2009, Tschumperle & Deriche 2005). The filtration-based approach introduces an additional smoothing or blur. The iterative schemas need a large number of iteration steps because usually they use small values of relaxation parameter.

Filter (8.19) with transient characteristic which is defined by equation (8.20) can be used as a denoising filter for prior image X_{pr} estimation. This filter bounds initial X and smoothed H^*X images. As can be seen in Figure 8.2, such a filter does not introduce additional smoothing. At the same time, it weakly sharpens the image surface in comparison with the filter with optimised transient characteristics (8.26). If the filter order is high, then it can eliminate noise influence by weighted accumulation of image matrix elements. An example of an image blurred and corrupted by the impulsive noise is shown in Figure 8.7. The PSF and IPSF G_{pr} were defined by equations (8.16) and (8.20), $P \times Q = 33 \times 33$, $L \times M = 17 \times 17$. The PSF was of the second type in Figure 8.1. Then, the PSF and the optimised IPSF (8.26) were defined using filtered image $X_{pr} = G_{pr} * X$ (the second one from the left in Figure 8.7). The PSF was of the first type in this case. Its parameters are same as in the prior one. There were primary (the third one in Figure 8.7) and two similar optimised image estimates obtained by the BVDR (on the right in Figure 8.7) and CS schemas. There were 20 iteration steps with the relaxation parameter $\delta t \sim 0.05$ that was restricted by the ratio (8.63). The result of optimisation of the image estimate without prior filtration was deblurred, but hardly corrupted by noise. The second and third images in Figure 8.7 show that the suggested denoising filter can be cascaded with the aim of eliminating noise influence. The image was not destroyed by the filter cascade because each next filter is adapted to the previous filtering result. The noise pulses of the size of some pixels did not spread in to spots, as? they? can be a result of smoothing.

5 CONCLUSION

The AR model is very well studied but its presentation in the manner of convolution operator **A** (8.8) opens its new ability to signal splitting. The AR model carries the physical sense of passing wave compensation by its own reflections. The direct AR operator compensates periodical processes and the conjugated operator compensates impulse processes. If a signal is a convolution of the two mentioned types of signals, then these signals can be separated because they have different structure and spectrums.

Numerical experiments have shown that:

- The iterative transform (8.31) essentially changes the PSF chosen heuristically. The PSF estimated as a conjugated null space is an invariant of transform (8.31). Thus we have obtained a (quasi) optimal PSF estimate in accordance with the ML criterion.
- The CNS method is appropriate to PSF estimation when a blur is characterised by a smooth convex function. Sharp image displacements are not available to estimate.
- The PSF size must agree with the blur level. If the PSF model order is less necessary, then this deficiency can be compensated by additional optimisation iterations. If the order is sufficiently greater than the required one, the restored image will be corrupted. In this case the IPSF has more than one dished maximum.
- Problem (8.26) has better convergence with regularisation functional (8.21) in comparison with the TV functional (8.33) and other known functionals with derivatives of the same order.
- The CS schema (8.53) is the most appropriate to optimisation of primary estimates in real time implementation. The required iteration steps for reaching a local minimum in functional (8.51) does not exceed 10 at $\delta t = 1$. As Figure 8.5 has shown, similar results were obtained by the CS and BVDR schemas using 5–6 and 10 iteration steps correspondingly. But only a metric tensor determinant is applicable for image regularisation in the case of the CS schema. At the same time, all known regularisation functionals can be used in the BVDR schema (8.45)–(8.46) with the aim of restriction of image gradient or fluctuation, noise elimination etc.

The suggested deblurring schemas reduce the number of required iterations more than 10 times in comparison with the LR schema when an image series is processed and the PSF changes slowly in time. No more than twenty convolution procedures are sufficient for the optimised image or its RGB component estimate finding. In many applications reconstruction of image colours is not required, and then a one-step convolution transform is sufficient. The image reconstruction can be implemented in real time by multicore processor arrays or graphic processor units in such conditions.

REFERENCES

Aogaki S., Moritani I., Sugai T., Takeutchi F. and Toyama F. M. 2006. Simple method to eliminate blur based on Lane and Bates algorithm. *Preprint* cs/0609165.

Babacan S.D., Molina R. and Katsaggelos A.K. 2009. Variational Bayesian blind deconvolution using a total variation prior. *IEEE Trans. Image Process.*, v. 18, 12–26.

Bar L., Brook A., Sochen N. and Kiryati N. 2007. Color image deblurring with impulsive noise. *IEEE Trans. Image Proc.*, v. 16, 1101–1111.

Bar L., Sochen N. and Kiryati N. 2007. Convergence of an iterative method for variational deconvolution and impulse noise removal. *SIAM Multiscale Modeling and Simulation,* v. 6, 983–994.

Biemond J., Lagedijk R.L. and Mersereau R.M. 1990. Iterative methods for image deblurring. *Proc. IEEE*, v. 78, 856–883.

Biemond J., Van der Putten F.G. and Woods J.W. 1988. Identification and restoration of images with symmetric noncausal blurs. *IEEE Trans. Circuits and Systems*, v. 35, 385–393.
Biggs D.S.C. and Andrews M. 1997. Acceleration of iterative image restoration algorithms *App. Opt.*, v. 36, 1766–1775.
Brito-Loeza C. and Chen Ke. 2010. Multigrid algorithm for high order denoising. *SIAM J. Imag. Sc.*, v. 3, 363–389.
Bronstein M.M., Bronstein A.M., Zibulevsky M. and Zeevi Y.Y. 2005. Blind deconvolution of images using optimal sparse presentations. *IEEE Trans. Image Process.*, v. 14, 726–736.
Cai J.F., Osher S. and Shen Z. 2009. Convergence of the linearized Bregman iteration for ℓ1-norm minimization *Math. Comput.*, v. 78, 2127–2136.
Carasso A.S. 2006. APEX blind deconvolution of color Hubble space telescope imagery and other astronomical data. *Opt. Eng.*, v. 45, 107004 1–15.
Chambolle A. 2004. An algorithm for total variation minimization and application. *J. of Math. Imaging and Vis.*, v. 20, 89–97.
Chan T.F. and Wong C. 1998. Total variation blind deconvolution. *EEE Trans. Image Proc.*, v. 7, 370–375.
Chan T.F., Esedoglu S., Park F. and Yip A. 2005. Recent developments in total variation image restoration. *The Handbook of Mathematical Models in Computer Vision* Ed. by: N. Paragios, Y. Chen and O. Faugeras (New York: Springer).
Dey N. et al. 2004. 3D microscopy deconvolution using Richardson-Lucy algorithm with total variation regularization. *INRIA preprint* 5272.
Donatelli M., Estatico C., Martinelli A. and Serra-Capizzano S. 2006. Improved image deblurring with anti-reflective boundary conditions and re-blurring. *Inverse Problems*, v. 22, 2035–2053.
Dubrovin B.A., Fomenko A.T. and Novikov S.P. 1992. *Modern Geometry—Methods and Applications Pt.1* (New York: Springer).
Fish D.A., Brinicombe A.M., Pike E.R. and Walker J.G. 1995. Blind deconvolution by means of the Richardson–Lucy algorithm. *J. Opt. Soc. Am.*, v. A 12, 58–65.
Han J., Han L., Neumann M. and Prasad U. 2009. On the rate of convergence of the image space reconstruction algorithm. *Operators and matrices*, v. 3(1), 41–58.
Hao Z., Yu L. and Qinzhang W. 2007. Blind image deconvolution subject to bandwidth and total variation constraints. *Optics Letters*, v. 32, 2550–2552.
Holmes T.J. 1992. Blind deconvolution of quantum-limited incoherent imagery: maximum likelihood approach. *J. Opt. Soc.Am.*, v. A 9, 1052–1061.
Jiang M. and Wang G. 2003. Convergence studies on iterative algorithms for image reconstruction. *IEEE Trans. Med. Imaging*, v. 22, 569–579.
Jiang M. and Wang G. 2003. Development of blind image deconvolution and its applications. *J. of X-Ray Sc. and Tech.*, v. 11, 13–19.
Katsaggelos A.K., Babacan S.D. and Tsai C.J. 2009. Iterative image restoration. *The Essential Guide to Image Processing* Ed. by A. Bovik (Elsevier).
Keren D. and Gotlib A. 1998. Denoising color images using regularization and correlation terms. *J. of Vis. Comm. and Image Repr.*, v. 9(4), 352–365.
Kimmel R., Malladi R. and Sochen N. 2000. Images as embedded maps and minimal surfaces: movies, color, texture, and volumetric medical images. *Int. J. of Computer Vision,* v. 39(2), 111–129.
Kundur D. and Hatzinakos D., 1996. Blind image deconvolution. *IEEE Signal Proc. Mag.* No. 5, 43–64.
Lagendijk R.L., Tekalp A.M. and Biemond J. 1990. Maximum likelihood image and blur identification: a unifying approach. *Opt. Eng.*, v. 29, 422–435.
Landweber L. 1951. An iterative formula for Fredholm integral equations of the first kind. *Am. J. Math.*, v. 73, 615–624.
Lane R.G. and Bates R.H.T. 1987. Automatic multidimensional deconvolution. *J. Opt. Soc. Am.*, v. A 4(1), 180–188.
Levin A., Weiss Y., Durand F. and Freeman W.T. 2011. Understanding blind deconvolution algorithms. *IEEE Trans. Patt. Anal. and Machine Intel.*, v. 33, 2354–2367.
Liang L. and Xu Y. 2003. Adaptive Landweber method to deblur images. *IEEE Signal Process. Lett.*, v. 10(5), 129–132.
Liao H. and Ng M.K. 2011. Blind deconvolution using generalized cross-validation approach to regularization parameter estimation. *IEEE Trans. Image Process.*, v. 20, 670–680.
Likas A.C. and Galatsanos N.P. 2004. A variational approach for Bayesian blind image deconvolution. *IEEE Trans. Signal Process.*, v. 52, 2222–2233.

Lucy L.B. 1974. An iterative technique for rectification of observed distributions. *Astronom. J.* v. 79, 745–574.
Lysaker M., Osher S. and Xue-Cheng Tai 2004. Noise removal using smoothed normals and surface fitting. *IEEE Trans. Image Process.*, v. 13, 1345–1357.
Michailovich O.V. and Tannenbaum A. 2007. Blind deconvolution of medical ultrasound images: a parametric inverse filtering approach. *IEEE Trans. Image Process.*, v. 16, 3005–3019.
Molina R., Mateos J. and Katsaggelos A. 2006. Blind deconvolution using a variational approach to parameter image and blur estimation. *IEEE Trans. Image Process.*, v. 15, 3715–3727.
Money J.H. and Kang S.H. 2008. Total variation minimizing blind deconvolution with shock filter reference. *Image and Vision Computing*, v. 26(2), 302–314.
Ng M., Chan R. and Tang W. 2000. A fast algorithm for deblurring models with Neumann boundary conditions. *SIAM J. Sci. Comput.*, v. 21, 851–866.
Pai H.-T. and Bovik A.C. 1997. Exact multi-channel blind image restoration. *IEEE Signal Process. Lett.*, v. 4, 217–220.
Pai H.-T. and Bovik A.C. 2001. On eigenstructure-based direct multichannel blind image restoration. *IEEE Trans. Image Process.*, v. 10, 1434–1446.
Pai H.-T., Bovik A.C. and Evance B.L. 1997. Multi-channel blind image restoration. *Turkish J. of Electrical Eng. & Computer Sciences*, v. 3, 79–97.
Richardson W.H. 1972. Bayesian-based iterative method of image restoration. *J of the Opt. Soc. of Am.*, v. 62, 55–59.
Rudin L.I., Osher S. and Fatemi E. 1992. Nonlinear total variation based noise removal algorithms Physica, v. D 60, 259–268.
Singh M.K., Tiwary U.S. and Kim Y.H. 2008. An adaptively accelerated Lucy-Richardson method for image deblurring. *EURASIP J. on Adv. in Signal Process.*, v. 2008, 365021.
Tschumperle D. and Deriche R. 2005. Vector-valued image regularization with PDE's: a common framework for different applications. *IEEE Trans. Patt. Anal. and Machine Intel.*, v. 27(4), 506–517.
Tzikas D.G., Likas A.C. and Galatsanos N.P. 2009. Variational Bayesian sparse kernel-based blind image deconvolution with Student's-t priors. *IEEE Trans. Image Process.*, v. 18, 753–764.
Wagner F. 2007. A quarter-century of H-mode studies. *Plasma Phys. Control. Fusion*, v. 49, B1–B33.
Yang W.Q., Spink D.M., York T.A. and McCann H. 1999. An image reconstruction algorithm based on Landweber iteration method for electrical capacitance tomography. *Meas. Sci. Technol.*, v. 10, 1065–1069.
You Y.-L. and Kaveh M. 1996. A regularization approach to joint blur identification and image restoration. *IEEE Trans. Image Process.*, v. 5, 416–428.
Zhu W. and Chan T. 2012. Image denoising using mean curvature of image surface. *SIAM J. Imaging Sci.* v. 5(1), 1–32.

CHAPTER 9

Biologically motivated approach to multistage image processing

L.I. Timchenko, N.I. Kokryatskaya & I.D. Ivasyuk
State University for Transport Economy and Technologies, Kyiv, Ukraine

T. Małecka-Massalska & Z. Omiotek
Lublin University of Technology, Lublin, Poland

B. Akhmetov
Kazakh National Technical University after K.I. Satpaev, Almaty, Kazakhstan

1 INTRODUCTION

Creating effective data analysis with efficient representation of complex hierarchical architectures is one of the key issues when developing novel computer systems. Therefore investigating structures with flexible, complexity dependent hierarchies is of great importance. The idea of using effective processing methods developed by nature has resulted in mathematical models which implement certain features of the cerebral cortex. The latest neurophysiological research, primarily of Professor Zeki, points towards a multistage structure for cortical processing (Zeki 1993). His important assumption is that it is not necessary to pass the data through all hierarchical transformational levels. Certain *pro tem* information about the input can be extracted after each of the early processing stages. In that way further processing involves less data and so becomes faster. In synthetic systems this approach is not sufficiently developed and not attached to real time. In the case of artificial neural networks (ANN), most of the structures implement fixed hierarchical mapping with numerous redundant connections, which slow down the process of output computation. In what way can the redundancy of the neural elements' interconnections be optimised to achieve a real-time performance? The concept of a multistage network proposed in this paper could be a possible answer. The main distinguishing feature of this approach is the introduction of a dynamics of successive transformations applied to spatial regions. This dynamics enables to extract specific temporally uncorrelated components after each transformation. This process represents the design of a multistage network or a part of a network. Parameters of the elements, participating in correlation and decorrelation processes, can have various physical properties, such as signal magnitude, frequency, phase, power spectrum, image brightness, texture, connectivity, etc. These are defined by the type of transformation, which must be chosen in accordance with the nature of the problem.

The paper presents the multistage methodology applied to image processing. The concept of parallel multistage image processing can be considered as a consecutive transformation of image components, which consist of elements grouped under a certain criterion. At each stage one component from each parallel channel is extracted and passed to the next processing level, thus reducing the entropy of the remaining image data on that level. In case of the simultaneous extraction from different parallel channels, the extracted components are passed onto the next hierarchical level for further processing. Otherwise, processing of these components is already completed, and they reflect the output result of the processing at the current stage. This procedure of image processing is applied at every level of the hierarchy iteratively until all components at that level are extracted. At each processing level some output information about the input data is extracted, representing a *pro tem* result. This enables a new view of real-time image analysis with the final result being obtained from the principal components uncorrelated in the spatio-temporal domain. The multistage output object description is represented as an activity pattern rather than as a set of connection weights. A very important distinction of the multistage model is the ability to make a closer definition of the input at each stage of the process.

This article offers a new approach to the creation of computing medium—parallel-hierarchical (PH) networks (Timchenko 2000), investigated in the form of a model of a neuro-like scheme of data processing. The approach has a number of advantages as compared with other formation methods of neuro-like media (for example, the already known methods of formation of artificial neural networks). The main advantage of this approach is using the dynamics of multilevel parallel interaction of information signals at different hierarchy levels of computer networks that allows to use such known natural features of computation organisation in the cortex as: topographic nature of mapping, simultaneity (parallelism) of signal operation, inlaid cortex, structure, rough hierarchy of the cortex, or the mechanism of perception and training spatially correlated in time. The formation of multi-stage PH networks assumes the process of sequential transformation of correlated elements, and the formation of time-decorrelated elements of neural networks at its transition from one stable state into another. The key feature of the approach offered is the analysis of the dynamics of the spatially correlated mechanism of current transformation and formation of the resultant elements of neural networks. Such a mechanism allows a new way of presenting the processing in neural networks as a process of parallel-sequential transformation of various components of image and a.c. The physical content of the input elements of neural networks, participating in correlation-decorrelation, such as, for example, the amplitude or frequency, phase or energy of signals, cohesion or texture of images, is determined by the type of cohesion or texture of images, by the type of transformation being used, the selection of which depends on the class of the problems being solved. In general, the multistage concept regarding image processing can be formulated in the following way. The image analysis presents a sequential transformation of concurrent image components and the detection of the time-discrepant ones at transition of neural networks elements from a current energy state with certain space coordinates into states with less energy and other space coordinates (Timchenko et al. 2002). Such process of image analysis occurs at many stages, each of which includes fulfilment of the above-stated procedure. The condition for transition of the image components at a higher level is the availability of the dynamics of mutual coincidence of the intermediate results of processing in time in parallel channels of a lower layer. The outcome of image analysis is formed from image components isolated in the time-space area.

The development of computing facilities starts with transition from conventional computing frames of von Neumann to "expert systems" and "smart" neuroengineering systems, imitating the intellectual cerebral activity of the human being—computing means of the sixth generation. We can state that the "ideal" converter unit of the optical information of parallel type is an eye, probably the most unique human sensory system. The human brain is a natural processor- which converts sensor information. But there is a problem. Is there a possibility to simulate the process of eye functioning—processor perception of the sensory information on neuroshaped circuits intended for data processing? The analysis of recent studies on neurobiology and publications on modelling neural mechanisms of sensor information perception has shown that some problems still remain obscure, namely: how the interaction of neurounits takes place in the cortex, their interaction on the level of natural local neural networks; how temporal integration of spatially-separated, neuroassemblies in horizontal and vertical routes takes place at the moment of coordinated action of numerous simultaneously acting irritants? That is why our research investigates a hypothetical model of special integration and structuralisation of information in the cortex of the human brain, concerning problems of perception, information storage and pattern recognition. To a great extent, the models considered in the articlepossess metaphorical similarity with computers; nevertheless they are supposed to provide a new, more elaborated approach to computer-based calculations. Proceeding from this approach new microprocessor-based systems and computers of new architecture could be created. Besides, the models will allow elaborating a new approach to biological systems. The prototype of the suggested approach can be considered to be the principles of collective computations in neuroshaped circuits intended for collective decision making, requiring corporate interaction of large quantity of simple solutions, as a result of which a complex solution is taken by means of data combining during any period of time. After analysis of neurobiological data regarding the theory of sensor information stratification in the human brain and the peculiarities of the computation system's a number of discrepancies concerning natural mechanisms of object perception and external environment were revealed. These discrepancies did not find a corresponding reflection in modern neuroshaped computation facilities, a fact considerably limiting their technical possibilities and preventing such facilities from meeting the main requirements relating to the intellectual means of information processing (Churchland & Sejnowski 1992).

In spite of attempts that have been made for over half a century, the problem of creating an artificial intelligence system based on the application of computers is still far from its solution, although some interesting theoretical results have been obtained. In this connection the report delivered in the White House by Professor Hogard, of Cambridge University, must be mentioned. Professor Hogard considers the creation of artificial intelligence to be the main scientific problem of the present millennium. Over the last 50 years computational modelling in the sphere of brain-like functioning has gone through enormous upheavals. From the early work by Rosenblatt ("Perceptron") to later research in learning methods and representational function ("Hopfield Networks", "Back Propagation") there has been no formal setting for the analysis of collective structures, like sets of neurons. Rather, there have been independent islands of research focused on memory, visual perception, speech recognition, handwriting recognition etc., as applications or focused models of cortical function in biological systems—typically in small circuits (lobster's gastro-intestinal system, motion detection circuits in crickets, etc.). Despite a few researchers such as Steve Grossberg, there are almost no claims to general principles how to organise and produce systematic results for neural networks? (Grossberg & Williamson 2001, Grossberg et al. 2000).

Using collections of neural computing units with homogeneous learning rules is hardly a means to understand the general system level function. The brain's dynamics is in orders of 1000s to millions of interacting subsystems (Kandel & Hawkins 1992), clearly the neuron is at the wrong level of analysis, but treating the brain as if it were independent insulated modules is patently false. This scientific work is unique in that it focuses directly on this kind of problem: formulation of methodology, theory of the system and circuit engineering of hierarchy structures with space-multilevel data presentation and time-network principles of their analysis. Fundamentally, this type of research is about collective decision-making and work is focused on the time-space dynamics of this phenomenon which is common to every type of decision making in human problem solving. Recently further development of similar hierarchical associative structures has been given a new impulse (Hirahara et al. 2000).

2 METHODS

2.1 *Mathematical description of multistage image processing*

This section presents a detailed mathematical description of the multistage image processing technique. The procedure of the multistage processing is hierarchical, and on the first level it includes temporal decomposition of the initial image data and transmission of the obtained components to the second level. At each following processing level consecutive operations of temporal decomposition, temporal aligning of the decomposed data, extraction of a principal component, and transmission of the remaining data to the next level are applied once. The processing terminates at the level which receives a single input component.

Let a still image M of the size $l \times m$ be symbolised as a set of elements $M = \{h_{ij} | i = 0,1,...,l-1; j = 0, 1,...,m-1\}$, where h_{ij} is a parameter of the image element. It can represent brightness, colour, etc. The image components are grouped from elements with similar parameter values. Then image M can be represented as a set of components $M = \{a_k | k = 0,1,...,R-1\}$, where R is the number of the components. A possible expression of the temporal decomposition of the still image can be shown to be (Svechnikov et al. 1987):

$$\sum_{i=0}^{l-1}\sum_{j=0}^{m-1} h_{ij} = \sum_{t=1}^{R}\left(\left(n-\sum_{k=0}^{t-1} n_k\right)(a_t - a_{t-1})\right),$$

where $n = l \times m$ is the number of elements in image M, n_k is the number of elements in the k-th component, t is the step of temporal decomposition, and a_t is the arbitrary element of the component a_k, with $a_0 = 0$ and $n_0 = 0$. The decomposed image M^1 consists of temporal components of the form:

$$M^1 = \left\{\left(n-\sum_{k=0}^{t-1} n_k\right)(a_t - a_{t-1}) \,\middle|\, t = 1, 2, ..., R\right\}. \tag{9.1}$$

Let the transformation (9.1) be denoted as $G(M) = M^1 = \{a^1_t | t = 1,2,...,R\}$. The initial image M is segmented into S segments each of them being allocated in a parallel channel. The temporal decomposition G is applied to each segment simultaneously. Then the decomposed s-th image segment is: $M^1_s = \{a1st | t = 1,2,...,R^1_s\}$, where $s = 1,2,...,S$, and R^1_s is the number of the components in the s-th segment (length of the decomposed segment sequence). Now the whole decomposed image can be represented as matrix A_1 of the form:

$$A_1 = \begin{bmatrix} M^1_1 \\ M^1_2 \\ \cdots \\ M^1_i \\ \cdots \\ M^1_S \end{bmatrix} = \begin{bmatrix} a^1_{11} & a^1_{12} & \cdots & a^1_{1R^1_1} & x & x & \cdots & x \\ a^1_{21} & a^2_{22} & \cdots & \cdots & a^1_{2R^1_2} & x & \cdots & x \\ \cdots & \cdots & \cdots & \cdots & \cdots & \cdots & \cdots & x \\ a^1_{i1} & a^1_{i2} & \cdots & \cdots & \cdots & \cdots & \cdots & a^1_{iR^1_i} \\ \cdots & \cdots & \cdots & \cdots & \cdots & \cdots & \cdots & x \\ a^1_{S1} & a^1_{S2} & \cdots & a^1_{SR^1_S} & x & x & \cdots & x \end{bmatrix},$$

where x denotes an empty position. The column index indicates the stage at which the component was extracted and the row index indicates the channel. In mathematical terms transmission of the decomposed data A_1 to the second level is represented as transposition T. That is, the initial matrix of the second level $A^T_1 = T(A_1)$. At the second level the temporal decomposition G discovers correlations between the components, which were simultaneously extracted from different channels of the first level. Transformation G is applied to the rows of A^T_1 to obtain the matrix A_2:

$$A_2 = G\left(A_1^T\right) = G\left(T\left(G\left(M\right)\right)\right) = \begin{bmatrix} a^2_{11} & a^2_{12} & \cdots & \cdots & a^2_{1R^2_1} & x & \cdots & x \\ a^2_{21} & a^2_{22} & \cdots & a^2_{2R^2_2} & x & x & \cdots & x \\ \cdots & \cdots & \cdots & \cdots & \cdots & \cdots & \cdots & x \\ a^2_{j1} & a^2_{j2} & \cdots & \cdots & \cdots & \cdots & \cdots & a^2_{jR^2_j} \\ \cdots & \cdots & \cdots & \cdots & \cdots & \cdots & \cdots & x \\ a^2_{R^1 1} & a^2_{R^1 2} & \cdots & a^2_{R^1 R^2_{R^1}} & x & x & \cdots & x \end{bmatrix},$$

where R^1 denotes the maximum length of the segments, $R^1 = max\{R^1_1, R^1_2, ..., R^1_s\}$. Matrix A_2 represents the process of temporal decomposition at the second level, in the way that each component a^2_{ij} is extracted at the stage $t = i + j - 1$. For further processing it is more convenient to adjust the image representation so that for each component the column index illustrates stage t when this component was extracted. Then at the next level the correlations between the components, which are simultaneously extracted from different channels, can be discovered in the same way as at the previous level. This adjustment is implemented as the horizontal offset of the A_2 rows, so that in each row the first nonempty element has its column index equal to the row index. The resultant matrix is denoted A'_2, and $A'_2 = P(A_2)$, where P is the offset transformation:

$$A'_2 = \begin{bmatrix} a^2_{11} & a^2_{12} & \dots & \dots & \dots & a^2_{1R^2_1} & x & \dots & \dots & \dots & \dots & x \\ x & a^2_{21} & a^1_{22} & \dots & a^2_{2R^2_2} & x & x & \dots & \dots & \dots & \dots & x \\ \dots & \dots & \dots & \dots & \dots & \dots & \dots & \dots & \dots & \dots & \dots & x \\ x & x & x & a^2_{j^1} & a^2_{j^2} & \dots & \dots & \dots & \dots & \dots & \dots & a^2_{jR^2_j} \\ \dots & \dots & \dots & \dots & \dots & \dots & \dots & \dots & \dots & \dots & \dots & x \\ x & x & x & x & x & a^2_{R^1 1} & a^2_{R^1 2} & \dots & a^2_{R^1 R^2_{R^1}} & x & \dots & x \end{bmatrix}.$$

According to the principle of multistage organisation of the result, component a^2_{11}, extracted at the first stage of the processing at the second level, is a principal component. It represents a *pro tem* result of the processing on that level. This extraction is performed by extracting the first matrix column. The remaining data is stored in matrix A''_2. In algebraic form this procedure appears as $A''_2 = L(A'_2)$. The initial matrix of the third level A^T_2 is obtained by transposing A''_2, that is $A^T_2 = T(L(P(A_2)))$. The procedure described is applied at each of the following hierarchical levels until the k-th level, where matrix A_K contains a single element. Then $T(L(P(A_k))) = \varnothing$. Let the consecutive use of transformations G, P, L, T be denoted by F:

$$F(A^T_j) = T(L(P(G(A^T_j)))) = A^T_{j+1}.$$

Successive applications of F are denoted as $F^j(A^T_1) = F^{j-1}[F(A^T_1)]$. Then the whole multilevel process can be represented below in algebraic form:

$$F^{k-1}\left[T\left(G\left(\bigcup_{S=1}^{S} M_S\right)\right)\right] = \{a^j_{11} \mid j = 2, 3, ..., k\}, \tag{9.2}$$

where M_s are the segments of the input image M, k is the number of processing levels, and a^j_{11} is the principal component extracted at the j-th level, starting from the second one. Thus the multistage image processing procedure can be considered as network processing which at the first level incorporates the consecutive use of the temporal decomposition G and the transposition T applied to each of the image segments. At each of the $(k-1)$ successive levels the complex transformation F is applied once. It involves consecutive operations of decomposition, offset, extraction and transposition.

2.2 *Hierarchical data mapping in cortical vs. artificial neural networks*

Perhaps the most serious problem in effective realisation of the multistage processing idea is the utilisation of the neuron-like mechanisms of sensory information analysis. This requires complex evaluation of the achievements in information theory, statistics, neurophysiology and knowledge representations in artificial intelligence. Another important problem is the implementation of the spatio-temporal correlations, which exist between cortical neural coalitions (Shatz 1990), in real-time operating ANNs. Most ANN architectures ignore the issue of how the real world is mapped into the deeper level of the cerebral cortex. The functioning of the known ANN structures in real time also presents considerable difficulties. These are caused by inconsistency between our knowledge of the functioning of the cortical neural nets and of their artificial analogies. Neurophysiological research so far (Hubel & Wiesel 1968) shows that the processes of visual perception and cognition are dispersed over a number of cortical areas, i.e. there is no single master area to which all specialised areas uniquely project. On the other hand, the presence of the output layer in the multiple layer perceptron (MLP) is equivalent to the existence of such cortical "master area" which integrates all incoming information. Considering the ANNs in this context, the contradiction of their architecture with the cortical organisation is clear. Therefore, although effective learning algorithms have been developed for the ANNs, such networks are not able to match the efficiency of the cortex.

When using MLP with several fully interconnected hidden layers, it is very difficult to say what each hidden layer represents. At the same time, research of Linsker (Linsker 1988) has shown that an artificial multilayered network, which develops its interlayer connections according to simple "Hebb-type" rules rather than by supervised learning, self-organises to preserve maximum information when transforming signals at each layer. By using only local connections with the neurons of the previous layer, as shown in Figure 9.1, each neural element tends to respond to the most significant features of the input. Such layered organisation leads to the formation of direction-selective cells, which exhibit very similar characteristics to those of the corresponding cells in the primary visual cortex.

Similar evolutionary approach can also be applied to the next stage of visual perception. Unlike the previous stage, where processing involves analysis of local characteristics within the image, the aim at this stage is to extract structural image properties.

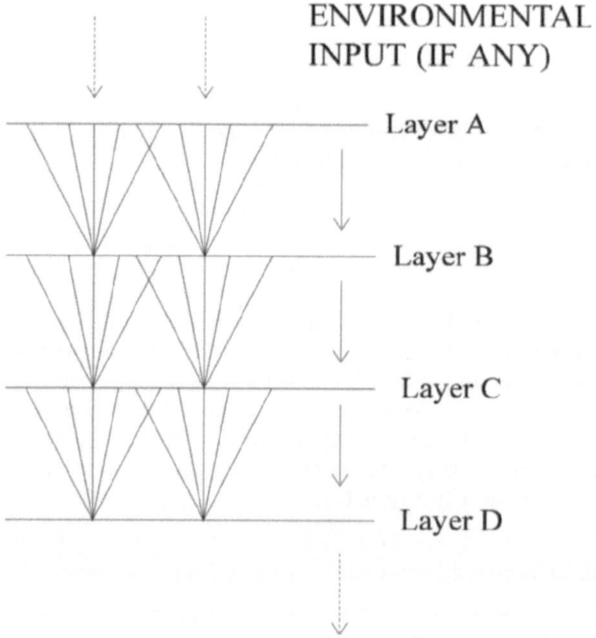

Figure 9.1 A layered self-adaptive network with local feed forward connections.

Structural components usually cannot appear in the image by chance, and therefore they represent some underlying principle. Grouping these components and investigating correlations between them on each consecutive hierarchical level results in the emergence of a more abstract structural representation. To do that, the multistage architecture uses the principle of flexible part-whole hierarchical mapping. This principle postulates subtasking of the problem with objects at one level being composed of inter-related objects at the previous level (Crick & Koch 1990). Structural objects of the real world are reconstructed during the latter stages of cortical sensor information analysis by means of combining maximally purified visual data. In the authors' terminology this is presented by the process of extracting the resulting principal components a^j_{11} from the matrices A'_j in the separate structures of k levels (Kozhemyako 2008). This methodology utilises certain neurophysiological principles, such as parallel channels for handling colour, shape and motion, multistage character of the processing in different cortical areas, spatio-temporal correlation between neural coalitions, and the mechanisms of associative learning (Livingstone & Hubel 1984).

3 RESULTS

3.1 *Realization of the multistage interactions*

Consider an example of spatio-temporal interaction and summation, with output results being uncorrelated in space and time analogously to the distribution of cortical results. On the contrary, intermediate results are correlated in a multistage way, in much the same manner as the formation of optimal neuronal coalitions on the basis of coincidence.

At each stage t in every processing channel the image component to be extracted is selected under the criterion $a_t = min\{a_1,a_2,...,a_R\}$, where R is the number of components. This procedure is analogous to the integration of information across space by extracting some common attribute.

Let the input to the parallel channels be given in the form of numerical fields M_1, M_2, and M_3:

$$M_1 = \begin{bmatrix} 2 \\ 3 \\ 5 \\ 7 \end{bmatrix}, \quad M_2 = \begin{bmatrix} 1 \\ 4 \\ 9 \\ 10 \end{bmatrix}, \quad M_3 = \begin{bmatrix} 3 \\ 15 \\ 20 \end{bmatrix}.$$

Applying equation (9.1) at the first hierarchical level, we obtain the temporal decomposition of the numerical fields:

$$G(M_1) = [8 \quad 3 \quad 4 \quad 2],$$
$$G(M_2) = [4 \quad 9 \quad 10 \quad 1],$$
$$G(M_3) = [9 \quad 24 \quad 5 \quad x],$$

where x denotes an empty position. Matrix A_1 is constructed by consolidating all $G(M_i)$ fields. The output result consists of the principal components extracted at the subsequent hierarchical levels:

$$A_1 = \begin{bmatrix} 8 & 3 & 4 & 2 \\ 4 & 9 & 10 & 1 \\ 9 & 24 & 5 & x \end{bmatrix},$$

$$A_2' = S\left(G\left(T\left(A_1\right)\right)\right) = \begin{bmatrix} 12 & 8 & 1 & x & x \\ x & 9 & 12 & 15 & x \\ x & x & 12 & 2 & 5 \\ x & x & x & 2 & 1 \end{bmatrix} \Rightarrow a_{11}^2 = 12,$$

$$A_3' = \begin{bmatrix} 16 & 1 & x & x & x \\ x & 3 & 22 & x & x \\ x & x & 6 & 13 & x \\ x & x & x & 2 & 4 \end{bmatrix} \Rightarrow a_{11}^3 = 16,$$

$$A_4' = \begin{bmatrix} 2 & 2 & x & x \\ x & 12 & 16 & x \\ x & x & 4 & 11 \\ x & x & x & 4 \end{bmatrix} \Rightarrow a_{11}^4 = 2,$$

$$A_5' = \begin{bmatrix} 4 & 10 & x & x \\ x & 8 & 12 & x \\ x & x & 8 & 7 \end{bmatrix} \Rightarrow a_{11}^5 = 4,$$

$$A_6' = \begin{bmatrix} 16 & 2 & x \\ x & 16 & 4 \\ x & x & 7 \end{bmatrix} \Rightarrow a_{11}^6 = 16,$$

$$A_7' = \begin{bmatrix} 4 & 14 & x \\ x & 8 & 3 \end{bmatrix} \Rightarrow a_{11}^7 = 4,$$

$$A_8' = \begin{bmatrix} 16 & 6 \\ x & 3 \end{bmatrix} \Rightarrow a_{11}^8 = 16,$$

$$A_9' = \begin{bmatrix} 6 & 3 \end{bmatrix} \Rightarrow a_{11}^9 = 6,$$

$$A_{10}' = \begin{bmatrix} 3 \end{bmatrix} \Rightarrow a_{11}^{10} = 3.$$

The result of the multistage spatio-temporal summation can be represented as an activity pattern:

$$F^9\left[T\left(G\left(\bigcup_{i=1}^{3} M_i\right)\right)\right] = (12 \quad 16 \quad 2 \quad 4 \quad 16 \quad 4 \quad 16 \quad 6 \quad 3).$$

It can further be processed as a variable length sequence by the recursive auto-associative memory (RAAM) (Pollack 1990).

3.2 *Image processing by multistage network*

When using the multistage approach for the representation of structural information within the image, there is no need to reconstruct the initial input from the obtained principal components. The main goal here is to discover some spatial regularities in order to interpret the image structure. However, reconstruction of the raw image is necessary in some applications, such as image coding and filtration. To apply the multistage approach to these tasks, information about the spatial transformations must be stored at each processing stage. Several transformations can be applied in the multistage network. Some possible examples include principal component analysis of local image patches (Rao & Ballard 1995), partial clusterisation of the Gabor coefficients (Daugman 1985), and the cosine transform. In this paper, analysis of the facial structure is performed using partial clusterisation of pixel connectivity. A three-level representation (White & Rohrer 1983, Kutaev 1989) of grey-scale facial image is used to specify a three-level pixel connectivity. The three connectivity levels are then processed using three multistage networks, each producing a pattern vector (Fig. 9.2).

In each network, the image components are clustered using the ISODATA algorithm (Hall & Ball 1965). Then, the newly organised clusters are graded on the basis of the uniformity of data in those clusters. Components with one output component are extracted. Thus, analysis of the output can be performed after the early stages of processing. The output pattern vectors highlight different structural organisation of each particular face.

At the same time, minor structural changes do not affect the first vector components, thus making the algorithm tolerant to slight changes in facial expression (Grudin et al. 1996[a], Grudin et al. 1996[b]). In the current realisation, the system may be viewed as performing a multistage sorting of the changing data. Even if the components are not correlated at the

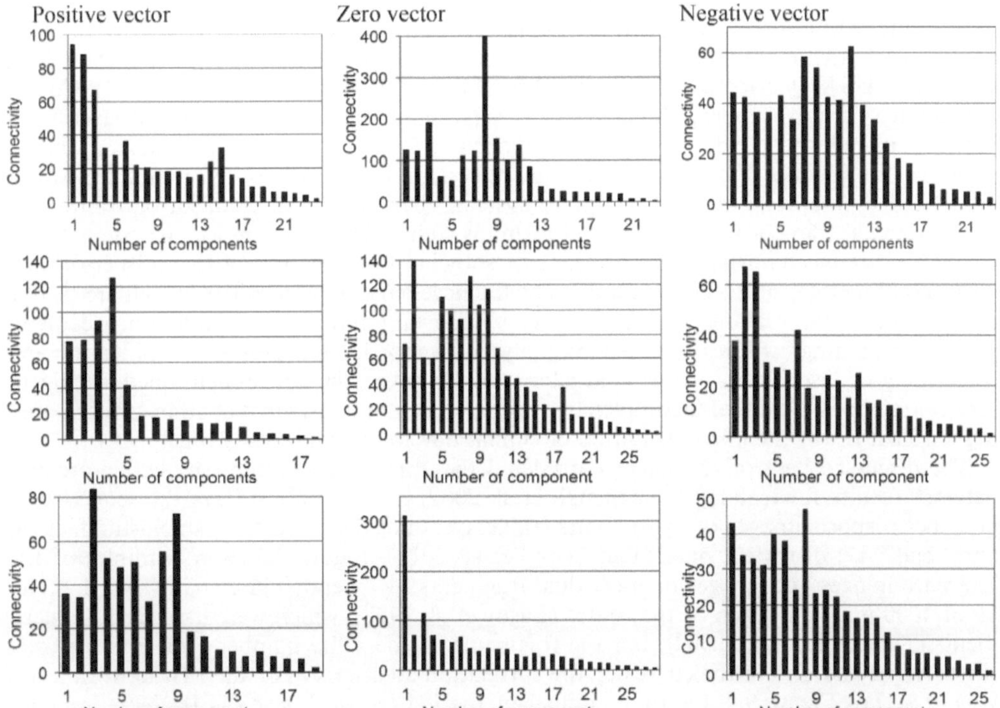

Figure 9.2 Pattern vectors generated by the multistage algorithm for three faces.

low levels of the multistage network, they can be found correlated at some higher levels. Any correlations affect the values of the remaining data and influence the output result (Grudin et al. 1997).

There are several factors, which contribute to the fast speed of this multistage processing:

1. Image data is segmented and fed into a number of parallel channels. Components from different segments may be only processed together at the higher levels, if they are assigned the same rank. Thus, the number of possible combinations is significantly reduced.
2. Calculations in the channels can be performed in parallel, for example, on our custom TMS320C40 image processing computer (Harvey et al. 1995).
3. Components of the output vector are extracted one at a time, with priority given to the more informative ones. Thus, the algorithm is robust to minor structural changes in the image.

Although at each level the more informative components are promoted in their processing, it is still possible to discover some very significant correlations at the later stages. The obvious example is the 0-th pattern vector of the first face, whose most significant component is extracted at stage 8. It is worth noting that the "winner takes all" approach is unable to detect this regularity at all. Calculation of the statistics of local coefficients also cannot emphasise it. Applications of the multistage approach include fast object identification and compact data representation.

3.3 *Experimental results of dynamic images of laser beam spots processing*

For variants of applied problems in scientific research, aimed at accurate determination of laser beam profile characteristics, as well as coordinate characteristics of laser route images with further possibility of forecasting laser images at arbitrary moments of time are promising. Much attention is paid to this scientific direction in Russia, for instance at the Federal State Unitary Enterprise "Scientific Industrial Astrophysics Association" (Basov et al. 1998) and in the USA, in some leading American corporations, such as Photon Inc. (San Jose, California, USA) (Carlos 2000), Spiricon Inc. (Logan, Utah, USA) (Roundy 1990), Coherent Auburn Group (Auburn, California, USA). The equipment of the systems of laser beam profiling includes as a rule such main components as: digital camera (with corresponding interface, for instance Fireware); travel camera system, based on the step motor controller, controlled by the user; modern computer system; chart of the mechanism of frame capture for signal transformation in digital form; as well as the software for the control of a frame capture mechanism chart by means of showing laser beam profiles and performing corresponding quantitative computations of the necessary characteristics, which are profile components. Additional service functions, very important in the authors' opinion, are intelligent programming facilities intended for analysis, diagnostics, recognition, classification and forecasting of laser beam profile characteristics. However, the above-mentioned intelligent service functions are either incompletely considered or not considered at all in modern analogues. That is why the implementation of similar developments is really timely.

The discussed part of the paper considered the application of the parallel-hierarchical network facility for training (Timchenko et al. 2002) and formation from the sequence of laser beam sports images of "good" images, i.e. ones not distorted by destabilising factors, and "bad", i.e. distorted, ones (Timchenko et al. 2011). Figure 9.3 shows samples of the reference images and images of individual fragments of extended laser paths No. 1 ÷ No. 10 of 1000 images in each of the routes (Basov et al. 1998), which were used in the experiments (Timchenko et al. 2002). For the fragments of the route number 1 of PH construct the network and obtain the curves of the correlation comparison of the PH network levels (Fig. 9.4). For Figure 9.4, the total number of the PH Network levels is 18. Next, we construct a graph of average levels of correlation coefficients (Fig. 9.5). Obtained: the average correlation coefficient of the PH network levels, amounting to 0.41, hence the tunnel is in the range of [0.41...1].

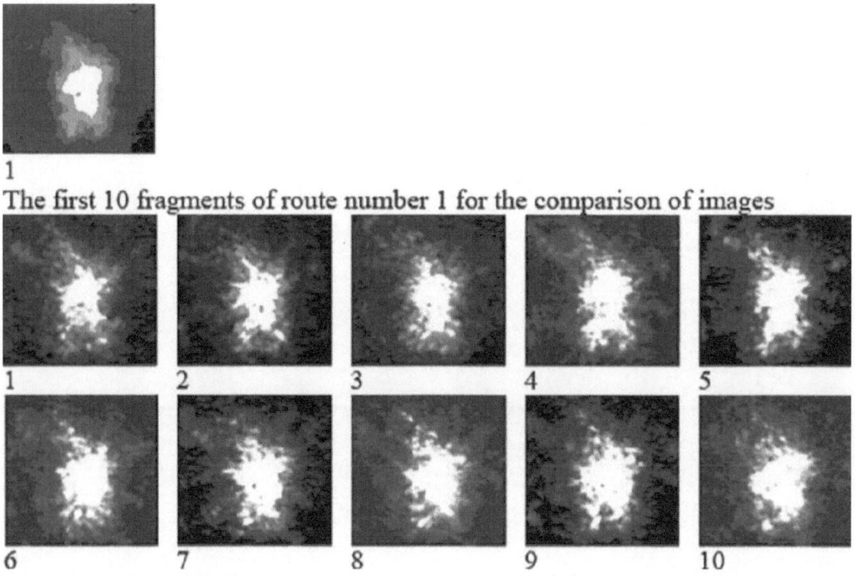

Figure 9.3 Samples of images and fragments of lines. Master image is formed of 10% of the fragments of route No. 1: [SCR_001.BMP…SCR_100.BMP].

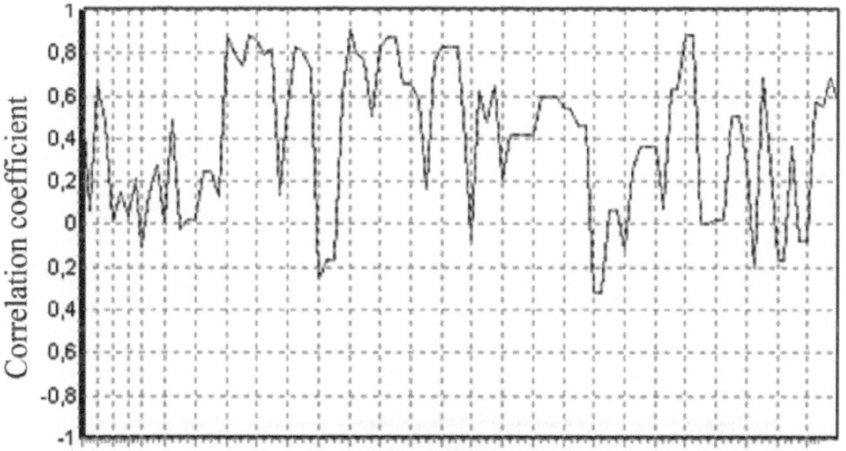

Figure 9.4 Example of correlation comparisons of the PH network levels.

Make optimisation of weights for the "good" image from the formula:

$$\begin{aligned} x_{ec} &= \frac{1}{M}\sum_{x=0}^{N-1}\sum_{y=0}^{N-1} w(f(x,y))\cdot(x+\delta_X), \\ y_{ec} &= \frac{1}{M}\sum_{x=0}^{N-1}\sum_{y=0}^{N-1} w(f(x,y))\cdot(y+\delta_y), \end{aligned} \tag{9.3}$$

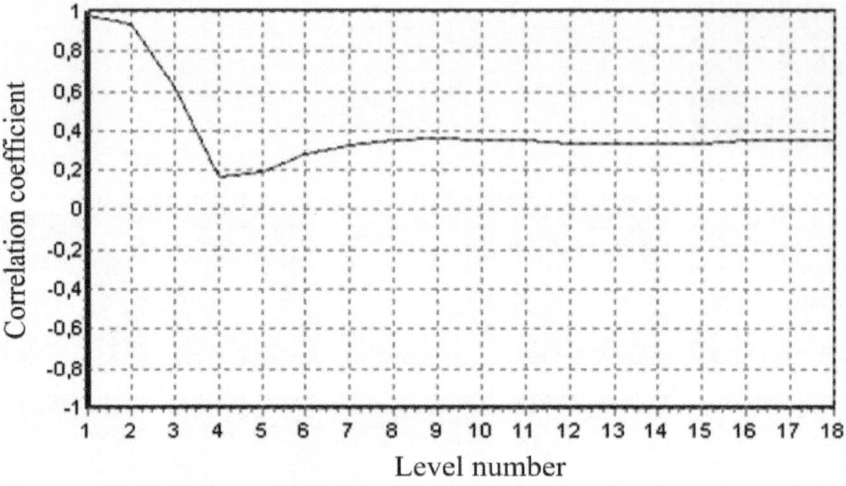

Figure 9.5 Graph of the average levels of correlation coefficients.

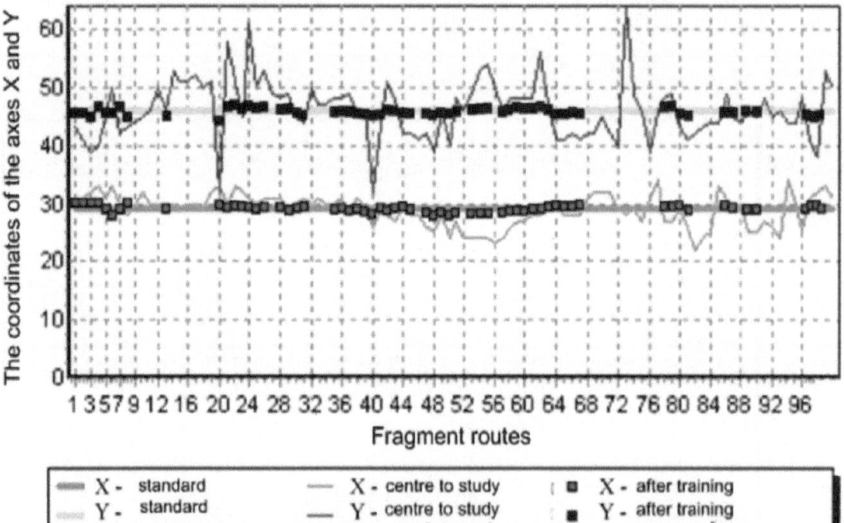

Figure 9.6 Graph of the coordinate determination of the energy centers of laser beam image spots before and after training the PH network.

where $M = \sum_{x=0}^{N-1}\sum_{y=0}^{N-1} w(f(x,y))$, $w = 1,2,...,N$, $f(x,y)$ – function of image brightness, $M(\cdot)$ – moment of inertia of the first order, $\delta_X = \frac{1}{N}\sum_{i=0}^{N-1}(\overline{x} - x_i)$ and $\delta_Y = \frac{1}{N}\sum_{i=0}^{N-1}(\overline{y} - y_i)$ are displacements of the centres of the axes X and Y accordingly, $\overline{x}, \overline{y}$ – are average values of the centre sample images of the axes X and Y accordingly, x_i, y_i – are coordinates of the centre of each "good" image. Define "good" image of route number 1, and optimise the weights of Formula (9.3), thereby calculating the coordinates of the energy centres of laser beam image spots (Fig. 9.6).

4 DISCUSSION AND CONCLUSION

The paper investigates the mapping of the part-whole hierarchies into the connectionist network in order to accomplish multistage information processing. Image elements are grouped into components, which are then consequentially passed to the higher levels of the hierarchy to participate in correlation processes. In this approach, the processing at the first level reveals and temporally separates the structural components in the image. Detection of structure reduces redundancy and, moreover, almost certainly illustrates some underlying principle.

A possible criterion for discovering structural relationships in the image is connectedness (Rock & Palmer 1990), which is one of the most informative visual characteristics. It explains a powerful tendency of the human visual system to perceive any uniform connected area as a single unit. The Gestalt law of connectedness is probably one of the most fundamental grouping principles. In the authors' opinion, formalization of the concept of connectedness in the spatio-temporal domain can help approach the complex problem of shape recognition. Processing at the successive levels of the multistage hierarchy investigates spatio-temporal interactions between the revealed structural components. The revealed components and the relationships between them will be represented throughout the hierarchical structure and will appear in some form in the output. In that way the output sequence reflects the structure of the input and can be compared with those of the previously processed images on the basis of the closest match.

The graph representation of the multistage network, shown in Figure 9.1, includes temporal components as well as spatial ones. Such implementation may result in the appearance of new procedures for unsupervised learning, which seek a compromise between two extreme approaches with clearly distributed (Linsker 1988) and clearly localised (Kohonen 1982) representations. The structure shown in Figure 9.1 implements five general properties, which are fundamental for the human visual perception:

- topographical character of calculations (Churchland & Sejnowski 1992);
- simultaneousness (parallelism) of signal actions (Hubel 1988);
- coarse cortical hierarchy (Kuffler et al. 1984);
- temporally correlated spatial mechanism of perception (Livingstone & Hubel 1984);
- mosaic structure of the cortex (Hubel & Wiesel 1968).

The strategy of multistage processing has several analogies in the cortical organisation. It conforms with the theory of multistage integration in the visual cortex (Zeki 1993), which states that integration does not occur simultaneously by virtue of the convergence of signals in a single master area. On the contrary, it is a parallel-hierarchical process in which each level directly contributes to the perception of incoming visual information. This process involves two major types of convergence operating at all levels. Topical convergence occurs within each visual pathway, accumulating information on a certain feature from different image locations. Confluent convergence occurs between the pathways and involves integration of the features of different nature. The proposed multistage architecture, shown in Figure 9.1, embodies both these convergence types. Application of this principle in synthetic systems will provide more effective processing methods. Some major features of the proposed structure are very similar to the mechanisms of pre- and postsynaptic coincidence, which are characteristic of the memory processes in neural cells. In the cortex, such processes implement spatio-temporal correlation of active neurons. Part of the neural cells tend to organise optimal coalitions, i.e. make calculations. Other neurons represent the results of those calculations. A question has been raised about the existence of neurons which directly exhibit the contents of symbolic consciousness (Crick & Koch 1990). Analysing Equation (9.2), it is clear that the output elements a^j_{1l} of the multistage network satisfy the criterion of such neurons.

The main application areas of this methodology are:

- methods of object detection and filtration;
- realisation of parallel coding;
- artificial neural network theory and creation of the formal apparatus for simulation of the cortical neural mechanisms of perception.

A number of artificial neural structures with effective learning algorithms have been developed, which implement certain principles of neural organisation of the cortex. However, the mechanisms of the formation of cortical coalitions and their joint actions are not fully understood. The task of experimentally observing interactions between different neural groups has proved to be extremely difficult (Hubel 1988). Therefore the attempt of simulating such interactions using mathematical knowledge is very pertinent and can help reveal the methods created by nature. The proposed method of automatic face recognition can be used for the following applications. They are: comparison of photographs on credit cards, driver's licenses, photo identification of customers for a variety of organisations to control access to various kinds of information that can be obtained in the computer network of organisations such as archives, banks, security agencies, etc., as well as in conducting financial transactions performed in the Internet computer network. When using a parallel hierarchical model for pattern recognition problems of dynamic images, training the network shows that among "good" fragment routes there were approximately 50% of the fragments of tracks for which weights were optimised. Optimisation of weight significantly increases the accuracy of the coordinates of the fragment centres of the laser beam spot image.

Experiments show that the spot image of laser beams as a result of various destabilising factors is impossible to measure accurately the coordinates of their energy centres, but the accuracy can be significantly improved by using trained PH network with their subsequent classification into "good" and "bad". The physical modelling method for determining the coordinates of image spots of laser beams using signal processor of TMS320S5510 type with 200 MHz and a capacity of 400 million operations per second shows that the processing of one image equals ~ 10.65 ms (Timchenko et al. 2001), which is quite sufficient for the realisation of television image processing of laser tracks.

The obtained results may find wide applications in different systems, where you want to correct automatically the distortions of the laser source of light radiation. This is, for example, an optical navigation system using lasers in conditions of reduced visibility in the atmosphere, the exact orientation of the system that make it possible to determine the spatial position of a moving object in different weather conditions, laser navigation systems. It is also a laser communication system and transmission of information, locations and remote measurement, tracing, etc. systems where the parameters of the laser beam, carrying useful information are affected by the atmosphere.

ACKNOWLEDGMENT

The authors express their gratitude to the scientific co-director of the work Yuri Kutaev for proposing the task and its practical realisation.

REFERENCES

Basov, N.G., Zemskov, E.M., Kutaev, Yu.F., et al. 1998. Laser Control of Near Earth Space and Possibilities for Removal of Space Debris from Orbit with Explosive Photo-Dissociation Lasers with Phase Conjugation. In *Proc. SPIE Symposium*: 219–228.

Carlos, B. 2000. *Roundy Current Technology of Laser Beam Profile Measurements*. Spiricon. Inc.

Churchland, P. & Sejnowski, T.J. 1992. *The Computational Brain*. The MIT Press/Bradford Books.

Crick, F. & Koch, C. 1990. Towards Neurobiological Theory of Consciousness. *Seminars in the Neurosciences* 2: 263–275.

Daugman, J. 1985. Uncertainty Relation for Resolution in Space, Spatial Frequency, and Orientation Optimized by 2D Visual Cortical Filters. *J. Opt. Soc. Amer. (A)* 2(7): 1160–1169.

Grossberg, S., Ross, W.D. & Mingolla, E. 2000. Visual cortical mechanisms of perceptual grouping: Interacting layers, networks, columns, and maps. *J. Neural Networks* 13: 571–588.

Grossberg, S. & Williamson, J.R. 2001. A neural model of how horizontal and interlaminar connections of visual cortex develop into adult circuits that carry out perceptual groupings and learning. *J. Cerebral Cortex* 11: 37–58.

Grudin, A.M., Harvey, D.M. & Timchenko, L.I. 1996[a]. Multistage hierarchy for fast image analysis. In *Proc. The European Symposium on Satellite Remote Sensing III* 2955: 120–128.

Grudin, A.M., Harvey, D.M. & Timchenko, L.I. 1997. Fast Face Recognition Method Using a Multistage Hierarchical Network. In *Proc. IEEE Intl. Conf. Acoust., Speech and Signal Proc.* 4: 2545–2548.

Grudin, M.A., Timchenko, L.I., Harvey, D.M. & Gel, V.P. 1996[b]. A System-Theoretical Approach to Multistage Hierarchical Image Processing. In *Proc. EUROPTO Symposium* 2785: 225–234.

Hall, D.J. & Ball, G.B. 1965. *ISODATA: A Novel Method of Data Analysis and Pattern Classification. Technical Report*. Menlo Park, California: Stanford Research Institute.

Harvey, D.M., Kshirsagar, S.P., Hobson, C.A., Hartley, D.A. & Moorehead, J.D. 1995. Digital Signal Processing Systems Architectures for Image Processing. In *Proc. The Fifth International Conference on Image Processing and Its Applications* 410: 460–464.

Hirahara, M., Oka, N. & Kindo, T. 2000. A cascade associative memory model with a hierarchical memory structure. *J. Neural Network* 13(1): 41–50.

Hubel, D.H. 1988. *Eye, Brain and Vision*. New York: Scientific American Library.

Hubel, D.H. & Wiesel, T.N. 1968. Receptive Fields and Functional Architecture of Monkey Striate Cortex. *J. Physiol.* 195: 215–243.

Kandel, R. & Hawkins, R. 1992. The Biological Basis of Learning and Individuality. *J. Scientific American* 267(3): 53–60.

Kohonen, T. 1982. Self-organized formation of topologically correct feature maps. *J. Biol. Cybern.* 43: 59–69.

Kozhemyako, V.P., Timchenko, L.I. & Yarovyy, A.A. 2008. Methodological Principles of Pyramidal and Parallel-Hierarchical Image Processing on the Base of Neural-Like Network Systems. *J. Advances in Electrical and Computer Engineering* 8(2): 54–60.

Kuffler, S.W., Nicholls, J.G. & Martin, A.R. 1984. *From Neuron to Brain*. Sunderland, Mass.: Sinauer Associates.

Kutaev, Yu.F. 1989. *Systems of correlative-extremal measurement of the coordinates, based on generalized Q-transform of images*. Ph.D. dissertation, Vinnytsia, Ukraine: Vinnytsia Polytechnic Institute.

Linsker, R. 1988. Self-Organization in a Perceptual Network. *J. Computer* 21(3): 105–117.

Livingstone, M.S. & Hubel, D.H. 1984. Anatomy in the Primate Visual Cortex. *J. Neurosci.* 4: 309–356.

Pollack, J.B. 1990. Recursive Distributed Representations. *J. Artif. Intell.* 46(1–2): 77–106.

Rao, R.P.N. & Ballard, D.H. 1995. Natural Basis Functions and Topographic Memory for Face Recognition. In *Proc. Intl. Joint Conf. on Artif. Intell.*: 10–17.

Rock, I. & Palmer, S. 1990. The Legacy of Gestalt Psychology. *J. Scientific American* 263(6): 48–61.

Roundy, C.B. 1990. The importance of beam profile. *J. Physics World* July: 65–66.

Shatz, C.J. 1990. Impulse Activity and the Patterning of Connection During CNS Development. *J. Neuron* 5(6): 745–758.

Sherrington, G.E. 1961. *The Integrative Action of the Nervous System*. New Haven, Conn.: Yale University Press.

Svechnikov, S.V., Kozhemiako, V.P. & Timchenko, L.I. 1987. *Logiko-Vremennyje Kvaziimpulsno-Potentsialnyje Optoelektronnyje Elementy i Ustrojstva*. Kiev: Naukova Dumka.

Timchenko, L.I. 2000. A multistage parallel-hierarchic network as a model of a neurolike computation scheme. *J. Cybernetics and systems analysis* 36(2): 251–267.

Timchenko, L.I., Kokryatskaya, N.I., et al. 2011. A method of organization of a parallel-hierarchical network for image recognition. *J. Cybernetics and systems analysis* 47(1): 140–151.

Timchenko, L.I., Kutaev, Yu.F., Gertsiy, A.A., et al. 2001. System of coordinates referencing for nonstationary signals. *J. of Russian Academy of Science, Series Physics* 6: 886–890.

Timchenko, L.I., Kutaev, Yu.F., Kozhemyako, V.P., et al. 2002. Method for Training of a Parallel-Hierarchical Network, Based on Population Coding for Processing of Extended Laser Paths Images. In *Proc. SPIE* 4790: 465–479.

White, J.M. & Rohrer, G.D. 1983. Image Thresholding for Optical Character Recognition and Other Applications Requiring Character Image Extraction. *J. Res. Develop.* 27(4): 400–411.

Zeki, S. 1993. *A Vision of the Brain*. Oxford: Blackwell Scientific Publication.

CHAPTER 10

Combined models of artificial immune systems

V.I. Lytvynenko
Kherson National Technical University, Kherson, Ukraine

W. Wójcik & A. Smolarz
Lublin University of Technology, Lublin, Poland

B. Suleimenov
K.I. Satpaev Kazakh National Research Technical University, Almaty, Kazakhstan

M. Junisbekov
M.Kh. Dulaty Taraz State University, Taraz, Kazakhstan

1 ARTIFICIAL IMMUNE SYSTEMS

Artificial Immune Systems (AIS), as defined by de Castro and Timmis (de Castro 2002) are: "Adaptive systems inspired by theoretical immunology and observed immune functions, principles and models, which are applied to problem solving". However, AIS are one of many types of algorithms inspired by biological systems, such as neural networks, evolutionary algorithms and swarm intelligence. There are many different types of algorithms within AIS and research to date has focused primarily on the theories of immune networks, clonal selection and negative selection. These theories have been abstracted into various algorithms and applied to a wide variety of application areas such as anomaly detection, pattern recognition, learning and robotics.

It is well known, that the algorithm of Negative Selection (NS) has some restrictions and limitations (Dasgupta 2006). It is not appropriate, for example, when the number of self samples is small and sparse. Some limitations of the binary-string representation in negative selection algorithms are as follows:

- binary matching rules are not able to capture the semantics of some complex self/non-self spaces,
- it is not easy to extract meaningful domain knowledge,
- in some cases a large number of detectors are needed to guarantee better coverage (detection rate),
- it is difficult to integrate the NS algorithm with other immune algorithms,
- the crisp boundary of "self" and "non-self" may be very hard to define.

In real-valued representation the detectors are represented by hyper-shapes in *n*-dimensional space. The algorithms use geometrical spaces and heuristics to distribute detectors in non-self space. Some limitations of the real-valued representation in negative selection algorithms are as follows:

- the issue of holes in some geometrical shapes, and the need of multi-shaped detectors,
- the curse of dimensionality,
- the estimation of coverage,
- the selection of distance measure.

Generation of a set of detectors in R at the training phase occurs casually. Nevertheless, during the experiments it was established that it is impossible to define in advance the minimum quantity of detectors necessary to provide the maximum quality of recognition. An increase in the number of detectors leads to the time-consuming recognition phase, and its reduction—to deterioration of algorithm performance. The latter is caused by an increased probability of the formation of "cavities", which are areas in "non-self" space which are not distinguished by any of detector. Thus, a research problem is working out a method of generating detectors able to adaptively select their options, number and arrangement. Further, one of the possible solutions is described—a hybridisation (combining) of negative selection algorithms, a clonal selection algorithm and an artificial immune network.

2 HYBRIDISATION OF ARTIFICIAL IMMUNE SYSTEMS

The idea of hybridisation based on the following fact: most paradigms contain information about them for a particular task, which requires the previous definition, which is a difficult task in itself as well (de Castro 2002). For example, a neural network needs the determination of its structure, i.e. the number of links, the number of neurons in the layer, and the number of layers. The evolutionary procedures need prior information about the number of chromosomes in the population, but then one of the main problems of fuzzy systems is to determine the number of linguistic variable terms. A special place in our consideration is the problem of adaptive tuning of parameters such as the probability of evolutionary operators, the form and parameters of membership functions, etc. These tasks can be essentially attributed to a class of combinatorial problems and their solution depends on the effective performance of computer systems in general. Artificial immune systems are heuristic procedures whose advantage is the ability to solve many problems quickly. Therefore logical integration approaches allow to obtain better final outcomes than the results obtained through the use of particular methods.

Formally, the problem of the development of immune algorithms can be represented as:

$$AIS = \langle \mathbf{\Sigma}, \mathbf{M}, \mathbf{A}, \mathbf{K} \rangle \tag{10.1}$$

where $\mathbf{\Sigma}$ is the set of components representing methods, $\mathbf{M}$ denotes the set of methods for the affinity evaluation, $\mathbf{A}$ is the set of procedures for adapting, and $\mathbf{K}$ is the set of criteria for AIS evaluation.

The techniques of formal representation of AIS allow to create abstract models of immune organs, cells or molecules. Evaluation mechanisms, which are called affinity functions, can quantify the interaction of these "artificial immune organs", and adapt the procedure presented as algorithms to achieve the goals and manage the dynamics of AIS. The evaluation criteria or a set of evaluation functions, taken from such computing paradigms as neural networks and evolutionary algorithms, can be used to evaluate the interaction of AIS individuals. At the same time, evolutionary algorithms are well suited to control the time variation of the states of cells and molecules of which an artificial immune system consists. In view of this, the process of AIS design can be divided into two main stages:

- selection of the appropriate form of representation of individuals and affinity measures;
- use of any existing algorithms (or the new algorithm) for the control of system states over time.

It should also be noted that the representation of individuals and affinity measure is fully determined by the problem domain in which one wants to use AISs as well as by the type of problems to be solved.

The main goal of hybridisation is the integration of the advantages of the latest information technologies. There are two approach combinations: a) the combined use of different types of immune algorithms, and algorithms with modified immune operators, and b) the combined use of several paradigms and soft computing algorithms: neural networks, fuzzy neural networks, evolutionary algorithms, artificial immune systems.

3 CANONICAL ALGORITHMS OF ARTIFICIAL IMMUNE SYSTEMS

As mentioned before, one of the possible solutions of the number of detectors is the combined use of different kinds of immune algorithms. This section is dedicated to introducing algorithms which will be used for hybridisation. The next sections will describe two types of hybridisation: a negative selection algorithm with a clonal selection algorithm as well as an artificial immune network algorithm of negative selection.

3.1 *The negative selection algorithm*

The negative selection of T-cells is responsible for eliminating the T-cells whose receptors are capable of binding with self-peptides presented by self-MHC (major histocompatibility complex) molecules. This process guarantees that the T-cells that leave the thymus do not recognise any self-cell or molecule. Forrest et al. (Forrest et al.1994) proposed a changed detection algorithm inspired by the negative selection of T-cells within the thymus. This procedure was called the negative selection algorithm and was originally applied in computational security. A single type of immune cell was modelled: T-cells were represented as bit strings of length *L*. The negative selection algorithm is simple. Given a set of self-peptides, named self-set **S**, the T-cell receptors will have to be tested for their capability of binding the self-peptides. If a T-cell recognises a self-peptide, it is discarded; otherwise it is selected as an immune-competent cell and enters the available repertoire **A** (Fig. 10.1).

The idea of the negative selection algorithm is to generate a set of detectors in a complementary set **N** and then to use these detectors for binary classification as "self" or "non-self" (Forrest et al., 1994). Formally, the negative selection algorithm can be represented as [10.6]:

$$NegA\lg = \left(\Sigma^L, L, \mathbf{S}, \mathbf{N}, r, n, s, pr\right) \tag{10.2}$$

where Σ^L denotes shape-space, L is receptor length; **S** is "self" detector set; **N** is "non-self" detector set; r denotes cross-reactive threshold; n is total number of appointed detectors; s is detector set size; pr denotes rule matching rows in adjacent positions.

The negative selection algorithm can be summarised as follows (Forrest et al., 1994):

- Define self as a collection $\boldsymbol{S}$ of elements in a feature space $\boldsymbol{U}$, a collection that needs to be monitored. For instance, if $\boldsymbol{U}$ corresponds to the space of states of a system represented

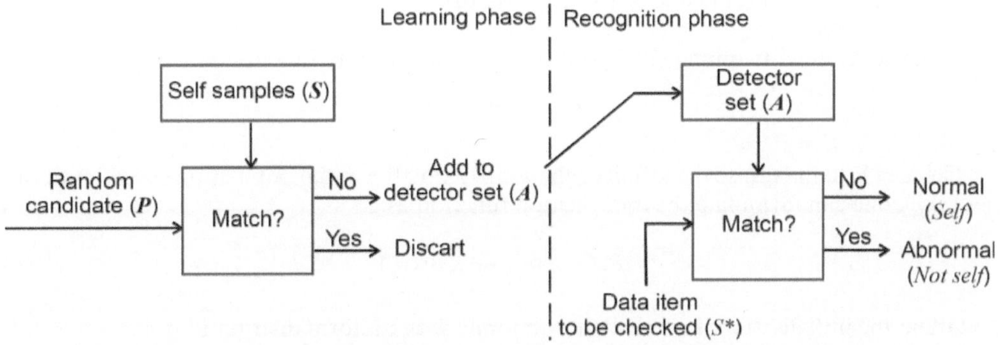

Figure 10.1 Negative selection algorithm (Dasgupta 2006).

by a list of features, ***S*** can represent the subset of states that are considered as normal for the system.

- Generate a set ***A*** of *detectors,* each of which fails to match any string in ***S***. An approach that mimics the immune system generates random detectors and discards those that match any element in the self set.
- Monitor ***S*** for changes by continually matching the detectors in ***A*** against ***S***. If any detector ever matches, then a change is known to have occurred, as the detectors are designed not to match any representative samples of ***S***.

3.2 *Clonal selection algorithm*

Formally algorithm of clonal selection can be represented as:

$$CLONALG = \left(\mathbf{P}^{l}, \mathbf{G}^{k}, l, k, m_{Ab}, \delta, \mathrm{f}, \mathrm{I}, \tau, \mathbf{AG}, \mathbf{AB}, \mathrm{S}, \mathrm{C}, \mathbf{M}, n, d\right), \tag{10.3}$$

where P^l is the search space (shape-space); G^k is space representation; l is the length of vector of attributes (dimension of search space); k is the length of antibody receptor; m_{Ab} is the dimension of antibody population; δ is the expression function; f is the affinity function; I is the initialisation function of the initial population of antibodies; τ is the completion condition of the algorithm work; AG is the subset of antigens; AB is the population of antibodies; S is the selection operator; C is the cloning operator; M is the mutation operator; n is the number of the best antibodies selected for cloning; d is the number of the worst antibodies subjected to substitution for new ones.

Consider the shape-space (P^l) phenotypes and their space images as antibodies (G^k) or genotype space [10.7]. The function:

$$\delta : P^{l} \rightarrow G^{k} \tag{10.4}$$

is a function of conversion options with P^l solutions to their internal image G^k in a population of individuals.

This function is otherwise called the expression function. It should be noted that in practice, for reasons of convenience, the development of AIS often imposes similar transformations the application of immune operators and calculate affinity individuals. For example, a vector of real attributes of dimension l can be transformed into a bit string of length k, which allows the mutation and affinity calculations of specific operators using different types of Hamming distance. Therefore, the terms "*genotype*", "*phenotype*" and "*expression*" in this description are borrowed from biology relatives by their functional structure and evolutionary algorithms, although more suitable for use in the context of the evolution of chromosomes than the molecular structure of antibodies. It is also assumed that for every solution $p \in P^l$ there is one and only one of its images $\delta(p) \in G^k$. Thus, in general, the opposite assertion is not correct.

Using generalised mapping [10.7], one can write the affinity function f as:

$$f : P^{l} \times P^{l} \rightarrow \Re^{+}. \tag{10.5}$$

The idea is to maximise the affinity function. Taking the initial population size of antibodies (m_{Ab}), one can formulate the initialisation function as:

$$I : G^{k} \times m_{Ab} \rightarrow AB\left(G^{k}\right). \tag{10.6}$$

Often, the initialisation is carried out randomly with uniform distribution.

Let the Q-nary operator perform a stochastic transformation on the set G^k, which uses the administering set K_Q to generate control parameters that determine the way to convert the current step of the procedure. For example, if mutations are expressed as a bit string, a bit mask can be used as a control parameter, which determines the position of individual numbers of the individual bits that undergo mutations. Thus, the functional entry operator Q can be represented as follows:

$$Q: G^k \times K_Q \rightarrow G^k. \tag{10.7}$$

The optimum solution of $Ab_{opt} \in G^k$ concerning the operator of Q and antigen $Ag \in AG,\ \ AG \subset G^k$ is called an individual, whose affinity cannot be increased by a further influence of the operator of transformation Q, i.e.

$$\forall k \in K_G : f\left(Q(Ab_{opt}, k), Ag\right) \leq f\left(Ab_{opt}, Ag\right). \tag{10.8}$$

The condition of shutdown (τ) is executed when the population of antibodies fully recognises the population of antigens, i.e.

$$\forall Ag \in AG : \exists Ab \in G^k \mid Ab = Ab_{opt}. \tag{10.9}$$

The selection operator S forms a subset of G_S individuals whose affinity is better in this generation. Thus, S together with the management set K_S represents the function:

$$S: G^k \times K_S \rightarrow \{0,1\}, \tag{10.10}$$

a set which is formed by the selection:

$$G_S = \{Ab \in G^k \mid S(Ab, k_S) = 1\}, \quad |G_S| = n. \tag{10.11}$$

Similarly, the selection is made of individuals in a population of memory cells. The cloning operator C increases the elements of the set G_S in a population and with the management set K_C can be written as:

$$C: G_S \times K_C \rightarrow G_S. \tag{10.12}$$

The mutation operator M with the operating set K_M can be written as:

$$M: G^k \times K_M \rightarrow G^k. \tag{10.13}$$

A metadynamic system is expressed as the substitution function of the worst antibody population:

$$R: G^k \times d \rightarrow AB_d\left(G^k\right). \tag{10.14}$$

The process of converting a population of antibodies by a clonal selection algorithm can be represented as a sequence of the following statements:

$$\begin{gathered} AB_t \xrightarrow{Selection(S)} G_S \xrightarrow{Cloning(C)} G_C \xrightarrow{Mutation(M)} \\ G_M \xrightarrow{\text{Repeat mutation}(S)} G_S \xrightarrow{\text{Replacement}(d)} AB_{t+1}, \end{gathered} \tag{10.15}$$

where t is the generation number, AB is the population of antibodies (detectors), G_S – the subset of selected best antibodies, G_C is the subset of clones and G_M is the subset of clones after mutation.

Let us show the generalised stepwise description of the algorithm.

1. *Initialisation.* Creation (usually by random generation) of the initial population of antibodies AB.
2. *Determination of affinity.* For every antibody AB_j, $AB_j \in AB$ determine its affinity relative to every antigen Ag_i, $Ag_i \in AG$. Write the result into the matrix of affinities $D: D=[|AG| \times m_{Ab}]$, and $d_{ij} = f(Ab_j, Ag_i)$, $d_{ij} \in D$.
3. *Clonal selection and propagation.* Select from population n of each the best antibodies for every row of the matrix D and place them into separate population of clones $AB_C, |AB_C| = n \cdot |AG|$. It is necessary to generate clones of elements of the population AB_C proportionally to their affinity, i.e. the greater it is, the greater number of clones is generated and vice versa.
4. *Affinity maturation.* Subject to mutation all the clones of a population AB_C with the probability inversely proportional to affinities, i.e. the probability of mutation is the greater, the lower is its affinity. Determine new affinity of every antibody AB_j, $AB_j \in AB_C$ similar to item 2 and obtain the matrix of affinities D_C. Select n antibodies from the population AB_C, for which the corresponding vector-column of the D_C matrix gives the best generalised result of affinity, and transfer them into the population of memory cells M_R.
5. *Metadynamics.* Substitute the worst d antibodies of the population AB by new random individuals.
6. Substitute n antibodies of the population AB by memory cells from M_R and pass to item 2 until the stoppage criterion is reached.

The peculiarity of the algorithm of clonal selection consists in the fact that in contrast to the immune network it supports a constant size of population of antibodies. In publication (Dasgupta 1999) the variety mechanism of antibodies is described and the hypothesis is suggested, according to which antibody Ab_1 is selected during the primary response, then subjected to hypermutations, after which follows selection. It makes possible for the system to investigate local zones around Ab_1 by small stages towards antibodies with high affinity, which results in a local optimum of Ab_1*. Since small-scale mutations are lost, the antibodies cannot perform the search from the local minimum/maximum. Editing the receptor (parameter d) makes it possible to realise the antibodies' great advance on the landscape of affinity, stopping at the place where affinity can be lower than (Ab_2). However, a random step will result in antibodies on the side of the vertex, a more promising region of ascent (Ab_3), which makes it possible to reach a practically arbitrary global maximum. From this place hypermutations, followed by selection, can bring antibodies to the topmost vertex (Ab_3*). It is necessary to note that hypermutations are useful for the investigation of local search domains, while editing (i.e., removing of antibodies with low affinity) can save the antibodies which hit the local optimum.

3.3 *Artificial immune network algorithm*

An immune network can be presented mathematically as a graph (moreover, not obligatorily fully connected), which consists of a set of nodes, i.e. network cells (antibodies) and a set of weighted edges, denoting connections between the cells (de Castro 2003). The value of an edge weight corresponds to the affinity of the connected cells. Two types of affinity in immune networks can be distinguished:

- affinity of connection "antigen-antibody" Ag-Ab is the degree of difference;
- affinity of connection "antigen-antibody" Ab-Ab is the degree of similarity.

The formalism of an immune network is similar to that of CLONALG, with the addition of several new operators and parameters:

$$immNET = (\mathbf{P}^l, \mathbf{G}^k, l, k, m_{Ab} \delta, \mathrm{f}, \mathrm{I}, \tau, \mathbf{AG}, \mathbf{AB}, \mathbf{S}, \mathbf{C}, \mathbf{M}, n, d, \mathbf{H}, \mathbf{R}), \tag{10.16}$$

where P^l is the search space (shape-space); G^k is the representation of space; l is the length of vector of attributes; k is the length of cell receptor; m_{Ab} is the size of cell population; δ is the expression function; f is the affinity function; I is the initialisation function of the initial population of network cells; τ is the algorithm completion condition; AG is the subset of antigens, AB is the population of network cells (antibodies); S is the selection operator; C is the cloning operator; M is the mutation operator; n is the number of the best cells selected for cloning, d is the number of the worst cells subject to substitution by new ones; H is the clonal removal operator and R is the network compression operator. In the given type of algorithm the operator H uses the threshold coefficient of death (σ_d) as the controlling parameter by reduction of network dimension by means of removal of unstimulated cells:

$$H : G^k \times G^k \times \sigma_d \rightarrow \{0,1\}. \tag{10.17}$$

The set of stimulated cells $G_{\bar{d}}$ can be defined as

$$G_{\bar{d}} = \{Ab \in G^k \mid \exists Ag \in AG : H(Ab, Ag, \sigma_d) = 0\}, \tag{10.18}$$

where

$$H(Ab, Ag, \sigma_d) = \begin{cases} 0, f(Ab, Ag) > \sigma_d; \\ 1, f(Ab, Ag) \le \sigma_d. \end{cases} \tag{10.19}$$

The network compression operator uses the threshold compression coefficient σ_S as the controlling parameter, also reducing the network dimension by means of removal of self-recognised (similar) cells:

$$R : G^k \times G^k \times \sigma_s \rightarrow \{0,1\}. \tag{10.20}$$

The compressed network is defined by the set G_R

$$G_R = \{Ab_i \in G^k \mid \forall i, j : R(Ab_i, Ab_j, \sigma_s) = 0\}, \quad i, j = \overline{1, m_{Ab}}, \tag{10.21}$$

where

$$R(Ab_i, Ab_j, \sigma_s) = \begin{cases} 0, & f(Ab_i, Ab_j) > \sigma_s \\ 1, & f(Ab_i, Ab_j) \le \sigma_s \end{cases}, \quad i \ne j. \tag{10.22}$$

The process of converting a population of antibodies by the artificial immune network algorithm can be represented as a sequence of the following statements:

$$\begin{gathered} AB_t \xrightarrow{\text{Selection } (S)} G_S \xrightarrow{\text{Cloning } (C)} G_C \xrightarrow{\text{Mutation } (M)} G_M \\ \xrightarrow{\text{Clonal removal } (H)} G_H \xrightarrow{\text{Clonal compression } (K^S)} G_{RC} \xrightarrow{\text{Nework compression}} AB_{t+1} \end{gathered} \tag{10.23}$$

The behaviour of an immune network in many respects differs from the behaviour of the algorithm of clonal selection, which is reflected in the algorithm, whose stepwise realisation is represented below. The process conversion model of the population of antibody states by the immune network is as follows:

1. Initialisation.
   1.1. Creation of the initial population of memory cells M_R.
   1.2. Creation of a population of antibodies (AB).

2. *Antigen presence.* Starting from this block, the algorithm realises one pass at a time for every antigen.
   2.1. *Determination of affinity.* Affinity is determined for all memory cells m_j, $m_j \in M_R$ for regular antigen Ag_i, $Ag_i \in AG$ and the best cell m_b, is selected.
   2.2. *Cloning.* The selected memory cell is cloned proportionally to its affinity with the generation of population of clones M_C.
   2.3. *Maturation of affinity.* Mutation of clones from M_C is performed. Changed clones are added to population of antibodies, i.e. $AB \leftarrow AB \cup M_C$. Affinity of the population of antibodies AB with the antigen Ag is determined.
   2.4. *Metadynamics.* Clonal removal of nonstimulated cells is done in accordance with the threshold σ_d.
   2.5. Repeated cloning of a part of antibodies from the population AB with generation of the clone population M_C and transition to items 2.3 if mean affinity of the population AB is lower than the given threshold value.
   2.6. From the population AB the cell-candidate (the best antibody) is selected to the population of memory cells Ab_b.
   2.7. Go to item 3 if $f(Ab_b, Ag_i) < f(m_b, Ag_i)$.
   2.8. Addition of antibody Ab_b to population M_R.
   2.9. *Cell-cell* interaction. Affinity of interaction of all cells of population M_R with each other is determined, i.e. $f(m_i, m_j), m_i, m_j \in M_R$.
   2.10. *Network* compression. Cells of population M_R recognising each other are removed according to the given threshold σ_s.
   2.11. Verification of the condition of blocking the algorithm and passing to item 2, if the condition does not hold.

4 THE COMBINED MODEL OF NEGATIVE AND CLONAL SELECTION

At the core idea of the combined system (Fig. 10.2) is the assumption that the association of clonal selection with the negative selection procedure will improve the level of detection (the level of coverage).

The execution of each negative selection procedure is different in the basic quantity of factors, such as:

a. quantity of detectors,
b. impact of the number of detectors on generation and detection efficiency,

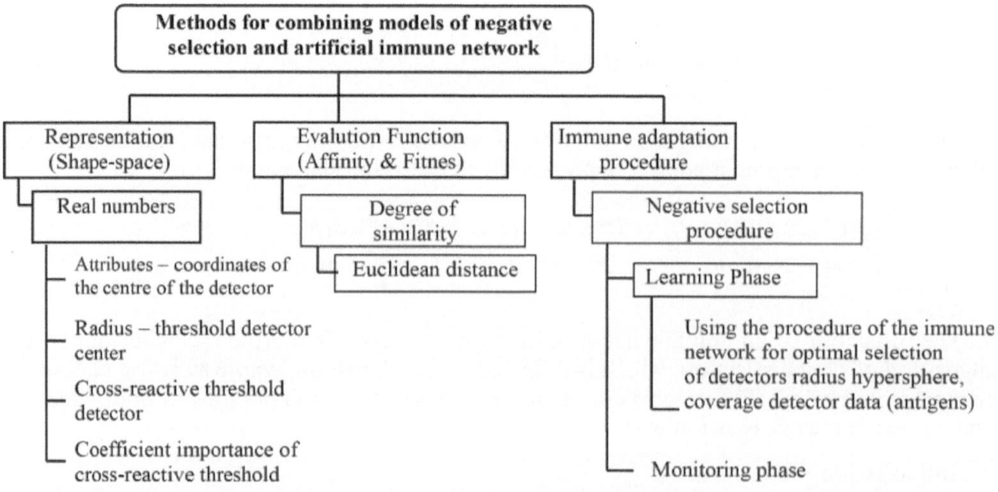

Figure 10.2 Combining of negative and clonal selection procedures.

c. coverage degree by sensor,
d. effect on detection accuracy.

The classic version of the negative selection model (Forrest 1992, Forrest et al. 1994, Hajela 1996), despite of its popularity, has some significant drawbacks. The set of detectors *A* is generated in the training phase at random, so it is impossible to determine a priori the minimum required number of detectors that will provide the highest quality of recognition. Increasing the number of detectors leads to a recognition phase slowdown, and its reduction to poor recognition performance. Small number of detectors increases the probability of creating "cavities", which are regions in space with "outsiders" that are not recognized by any detector. In some cases, a huge number of detectors is required to provide better coverage (the detection level). It is believed that it is difficult to combine the negative selection with other immune models, and that it is difficult to define a clear boundary between "self" and "non-self". Therefore, the objective is to develop advanced methods of generation of detectors able to adaptively select their adjustment, number and location. The use of artificial immune network has been proposed.

4.1 *Solution for the number of detectors problem*

In continuation, the efficiency of immune classifiers is studied. A classifier, in general, is a function that for a given vector of object attributes should decide to which class it belongs (Gonzalez 2003):

$$F:\Re^n \to Y. \tag{10.24}$$

Function *F* represents the space of sign vectors in the space of class labels *Y*. In the case of two classes $Y=\{0,1\}$, '1' is the corresponding case of the detection event, '0' – the event is not detected. We consider the variant of training with a teacher (supervised learning), when the classifier training available to us is a set of vectors $\{x\}$ for which is known their valid membership in one of the classes.

In binary classification class identifiers can be interpreted as the system states (active or passive, normal or abnormal) represented by a number of properties.

Definition 1. The space of states of the system (Gonzalez 2003). System status is determined by vector properties. Each state $x^i=(x_1^i,\ldots,x_n^i)\in[0,1]^n$ is represented by set $U\subseteq[0,1]^n$. The elements of the vector properties can be scaled or normalised in the range [0,1].

Definition 2. The normal subspace (Gonzalez 2003). The set of vectors of properties $Positiv \subseteq U$ that represent the normal system state. Its complement is called *Negativ* and determine how $Negativ = U - Positiv$. In some cases, we will define a set *Positiv* (or *Negativ*), using its characteristic function $\chi_{Positiv}:[0,1]^n \to \{0,1\}$.

$$\chi_{Positiv}(\vec{x})=\begin{cases}1 & \text{if } \vec{x}\in Positiv\\ 0 & \text{if } \vec{x}\in Negativ\end{cases} \tag{10.25}$$

Definition 3. The problem of binary classification (Gonzalez 2003). For a given set of positive examples $Positiv' \subseteq Positiv$ to evaluate the characteristic function ($\chi_{Positiv}$) normal space, which is due to have the ability to decide whether the observed state is normal or abnormal.

The proposed model address the problem of developing an improved method of generation of detectors capable to adaptively adjust their size and location. Modification in a training phase to optimise coverage by detector set of "non-self" is proposed (Forrest 1992, Perelson1996, Hajela 1996) via the mechanism of clonal selection. Solution of the problem requires modification of the antibody as shown in Figure 10.3).

In this view, attributes are the coordinates of the centre of the detector and the radius—the threshold sensitivity of the detector (cross-reactive threshold). Thus, each antibody encodes a possible alternative arrangement of detectors in "non-self" space. By manipulating the

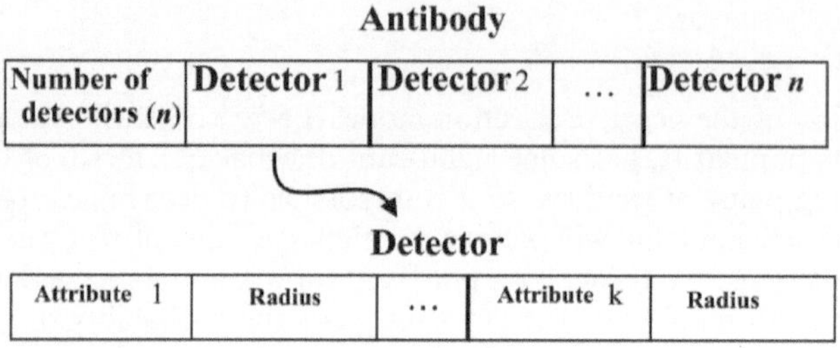

Figure 10.3 View of clonal negative model antibody.

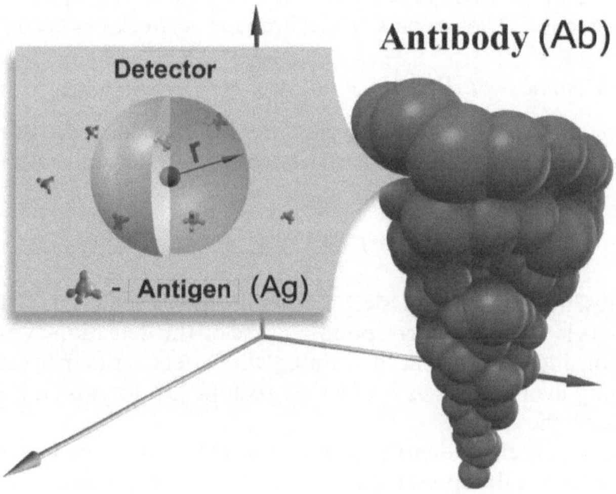

Figure 10.4 Graphical representation of antibodies and detectors of negative clonal model.

population of antibody-like structure is the best option scheme covering. A block diagram of the proposed procedure is shown in Figure 10.4.

4.2 *Methodology and benchmarks*

For evaluation of classifiers consider two test examples used in scientific practice for comparative tests of developed methods and models, i.e. the Breast Cancer Wisconsin (Mangasarian et al. 1995) and observations of the ionosphere by radar (Lichman 2013).

The purpose of the former one is classification of survey data of women for the presence of benign or malignant breast tumour on the basis of cytological studies obtained by biopsy (size and shape uniformity of cells, the presence of chromatin and mitotic cells). Totally nine attributes were used as input parameters to form two outputs (benign or malignant tumour). The dataset contains 699 examples. These were randomly mixed and divided into training set and test set. The first 458 (65.5%) examples were used for training and the remaining 241 (34.5%) for testing.

The second example contains observations of the ionosphere by radar. The purpose of the observation was the presence of free electrons in the ionosphere. The signals from radar, returning, gave the details of two types: a positive signal contained evidence proving the existence of structures in the ionosphere, a negative signal did not contain such evidence.

Table 10.1 Parameters of the combined model of clonal and negative selection.

Setup parameters	Values of model parameters negative selection	Parameter values of the combined model of clonal and negative selection
Algorithm for generating detectors	Generation and Testing	Generation and Testing
Size limit zone recognition detectors	50%	50%
Type of mutation	No	Simple
Probability of mutation	No	80%
Number of changing attributes	No	50
Number of changing forms	No	50
Hotel selection	No	70%
The replacement ratio	No	30%
Distance calculation method	Euclidean/Manhattan	Euclidean/Manhattan
Size of detector set	15/30	15/30
Size of population of antibodies	No	80
Number of generations (iterations)	100	100

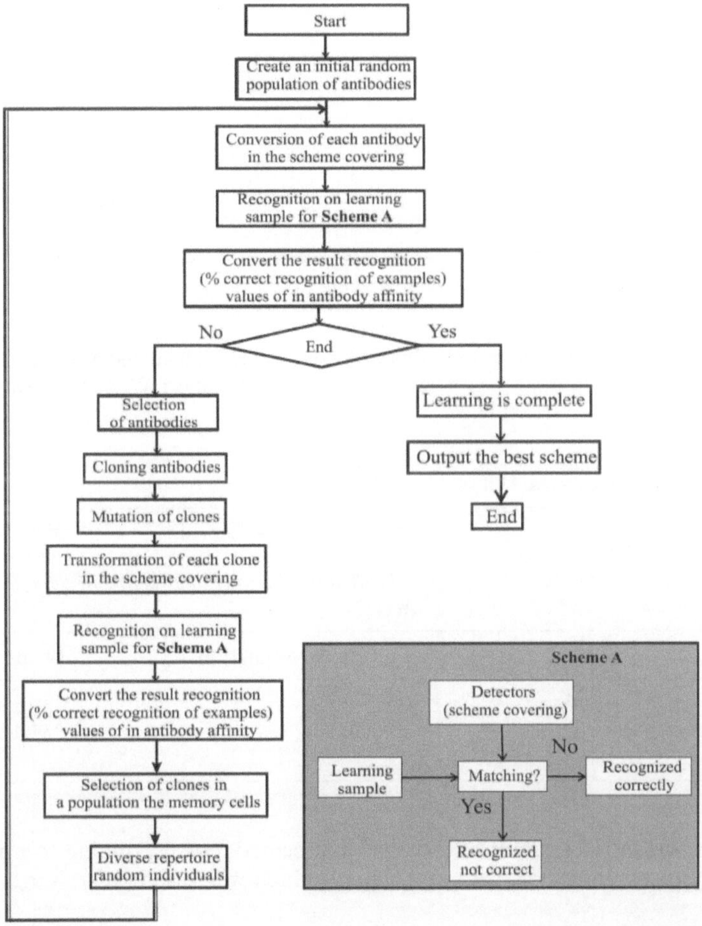

Figure 10.5 Block diagram of clonal selection with a modified phase learning method of negative selection.

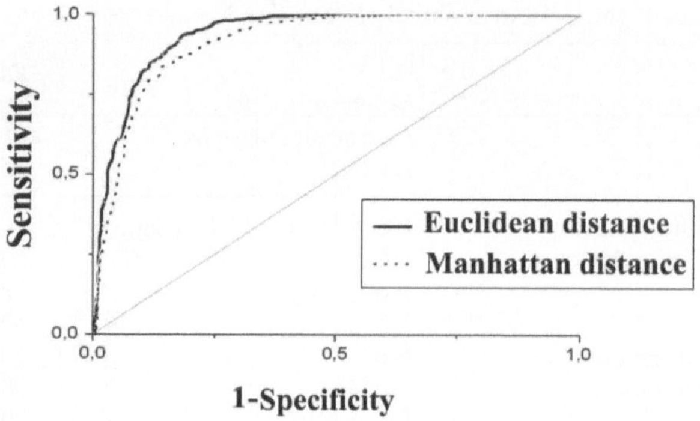

Figure 10.6 Comparison of ROC-curves obtained using the Euclidean and Manhattan distance when comparing test data vectors from the reference dataset Breast Cancer Wisconsin using the combined model of clonal and negative selection.

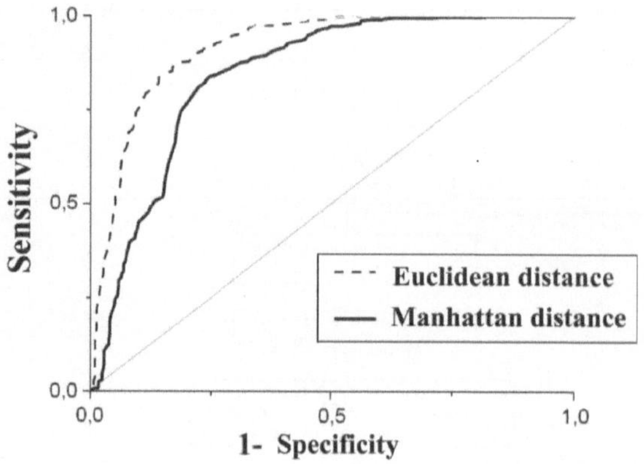

Figure 10.7 Comparison of ***ROC***-curves obtained using the Euclidean and Manhattan distance when comparing test data vectors from the reference dataset Breast Cancer Wisconsin using the combined model of clonal and negative selection.

Table 10.2 Comparison of area AUC.

	Breast Cancer Wisconsin	Signals of ionosphere
Data type	*The distance between the vectors of detectors and data vectors*	
Methods	Euclidean/Manhattan	Euclidean/Manhattan
The model of negative selection	0.935/0.924	0.916/0.831
Modified model of negative clonal selection	0.907/0.878	0.900/0.801

After signal processing 34 attributes have been allocated, corresponding to one of two possible classes. These include 351 examples, 200 of which were used for training, and 151 – for testing.

The clonal negative selection was benchmarked using the standard set of test problems, in comparison with the procedure of negative selection and combined models. To evaluate the

Table 10.3 The results of comparative studies of the effectiveness of the developed models from the reference data set "Breast Cancer Wisconsin".

Method	Classification accuracy, %
Combined model of negative clonal selection (Euclidean distance)	98.7 ± 1.5
Bayesian network	97.5 ± 1.8
The method of support vector	97.2
Naive Bayesian classifier	97.1
The method of k-nearest neighbors	97.1
Mixed Hausovskyy classifier	97.0 ± 2.1
Combined model of negative clonal selection (Manhattan distance)	97.0 ± 2.5
Modified model of negative selection (Euclidean distance)	96.9 ± 1.1
Algorithm for FSM (Feature Space Mapping)	96.9 ± 1.4
Fisher? linear discriminant Fisher? analyser	96.8
Multilayer perceptron	96.7
The modified model of negative selection (Manhattan distance)	96.7 ± 1.4
LVQ-network	96.6
SNB—semi-naive Bayes classifier	96.6
Decision Tree	96.2
RBF neural network	95.9
Algorithm for constructing decision trees C4.5	93.4

Table 10.4 The results of comparative studies of the effectiveness of the developed models from reference data set "signals ionosphere".

Method	Classification accuracy, %
Three neural networks	98.7
Combined model of negative clonal selection (Euclidean distance)	**97.9 ± 1.2**
Algorithm for constructing decision trees IB3	96.7
Combined model of negative clonal selection (Manhattan distance)	96.7 ± 1.4
Single layer perceptron	96.0
Modified model of negative selection (Euclidean distance)	96.0
Modified model of negative selection (Manhattan distance)	96.0 ± 1.4
Algorithm for constructing decision trees C4.5	94.9
The method of support vector	93.2

obtained groups of binary classifiers, *ROC*-curves are used (Fig. 10.6 and Fig. 10.7). In this case *AUC* (the area under curve) is the numerical index area under the curve and the percentage of correctly recognised objects in the test set.

One class is called the class with positive outputs, the other—with negative outputs. ROC-dependent curve shows the number of correctly classified positive examples of the number of incorrectly classified negative examples.

Comparative experiments of the effectiveness of the developed models with some well-known classifiers were conducted to estimate them by the AUC space (Tables 10.2, 10.3 and 10.4). Each experiment was done in 10 runs.

5 COMBINED IMMUNE NETWORK AND NEGATIVE SELECTION MODEL FOR SOLVING OF ANOMALY DETECTION PROBLEMS

As an alternative approach to solving problems of anomaly detection, this study addresses the problem of developing improved methods of generating detectors capable of adaptively choosing their adjustment, number and location. As a method it is proposed to use an artificial immune network structure and mechanism of which is discussed above.

5.1 *Modification of the learning phase in the model of negative selection*

Solving a specific problem with the help the generalised m requires specific descriptions of some operators and functions. In this case, the immune network uses encryption antibodies with the help of real numbers, while to calculate the distance Euclidean metric is used. This antibody forms around a radial *l*-dimensional region recognition with a radius *r*, called the cross-reactive threshold (Fig. 10.8). As shown in Figure 10.9, the cross-reactive threshold was included in the structure of antibodies, which enables adaptive setting of its value. Thus, the immune network fills the "non-self" space, which is recognised by hyper spheres of a different radius; that enables its more complete coverage.

In order to calculate the affinity values of the relationship "antigen-antibody" the following ratio is used:

$$f_{Ab-Ag} = \frac{k_r}{r} + D_{E(Ab-Ag)}, \tag{10.26}$$

r	Ab_{i1}	Ab_{i2}	...	Ab_{il}

Figure 10.8 Immune network antibody structure.

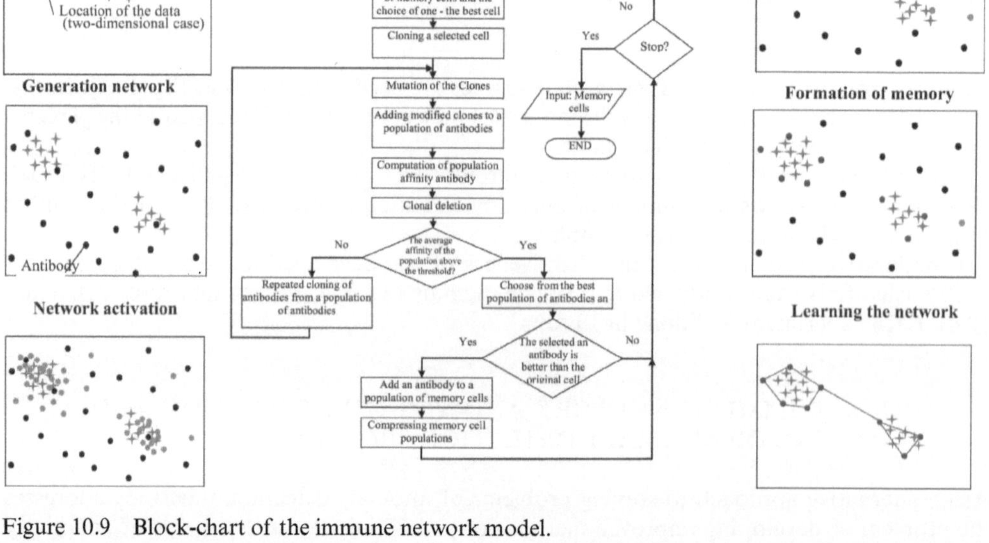

Figure 10.9 Block-chart of the immune network model.

where r is the cross-reactive antibody (detector) threshold, k_r – coefficient of importance of cross-reactive threshold (parameter settings). Parameter k_r is a very important study parameter. It manages the robustness of the resulting solution. Increasing this parameter causes the immune network to maintain larger radius detectors, which gives coarser, but more sustainable solutions. However, excessive increase of k_r negatively affects he accuracy of solutions. Figure 10.11 demonstrates the impact of parameter k_r on the way of detector generation.

Compression of immune network is based on self-recognition cells that is numerically expressed as affinity relationship of antibodies with each other. To calculate the values of the "antibody-antibody" affinity relationship the following formula is proposed:

$$f_{Ab-Ab} = -\frac{D_{E(Ab_1-Ab_2)} - (r_{Ab_1} + r_{Ab_2})}{2 \cdot \min(r_{Ab_1}, r_{Ab_2})}, \tag{10.27}$$

This possible interpretation of such values of f_{Ab-Ab} (Fig. 10.11) is as follows: ≤0 – recognizing hypersphere detectors do not overlap. This option does not require compression, because the antibodies do not recognise each other; (0,1) – hypersphere overlapped by shells, namely the value is the degree of overlap. This compression is dependent on the value of the parameter of threshold compression σ_s, which is a parameter of study; ≥1 – hypersphere smaller radius (r) is completely inside the hypersphere's larger radius. In this case, compression is definitely needed, because there is redundancy in recognising elements. This operator H of clonal deletion acts only on those antibodies that recognise at least one antigen. Thus, the resulting immune network at the end of each generation is guaranteed not to contain detectors that recognise "their" antigens.

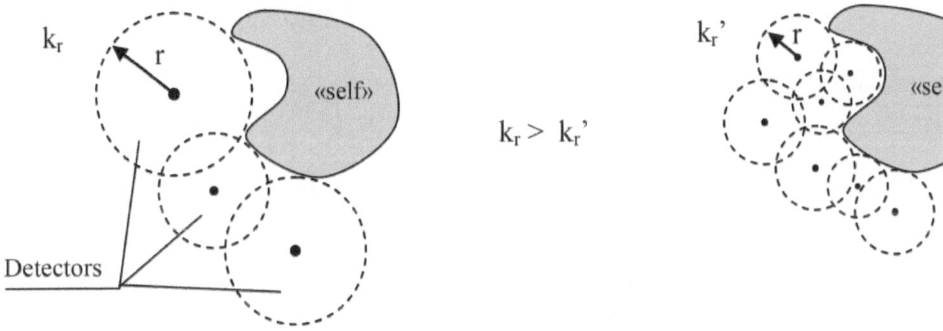

Figure 10.10 The influence of parameter value k_r on the way of detector generation.

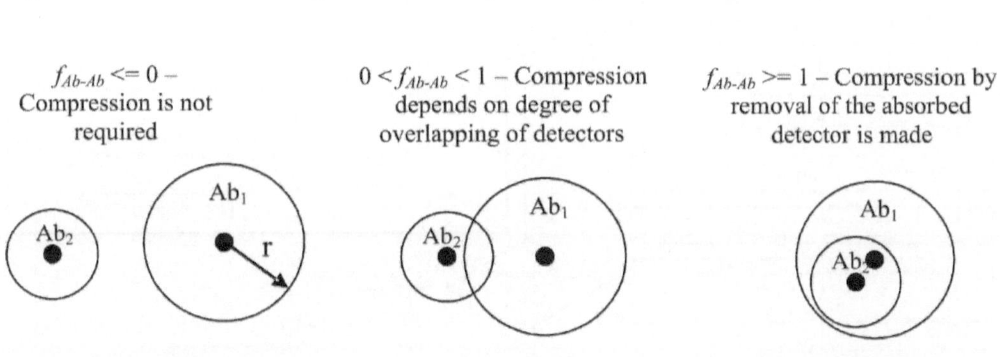

Figure 10.11 Different mutual arrangements of recognizing the hyper sphere of detectors depending on the value f_{Ab-Ab}.

5.2 *Solving the anomaly detection problem*

In general, the problem of anomaly detection in the hybrid procedure (Fig. 10.12) can be represented as follows (Dasgupta 2002, Gonzalez 2003). Let this discrete time series variables of the process be given as: $y_1, y_2, \ldots, y_n$. Assumed that the discrete control variable $y(t)$ is carried out on the range $[t_1, t_n]$. Let us chose a temporal window of width of k measurements ($k < n$). The values of time series, which is included inside the time window, form a feature vector $Y_t(y_t, y_{t-1}, \ldots, y_{t-k+1})$. The feature vector is assigned membership in one of two classes: *normal*(1) if the sample time series corresponding to this vector does not contain anomalies (i.e., belongs to the class of "self"), *abnormal*(0) otherwise. Temporary window shifts (slips) along the time series on the value steps of Δl, forming a set of vectors that divide the attribute space into two parts, with or without abnormalities. The problem lies in attributing any vector Y_j formed by the sliding time window to one of two selected classes. On the other hand, if we consider the study process as a dynamic system, a set of vectors is obtained by sliding window, phase portrait of dynamical system is the restored, and the same vectors—points that are phase trajectories of the system.

In normal behaviour, this trajectory can be interpreted as a reference image, whatever deviation from which is a sign of abnormality (Figure 10.13). It should be emphasised that the use of negative selection is not necessary to include in the training sample vectors corresponding to the anomalous behaviour that makes it possible to fix any, even unknown anomaly.

For an experimental verification of the method in solving the problem of detecting anomalies two test examples were selected. The first experiment used a periodic signal, the chart is presented in Figure 10.14. The study sample consisted of a range of 200 values. The training signal contains no anomalies. To create a training sample the sliding window width of two values were used. In this case, the attribute was two-dimensional space: (y_t, y_{t+1}).

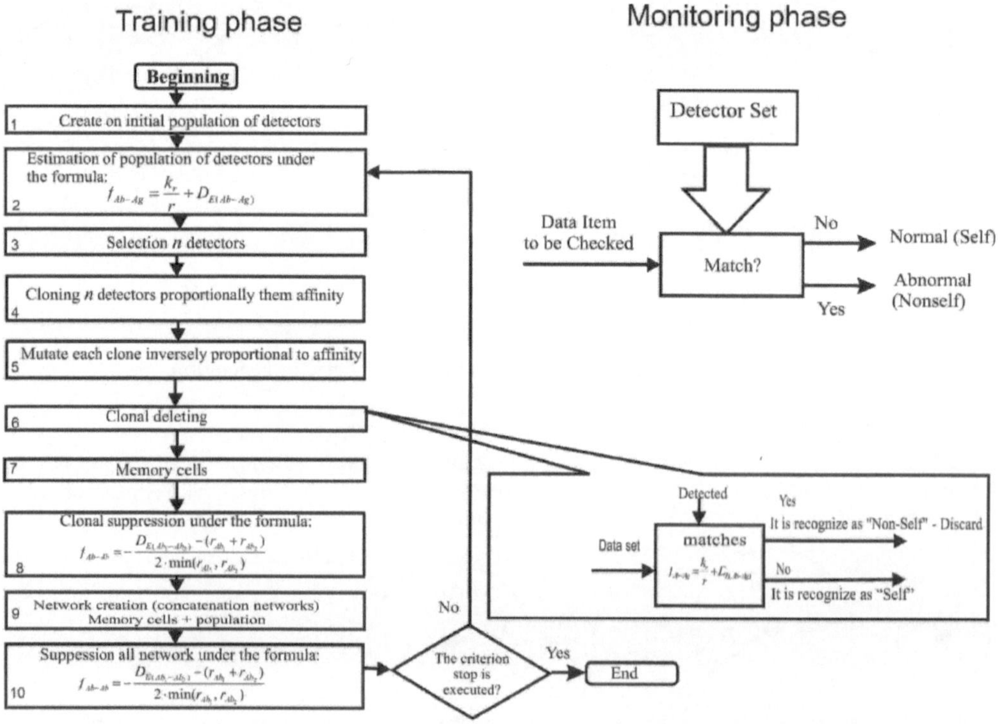

Figure 10.12 Generalised block-diagram of the hybrid procedure of the immune network with a negative selection.

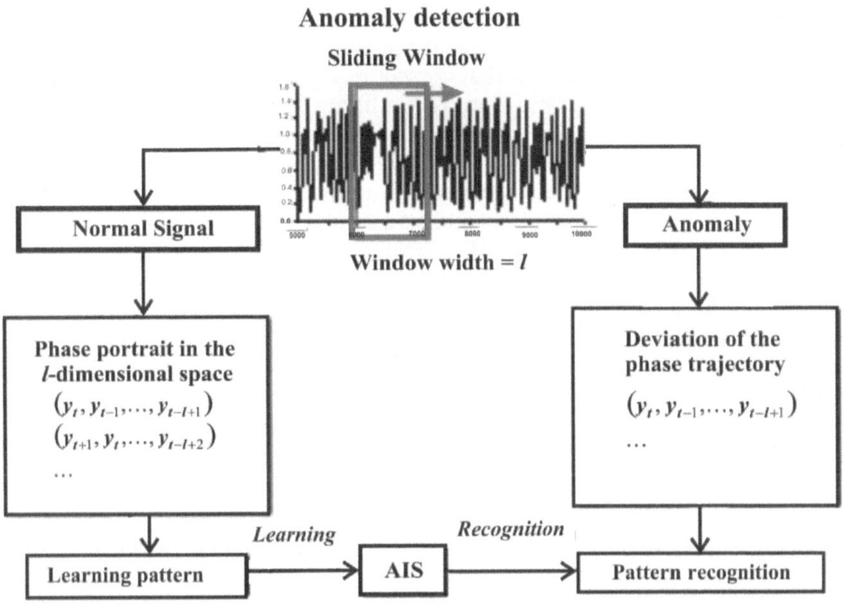

Figure 10.13 The task of anomaly detection.

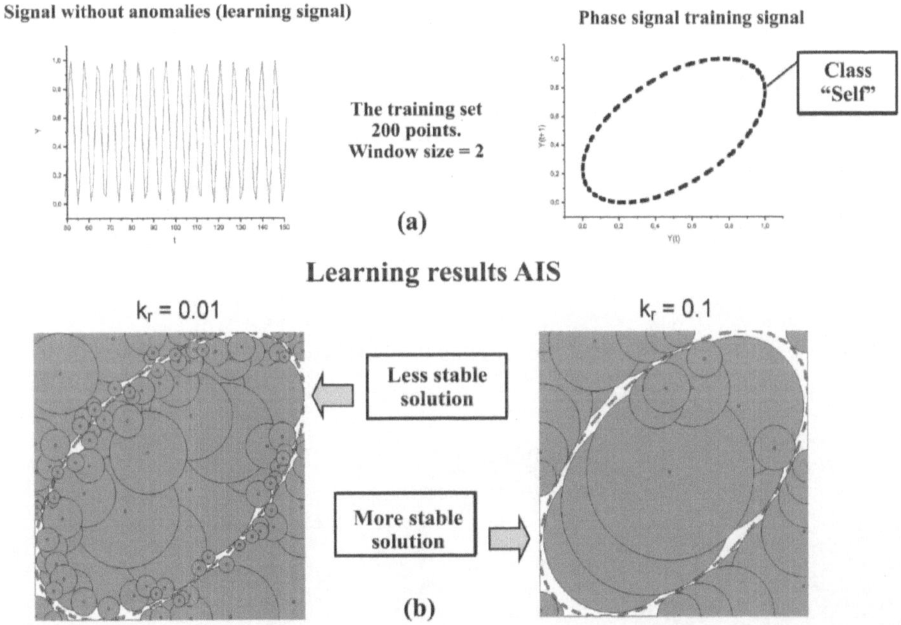

Figure 10.14 Test signal (a) is the signal chart containing no anomalies and the signal phase portrait renewed that does not contain the anomalies, (b) is the configuration of the immune network trained for two values of the parameter k_ε at: $k_\varepsilon = 0.01$ and when $k_\varepsilon = 0.1$.

The exterior using a periodic signal and its reconstructed phase portrait are shown in Figure 10.14(a). As seen from the figure, the phase trajectory of this dynamic system is not dense everywhere, so that the training sample is limited to 200 values.

The geometrical figure shown in Figure 10.14(a) (right) reflects data class "Self" and can be used as a training image for an artificial immune network. The only difficulty here is the presence of gaps on the restored path that correct recognition of the normal signal requires obtaining a sustainable solution. Below, study results are shown of artificial immune network for two values of the parameter importance of cross-reactive threshold k_ε that controls the stability of the solution.

Figure 10.14(b) (left) shows a less stable solution, as of the plane part, corresponding to the missed phase trajectory elements, is blocked by the detectors. This leads to the incorrect work. The solution in Figure 10.14(b) (right) is more stable and taken for further testing.

Now, the signal contains a local anomaly (Figure 10.15a), which found its reflection in the phase portrait as shown in Figure 10.15(b). In this case, the two points from the phase trajectories deviated and were recognised by appropriate detectors. It is possible to recognise multiple anomalous phenomena by just a few detectors Figure 10.16(a). The histogram in Figure 10.16(b) shows the number of detectors, which are activated at the presence of abnormality detection by a sliding window in the time series signal.

The second experiment demonstrates the ability to detect abnormal changes in the parameters of the mathematical relationships describing the behaviour of the system. This method is very useful for early detection of drift parameters controlled by the running system. In this case, the logistic equation $y_{t+1} = \lambda \cdot y_t(1 - y_t)$ was used as the study model, with the normal

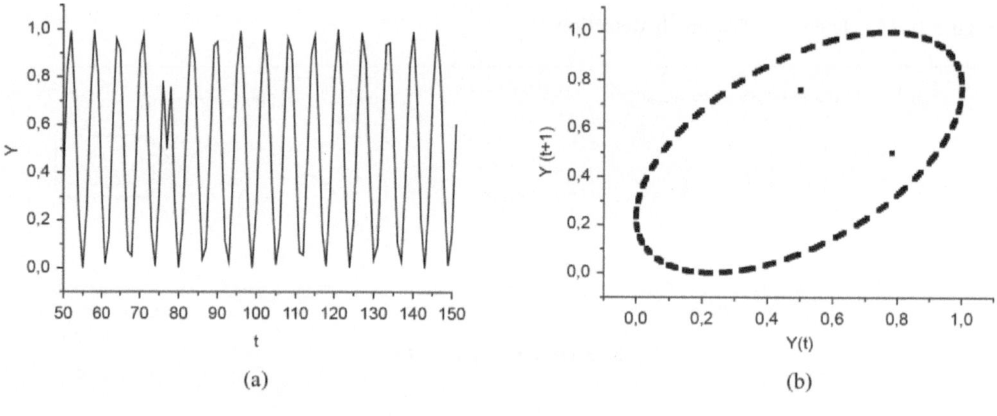

Figure 10.15 A test signal with a local anomaly and its phase portrait.

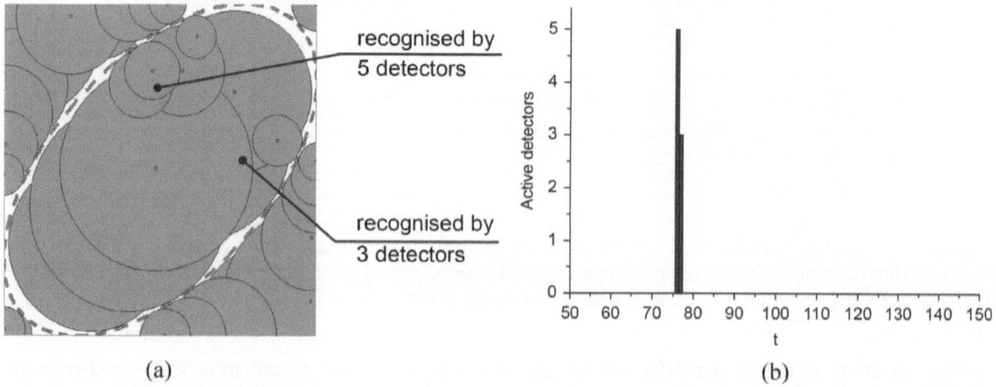

Figure 10.16 Recognition of abnormal vectors (a) and a histogram of detector activation (b).

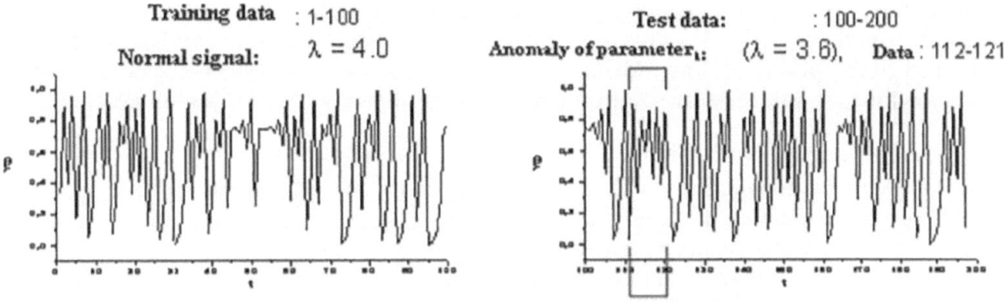

Figure 10.17 Normal signal with parameter $\lambda = 4.0$ (a); signal containing anomaly of parameter $\lambda = 3.6$ (b).

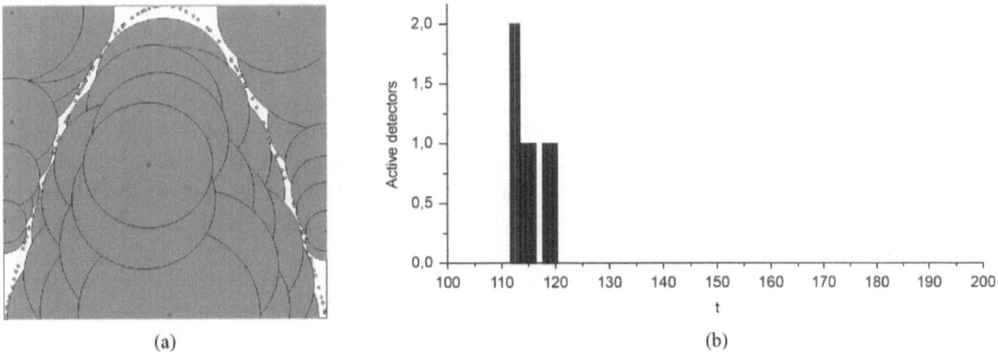

Figure 10.18 Structure of a trained artificial immune network (a), activation detectors in the presence of anomalies (b).

parameter of $\lambda = 4.0$. A graph of the normal signal is shown in Figure 10.17(a). At some point in time the value abruptly changed to 3.6, and was then restored to normal size, as shown in Figure 10.17(b). The study sample in this experiment was 100 of the first row of values. In the test sample the interval from 112 to 121 represents the value anomaly. The structure of trained artificial immune network is shown in Figure 10.18(a). The immune network observed anomalous variation of the parameter by activating the appropriate detectors Figure 10.18(b). As seen in Figure 10.18(b), activation detectors have no delay in time, which is an essential advantage of this method.

6 USING HYBRID NEGATIVE SELECTION ALGORITHM WITH ARTIFICIAL IMMUNE NETWORKS FOR INDUSTRIAL DIAGNOSTICS

6.1 *Test methodology and facility*

Combustion of pulverised coal was examined through optical methods, which were based on analysis of wide spectrum radiation emitted by the flame. The analysis also takes into account spatial features of such radiation source. Combustion of pulverised coal in the power burner takes place in a turbulent flow. At each point of it local fluctuations of both fuel and gaseous reagent concentrations, as well as temperature, occur. This leads to permanent local changes in the combustion process intensity, which results in continuous changes in flame luminosity that can be observed as flame flicker. As the combustion process affects the turbulent movement of its products and reagents, it determines the way the flame flicker parameters such as mean luminosity and luminosity frequency spectrum. A number of combustion supervision and flame-fault protection systems use information contained within flame flicker. The multichannel fibre-optic flame monitoring system developed at the Lublin University of Technology belongs to this class of solutions, additionally allowing observation of selected areas of the flame (Wójcik et al. 2001).

Experiments were made on a test rig located in the Institute of Power Engineering in Warsaw. It is a combustion chamber with a single pulverised coal swirl burner made in 1:10 scale in relation to a low-emission industrial burner. This object was chosen because of the opportunity to perform experiments with a single burner, being a suitable class of instrumentation. All measured quantities are visualised and recorded by the data acquisition system. The sampling period is 1 s. The combustion chamber was equipped with the above-mentioned optical fibre probe which allowed observation of five different areas of the flame. Figure 10.3 shows a section of part of the chamber with marked areas of view.

6.2 *Measurements*

The experiment begins with bringing the chamber to the proper temperature. When the temperature stabilises, a series of measurements are performed with changing air and fuel flows. During an individual measurement the amounts of fuel and air are kept constant. A single measurement lasts approximately 300 seconds. Such a measurement method is to eliminate the impact of the transport delay of gas analysers. It is assumed that during the measurement the conditions are fixed and the emission values stabilised. The tests were made at three different thermal loads, for pure pulverised coal and 10% blend with biomass (shredded straw). The amount of secondary air was being changed in order to achieve the air excess corresponding to normal operation, too high and too low conditions. Voltage signals

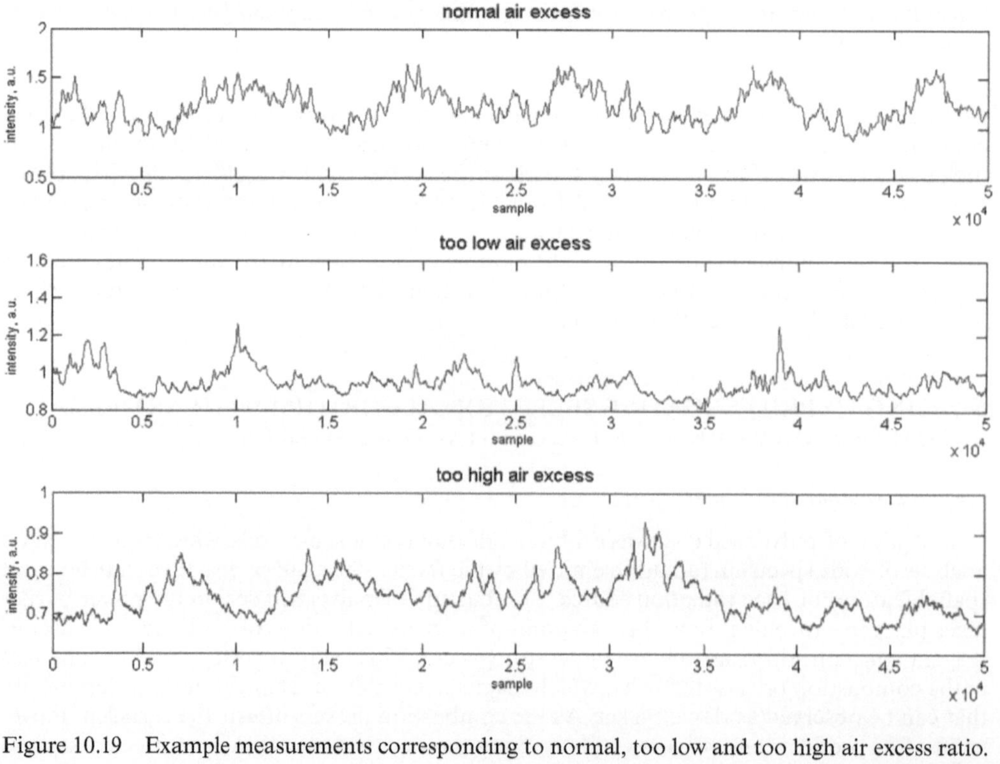

Figure 10.19 Example measurements corresponding to normal, too low and too high air excess ratio.

corresponding to the instantaneous brightness of the flame of the areas observed by individual optical fibres were sampled at the rate of 8 KS/s and saved by a dedicated system. Figure 10.19 shows example measurements corresponding to normal, too low and too high air excess ratio. A set of features was randomly divided into learning and testing subsets by 30%/70% and 70%/30%.

In order to avoid the bias associated with the random sampling of the training data the k-fold cross-validation was also performed. In k-fold cross-validation, the data is partitioned into k subsets of approximately equal size. Training and testing the algorithm is performed *k* times. Each time, one of the *k* subsets is used as the test set and the other *k*–1 subsets are put together to form a training set. Thus, *k* different test results exist for the algorithm. However, these *k* results are used to estimate performance measures for the classification system. Table 10.5 contains class distribution of the data points in the training and testing datasets.

The common performance measures used in diagnostics are accuracy, sensitivity and specificity. Accuracy expresses the ability of the classifier to produce accurate diagnosis. The measure of the ability of the model to identify the occurrence of a target class accurately is determined by sensitivity. Specificity is determined by the measure of the ability of the algorithm to separate the target class. The accuracy can be expressed as:

$$Accuracy(Z) = \frac{\sum_{i=1}^{|z|} Assess(z_i)}{|Z|}, \quad Assess(z) = \begin{cases} 1, & if\ calssify(z) = z.c \\ 0, & \text{otherwise} \end{cases} \tag{10.28}$$

where z denotes the patterns in testing set to be classified, $z.c.$ is the class of pattern z, *classify*(z) returns the classification of z by the classification algorithm. For sensitivity and specificity analysis, the following equations can be used:

$$Sensitivity = \frac{\mathrm{TP}}{\mathrm{TP}+\mathrm{FN}}, \quad Specificity = \frac{\mathrm{TN}}{\mathrm{TN}+\mathrm{FP}} \tag{10.29}$$

where TP, TN, FP i FN denote, respectively, true positive, true negative, false positive and false negative classification.

Many discriminative methods, including Support Vector Machine, neural network and classifiers based on the artificial immune systems, are often most accurate and efficient when dealing with two classes only (they can deal with more classes, but usually at reduced accuracy

Table 10.5 Class distribution of the data points in the training and testing datasets.

Class	Training set	Testing set	Total
λ too high	720	1680	2400
λ correct	720	1680	2400
λ too low	720	1680	2400
Total	2160	5040	7200
λ too high	1680	720	2400
λ correct	1680	720	2400
λ too low	1680	720	2400
Total	5040	2160	7200
λ too high	1920	480	2400
λ correct	1920	480	2400
λ too low	1920	480	2400
Total	5760	1140	7200

and efficiency) (Ding 2004). For a large number of classes, higher-level multi-class methods are developed that utilise these two-class classification methods as the basic building blocks. To solve our problem, we used the strategy of one-versus-all based on the hybrid algorithm we developed the negative selection and artificial immune network. The simplest approach is to reduce the problem of classifying among K classes into K binary problems, where each problem discriminates a given class from the other K minus 1 classes. For this approach, we require N = K binary classifiers, where the *k*-th classifier is trained with positive examples belonging to class k and negative examples belonging to the other K minus 1 classes. When testing an unknown example, the classifier producing the maximum output is considered the winner, and this class label is assigned to that example. Rifkin and Klautau state that this approach, although simple, provides performance that is comparable to other more complicated approaches when the binary classifier is well-tuned (Rifkin & Klautau 2004).

6.3 *Results*

Classification tests using modification of the learning phase in the model of negative selection were made according to the algorithm shown in Figures 10.20 and 10.21. Table 10.6 contains the results of the performance analysis. Average accuracy was about 98,99%. Classification accuracy obtained using fuzzy networks (TSK) was about 96,4% (Smolarz 2016). Normalised execution time of both algorithms was similar.

Optical signal can be used for operation status detection of an individual burner. The optical signal is the fastest and provides a selective way of getting information about the quality of combustion. Its interpretation, however, poses many difficulties.

The modification of the learning phase in the model of negative selection that uses optimisation as well as the artificial immune network for optimisation parameters detectors are developed. A distinctive feature of this procedure is a modification of the learning process, due to which the adaptive selection settings, the number and location of detectors are implemented. Experimental studies have shown a high efficiency of the proposed procedure, which is evident in its stability through the adaptive value of the cross-reactive threshold; its optimality due to the adaptive immune network configuration size, i.e. the number of detectors required; and its accuracy by reducing the number and size of the "cavities" created.

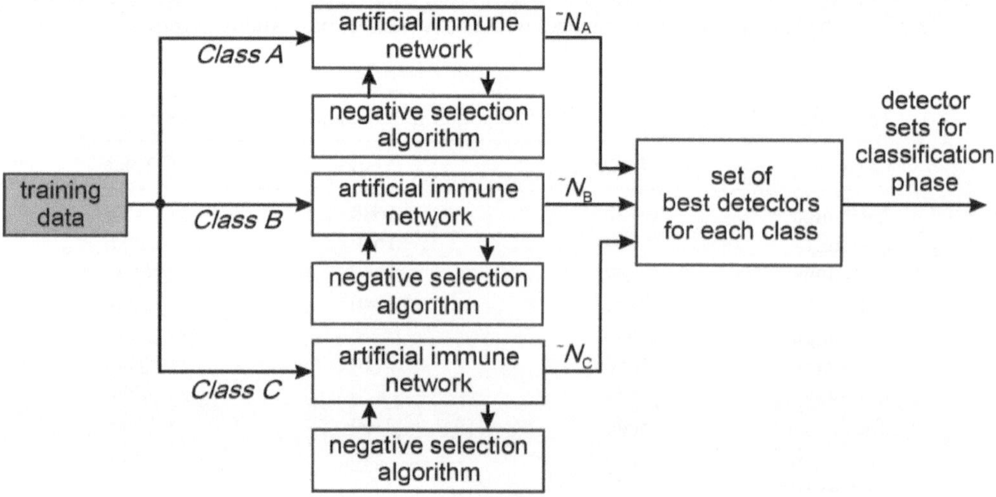

Figure 10.20 Synthesis of adaptive binary classifiers—learning phase in negative clonal selection algorithm.

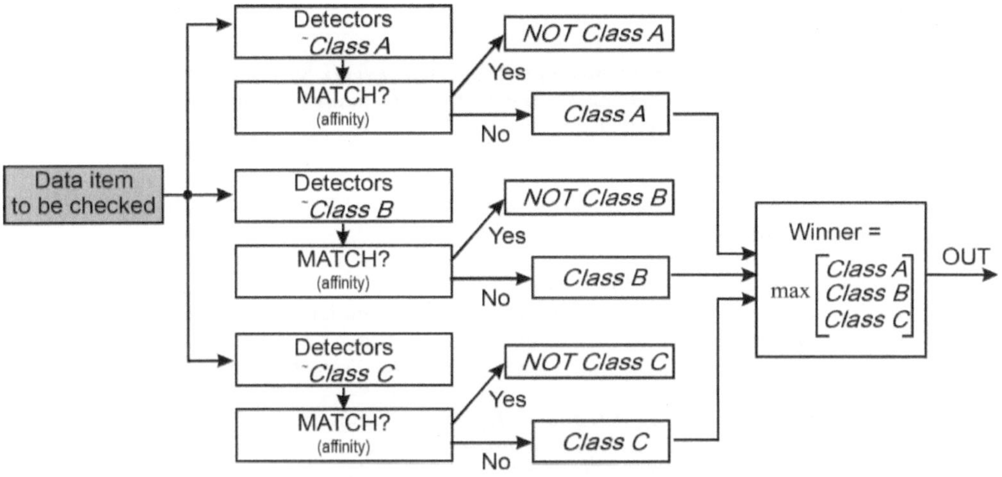

Figure 10.21 Classification phase in negative clonal selection algorithm.

Table 10.6 Performance measures for negative clonal selection algorithm.

Learning set/testing set distribution	Accuracy	Sensitivity	Specificity
40/60	98.95	99.25	99.10
60/40	99.18	99.20	99.45
80/20 5-fold cross-validation	98.85	98.75	99.25
Mean	98.99	99.07	99.27

The classification accuracy of the modification of the learning phase in the model of negative selection was better than the one of the fuzzy (TSK) algorithm when applied to the problem of detecting the excess ratio of anomalies in air using an optical system. Considering similar computational complexity of the above-mentioned algorithms, the advantage of the former one is clear. The modification of the learning phase in the model of negative selection combined with optical methods can then be used for the diagnostics of correct co-firing of pulverised coal blends with biomass in individual PC burners.

7 CONCLUSIONS

In this chapter the advantage of the proposed procedure of the clonal negative selection on the test data is shown by modifying ways of presenting the data and changing the mechanisms of generation and elimination of detectors which optimally chooses the detector size for solving binary classification problems.

A modified negative selection procedure that uses optimisation as well as an artificial immune network for the optimisation of detector parameters are developed. A distinctive feature of this procedure is a modification of the learning process, through which the number and location of detectors is implemented to adaptive selection settings.

A distinctive feature of this procedure is a modification of the learning process through which the adaptive selection settings, the number and location of detectors are implemented. Experimental studies have shown a high efficiency of the proposed procedure, which is evident in its stability through the adaptive value of the cross-reactive threshold; its optimality due to the adaptive immune network configuration size, i.e. the number of required detectors; and its accuracy by reducing the number and size of created "cavities".

REFERENCES

Dasgupta, D. 1999. *Artificial Immune Systems and Their Applications*, Springer-Verlag, Inc.

Dasgupta, D. 2002. Anomaly Detection in Multidimensional Data using Negative Selection Algorithm *IEEE World Congress on Computational Intelligence*:1039–1044.

Dasgupta, D., 2006, Advances in Artificial Immune Systems, *IEEE Computational Intelligence Magazine* 2006: 40–49.

De Castro, L.N. & Timmis, J. 2002. *Artificial Immune Systems: A New Computational Intelligence Approach*, London: Springer.

De Castro, L.N. & Timmis, J. 2003. Artificial Immune Systems as a Novel Soft Computing Paradigm. *Soft Computing Journal*. 7(7): 526–544.

Ding, C.H.Q. & Dubchak, I. 2004. Multi-class protein fold recognition using support vector machines and neural networks. *Bioinformatics* 17(4): 349–358.

Forrest, S. 1992. Computation and the Immune System. *IGBIO Newsletter, Association for Computing Machinery* 12(2): 52–57.

Forrest, S., Perelson, A.S., Allen L. & Cherukuri, R. 1994. Self-nonself discrimination in a computer, *Proceedings of the Symposium IEEE Computer Society on Research in Security and Privacy*: 202–212.

Gonzalez, F. 2003. *A Study of Artificial Immune Systems Applied to Anomaly Detection* [Ph.D. thesis]. USA The University of Memphis.

Hajela, P. 1996. Constramed Genetic Seach via Schema Adaptation: An Immune Network Solution. *Structural Optimisation* 12(1): 11–15.

Lichman, M. 2013. UCI Machine Learning Repository [http://archive.ics.uci.edu/ml]. Irvine, CA: University of California, School of Information and Computer Science.

Mangasarian, O.L., Street, W.N. & Wolberg, W.H. 1995. Breast cancer diagnosis and prognosis via linear programming. *Operations Research* 43(4): 570–577.

Perelson, A.S. 1996. Evolution and Somatic Learning of V-Region Genes. *Research in Immunology* 147: 202–208.

Rifkin, R & Klautau, A. 2004. Parallel networks that learn to pronounce english text. *Journal of Machine Learning Research*: 101–141.

Smolarz, A., Wójcik, W., Gromaszek, K., Komada, P., Lytvynenko, V.I., Mussabekov, N., Yesmakhanova, L. & Toigozhinova, A. 2016. Artificial intelligence methods in diagnostics of coal-biomass blends co-combustion in pulverised coal burners. *Environmental Engineering V*: 311–318.

Wójcik, W., Surtel, W., Smolarz, A., Kotyra, A., Komada, P. 2001. Optical fiber system for combustion quality analysis in power boilers. *Proceedings of SPIE* 4425: 517–522.

Author index